Guide to the
Canadian Family Medicine Examination

SECOND EDITION

Editors

Angela Arnold, BASc, MEng, MD, CCFP (EM)

Family Medicine and Emergency Medicine
University of Saskatchewan, Regina
Regina, Saskatchewan, Canada

Megan Dash, BSc, MD, CCFP (SEM), Dip Sport Med

Family Medicine and Enhanced Skills: Sports and Exercise Medicine
University of Saskatchewan, Regina
Regina, Saskatchewan, Canada

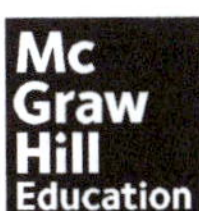

McGraw Hill Education

New York / Chicago / San Francisco / Athens / London / Madrid / Mexico City
Milan / New Delhi / Singapore / Sydney / Toronto

Guide to the Canadian Family Medicine Examination, Second Edition

1 2 3 4 5 6 7 8 9   LOV   22 21 20 19 18 17

ISBN 978-1-259-86186-4
MHID 1-259-86186-4

This book was set in Minion Pro by Cenveo® Publisher Services.
The editors were Amanda Fielding and Kim J. Davis.
The production supervisor was Catherine Saggese.
Project management was provided by Jyotsna Ojha, Cenveo Publisher Services.

Library of Congress Cataloging-in-Publication Data

Names: Arnold, Angela, 1968- editor. | Dash, Megan, editor.
Title: Guide to the Canadian family medicine examination / editors, Angela
   Arnold, Megan Dash.
Description: Second edition. | New York : McGraw-Hill Education, [2018] |
   Includes bibliographical references and index.
Identifiers: LCCN 2017025437 (print) | LCCN 2017026759 (ebook) | ISBN
   9781259861857 (Ebook) | ISBN 1259861856 (Ebook) | ISBN 9781259861864
   (pbk.: alk. paper)
Subjects: | MESH: Family Practice | Canada | Outlines | Examination Questions
Classification: LCC R834.5 (ebook) | LCC R834.5 (print) | NLM WB 18.2 | DDC
   616.0076—dc23
LC record available at https://lccn.loc.gov/2017025437

Guide to the
Canadian Family Medicine Examination

SECOND EDITION

Contents

Contributors

Malyha Alibhai, BMedSci, MBBS (Hons), CCFP
Clinical Assistant Professor
University of Saskatchewan
Regina, Saskatchewan, Canada
Chapter 5: Pediatrics

Angela Arnold, BASc, MEng, MD, CCFP (EM)
Family Medicine and Emergency Medicine
University of Saskatchewan, Regina
Regina, Saskatchewan, Canada
Chapter 14: Social Medicine/Psychology
Chapter 15: Preparation for the SOO

William Baldwin, MD
Family Medicine Resident
University of Saskatchewan
Regina, Saskatchewan, Canada
Chapter 16: SAMPs

Leanne Baumgartner, MD
Family Medicine Resident
University of Saskatchewan
Regina, Saskatchewan, Canada
Chapter 4: Surgery

Lourens Blignaut, MBChB, MCFP
Family Physician
Clinical Assistant Professor
University of Saskatchewan
Regina, Saskatchewan, Canada
Chapter 2: Internal Medicine

Matthew Butz, MD
Family Medicine Resident
University of Saskatchewan
Prince Albert, Saskatchewan, Canada
Chapter 6: Psychiatry

Megan Clark, MD, CCFP
Assistant Professor of Medicine
University of Saskatchewan
Regina, Saskatchewan, Canada
Chapter 13: Travel Medicine

Danielle Cutts, BA, MD, CCFP, FCFP
Assistant Clinical Professor
University of Saskatchewan
Regina, Saskatchewan, Canada
Chapter 9: Sexual Health

Megan Dash, BSc, MD, CCFP (SEM), Dip Sport Med
Family Medicine and Enhanced Skills: Sport and Exercise Medicine
University of Saskatchewan, Regina
Regina, Saskatchewan, Canada
Chapter 11: Musculoskeletal Medicine
Chapter 14: Social Medicine/Psychology

Taegen Fitch, MD
Family Medicine Resident
University of Saskatchewan
Regina, Saskatchewan, Canada
Chapter 7: Chronic Disease

Lisa Harasen, MD, CCFP
Family Medicine Resident
University of Saskatchewan
Regina, Saskatchewan, Canada
Chapter 8: Preventative Medicine

Andrew Houmphan, MD
Family Medicine Resident
University of Saskatchewan
Regina, Saskatchewan, Canada
Chapter 10: Women's Health

Elliott Hui, MD, CCFP
Community Family Physician
Regina, Saskatchewan, Canada
Chapter 12: Care of the Elderly

Kaalyn Humber, MD, CCFP
Family Medicine Resident
University of Saskatchewan
Regina, Saskatchewan, Canada
Chapter 7: Chronic Disease
Chapter 11: Musculoskeletal Medicine

William Denovan Johnston, MD, BSc
Associate Clinical Professor
University of Saskatchewan
Swift Current, Saskatchewan, Canada
Chapter 6: Psychiatry

Bradley Joss, MD, BSc
Family Medicine Resident
University of Saskatchewan
Regina, Saskatchewan, Canada
Chapter 5: Pediatrics

Rejina Kamrul, MBBS, CCFP
Associate Professor
Academic Family Medicine (Regina)
University of Saskatchewan
Regina, Saskatchewan, Canada
Chapter 7: Chronic Disease

Aaron Kastelic, MD, BComm
Family Medicine Resident
University of Saskatchewan
Regina, Saskatchewan, Canada
Chapter 3: Infectious Diseases

Jennifer Kuzmicz, MD, CFPC, FCFP
Assistant Professor of Family Medicine
University of Saskatchewan
Regina, Saskatchewan, Canada
Chapter 8: Preventative Medicine

Tara Lee, MD, BSc (Hons), CCFP
Clinical Associate Professor
University of Saskatchewan
Swift Current, Saskatchewan, Canada
Chapter 3: Infectious Diseases

M. Antoinette le Roux, MBChB, MPraxMed, CCFP
Clinical Assistant Professor
Department of Family Medicine
University of Saskatchewan
Saskatoon, Saskatchewan, Canada
Chapter 13: Travel Medicine

Sarah Liskowich, MD, CCFP
Assistant Professor of Medicine
University of Saskatchewan
Regina, Saskatchewan, Canada
Chapter 7: Chronic Disease

Kish Lyster, MD, CCFP (EM)
Clinical Assistant Professor
University of Saskatchewan
Regina, Saskatchewan, Canada
Chapter 1: Emergency Medicine
Chapter 2: Internal Medicine

Kyle MacDonald, MD
Family Medicine Resident
University of Saskatchewan
Regina, Saskatchewan, Canada
Chapter 6: Psychiatry

Sally Mahood, MD, CCFP, FCFP
Associate Professor Family Medicine
University of Saskatchewan
Regina, Saskatchewan, Canada
Chapter 10: Women's Health

Raenelle Nesbitt, MD, CCFP
Emergency Medicine Physician/Family Physician
Clinical Assistant Professor
Department of Academic Family Medicine
University of Saskatchewan
Regina, Saskatchewan, Canada
Chapter 1: Emergency Medicine

Stephanie Nyberg, MD
Family Medicine Resident
University of Saskatchewan
Regina, Saskatchewan, Canada
Chapter 9: Sexual Health

Jared Oberkirsch, MD, CCFP
Clinical Assistant Professor
University of Saskatchewan
Weyburn, Saskatchewan, Canada
Chapter 2: Internal Medicine

Tiann O'Carroll, MD, CCFP (EM)
Faculty, Department of Emergency Medicine
University of Saskatchewan
Regina, Saskatchewan, Canada
Chapter 6: Psychiatry

Jeremy Reed, MD, FRCSC
Orthopaedic Sports Surgeon
Clinical Associate Professor of Surgery
Adjunct Professor of Graduate Studies
University of Saskatchewan
ATLS Course Director
Regina, Saskatchewan, Canada
Chapter 1: Emergency Medicine
Chapter 11: Musculoskeletal Medicine

Olivia Reis, MD, CFCP
Family Medicine Resident
University of Saskatchewan
Regina, Saskatchewan, Canada
Chapter 2: Internal Medicine

Babak Salamati, MD, CCFP
Family Medicine Resident
University of Saskatchewan
North Battleford, Saskatchewan, Canada
Chapter 14: Social Medicine/Psychology

Sheila Smith, MD, CCFP (EM), FCFP
Clinical Assistant Professor
University of Saskatchewan
Regina, Saskatchewan, Canada
Chapter 4: Surgery

Andrea Vasquez, MD
Family Medicine Resident
University of Saskatchewan
Regina, Saskatchewan, Canada
Chapter 12: Care of the Elderly

Robert Weitemeyer, BSc, BA, BMBS
Family Medicine Resident
University of Saskatchewan
Regina, Saskatchewan, Canada
Chapter 1: Emergency Medicine

Christopher Young, MD
Family Medicine Resident
University of Saskatchewan
Regina, Saskatchewan, Canada
Chapter 1: Emergency Medicine

Cheryl Zagozeski, BSc, MD, CCFP, FCFP
Family Physician
Regina Community Clinic
Regina, Saskatchewan, Canada
Chapter 2: Internal Medicine

Lucas Zahorski, CCFP
Family Medicine Resident
University of Saskatchewan
Regina, Saskatchewan, Canada
Chapter 2: Internal Medicine

Preface

"The life so short, the craft so long to learn."

— Hippocrates

Dr. Arnold and I feel this quote encompasses the never-ending learning process—medicine. We have collaborated with many for this book, with the idea to assist individuals in studying for what may be the biggest exam of their life. It is not intended to be the only resource, but to aid in relieving some of the stress that this exam can, and likely will, create.

This book has been originated from handwritten notes, scribbled in the wee hours of the night, while Angela and I prepared for our exam. When finished we placed the notes in a giant orange binder, thus it was appropriately nicknamed *The Orange Book*. My original copy is sitting in the drawer at my office desk and I still pull it out every once in a while. I still remember the day Angela told me she thought we should submit our notes for publication. I laughed skeptically, but said I was up for the challenge. And now here we are! The book is no longer orange and has glossy pages and fancy tables, but the content and purpose of the book is largely unchanged.

The second edition has been updated to make sure that all the information is aligned with current practice guidelines, and a chapter of example SAMPs created to help you in your preparations for the Canadian family medicine examination. We've also tried to leave a lot of margin space so you have room to annotate.

Thanks to all the doctors and residents who gave their time to assist in the editing of this second edition. Your expertise and effort is highly valued.

To the reader, we hope you find this resource as useful as it was for us. Happy studying!

Megan Dash

Acknowledgements

Special thanks to Angela, for putting up with me and studying with me all those late nights, my husband Dr. Jeremy Reed for all your advice and support, and to our new little one Kendall Grace, for letting me edit this new edition while breastfeeding!

Megan Dash

Thanks to Megan for agreeing to the second edition. We've come a long way and I always appreciate the collaboration and how the book keeps us connected! I also want to acknowledge that being able to practice medicine is truly a privilege and I am grateful for all my colleagues and the people who have helped in this never-ending learning process.

Angela Arnold

Abbreviations

<	less than		CRP	C-reactive protein
A1C	glycated hemoglobin		CT	computed tomography
AAA	abdominal aortic aneurysm		CVD	cerebrovascular disease
ABPM	ambulatory blood pressure measurement (24-hour blood pressure monitoring)		CVS	cardiovascular system
			D&C	dilation and curettage
ACE-I	angiotensin converting enzyme inhibitor		DM	diabetes mellitus
AE	adverse effects		DVT	deep venous thrombosis
AFib	atrial fibrillation		DWI	diffusion weighted imaging
AIS	adenocarcinoma insitu		ECG	electrocardiogram
ALP	alkaline phosphatase		Eg	for example
ALT	alanine transaminase		EM	erythema multiforme
ARB	angiotensin receptor blocker		ENT	ear, nose, and throat
ASA	acetylsalicylic acid		FH	family history
ASC-US	atypical squamous cells of undetermined significance		FIT	fecal immunochemical test
			FNA	fine needle aspiration
AST	Aspartate transaminase		FOBT	fecal occult blood test
BCC	basal cell carcinoma		FPG	fasting plasma glucose
BMI	body mass index		FRAX	Fracture Risk Assessment Tool
BNP	B-type natriuretic peptide		FT_4	free thyroxine
BP	blood pressure		GBS	group B streptococcus
BPH	benign prostatic hyperplasia		GDM	gestational diabetes mellitus
BPM	blood pressure measurement		GERD	gastroesophageal reflux disease
BSA	body surface area		GGT	gamma-glutamyl transferase
C&M	cross and match		GHTN	gestational hypertension
CAD	coronary artery disease		HAART	highly active antiretroviral therapy
CAROC	comprehensive fracture risk assessment tool		HBV	hepatitis B virus
			HF	heart failure
CDA	Canadian Dermatology Association		HIDA scan	hepatobiliary scintigraphy
CHF	congestive heart failure		HIV	human immunodeficiency virus
CI	contraindicated		HOCM	hypertrophic obstructive cardiomyopathy
CKD	chronic kidney disease			
CN	cranial nerve		HR	heart rate
CNS	central nervous system		HRT	hormone replacement therapy
COMT	catechol-O-methyltransferase		HSIL	high-grade squamous intraepithelial lesion
COPD	chronic obstructive pulmonary disease		HTN	hypertension

IUGR	intrauterine growth restriction	PV	per vaginum
IV	intravenous	QOL	quality of life
LLDP	left lateral decubitus position	R/O	rule out
LOC	loss of consciousness	RAI	radioactive iodine
LSIL	low-grade squamous intraepithelial lesion	RAIU	radioactive iodine uptake scan
LT_4	l-thyroxine, levothyroxine	RCT	randomized controlled trial
MAO-I	monamine oxidase inhibitor	RS	respiratory system
MCV	mean corpuscular volume	rTPA	Recombinant Tissue Plasminogen Activator
MDD	major depressive disorder	RUQ	right upper quadrant
MI	myocardial infarction	Rx	treatment
MMI	methimazole	SCC	squamous cell carcinoma
MRI	magnetic resonance imaging	SE	side effects
MS	multiple sclerosis	SERM	selective estrogen receptor modulator
NNT	number needed to treat	SES	socio-economic status
NSAIDs	non-steroidal anti-inflammatory drugs	SJS	Stevens-Johnson syndrome
OGTT	oral glucose tolerance test	SSRI	selective seretonin reuptake inhibitor
OH	orthostatic hypotension	STI	Sexually transmitted infection
OSA	obstructive sleep apnea	T_3	triiodothyronine
PCOS	polycystic ovarian syndrome	T_4	thyroxine
PD	Parkinson disease	TCA	tricyclic antidepressants
PE	pulmonary embolism	TDaP	tetanus, diptheria, and acellular pertussis
PG	plasma glucose	TEN	toxic epidermal necrolysis
PHQ-9	preventative health questionnaire 9; a screening questionnaire for depression	TIA	transient ischemic attach
		TOP	termination of pregnancy
PMH	past medical history	TPO	thyroid peroxidase
PNS	peripheral nervous system	TRAP	tremor, rigidity, akinesia, postural instability
PO	oral route		
PPD	post partum depression	TRH	thyrotropin releasing hormone
PPG	post-prandial plasma glucose	TSH	thyroid stimulating hormone
PPROM	Preterm PROM (less than 37 weeks)	TSI	thyroid stimulating immunoglobulin
PPT	postpartum thyroiditis	U/S	ultrasound
PROM	premature (before the onset of labour) rupture of membranes	UE	upper extremities
		VZV	varicella zoster virus
PTU	propylthiouracil	WBC	white blood cells

Top Ten Tips for Writing SAMPs

1. Ensure that you read the questions thoroughly. Sometimes the answer is given within the question.

2. CBC is not an appropriate answer. You must state hemoglobin, white blood cell count, etc. This is the same for all laboratory investigations.

3. Take your time. You will have plenty of time to complete all the questions.

4. Be aware of the environment in which the question places you. Your answer may be different if you are in your office versus the emergency room.

5. Know classes of medications and ensure that you know a few options for each condition. For example, classes of medications to treat hypertension include calcium channel blockers, diuretics, beta blockers, and so on.

6. Be specific. Answers usually require only a few words.

7. Go with your gut. The questions are not trying to trick you.

8. Use generic names of medications, not trade names.

9. A table of normal laboratory values is provided on the exam, so do not waste your time memorizing those ranges.

10. Visit the CFPC Web site at http://www.cfpc.ca/EvaluationObjectives to review the objectives for the exam.

CHAPTER 1

Emergency Medicine

ACLS

Priority Topic 1

- Please refer to ACLS guidelines for a comprehensive review of ACLS algorithms for ACS, cardiac arrest, and arrhythmias (American Heart Association, 2015).
- Arrhythmias are a frequent problem encountered in the emergency room (ER). A general approach to arrhythmias is essential (Tables 1-1 and 1-2).

TABLE 1-1	Arrhythmias—Approach and Characteristics		
PATHOLOGY	**RHYTHM/CAUSE**	**CHARACTERISTICS**	**MANAGEMENT**
Tachycardia (HR >100)	Afib	• Narrow complex • Irregularly irregular • No P waves • With or without rapid ventricular response	ACLS protocol • if hemodynamically unstable electrical cardioversion • if stable medical rate conversion • follow with expert consultation
	SVT	• Narrow complex (**<0.12 s**) • Aberrant pacemaker can be atrial, AV node, ectopic • Various P wave anomalies (varied timing, morphology)	• Vagal manoeuvres • Adenosine 6 mg IV push; then 12 mg (only if regular). • If does not convert, consider beta-blocker or diltiazem. (Expert consultation) • If unstable synchronized cardioversion.
	V Tach	• Wide (**>0.12 s**) complexes • Greater than three ventricular complexes with rate >100	• *With pulse*; consider adenosine (as above) only if monomorphic and regular. Give amiodarone 150 mg IV over 10 min. If unstable synchronized cardioversion. (Expert consultation) • *If pulseless*; Follow PEA protocol. CPR, Epinephrine 1 mg q 3-5 min. If refractory amiodarone 300 mg IV may replace second dose of epinephrine. May repeat amiodarone one time of 150 mg.
	V Fib	• No clear QRS complexes • No pulse (too disorganized)	• Start CPR immediately, defibrillate. • Epinephrine 1 mg IV q 3-5 min. • Amiodarone 300 mg IV (may replace second dose of epinephrine), may repeat amiodarone one time of 150 mg.
Bradycardia (HR <60)	**Various:** Search for causes = 6 Hs and 5 Ts	• Heart rate <60 • May or may not be symptomatic • Rx only if clinically inadequate perfusion	• Transcutaneous pacing (titrate mA to 10% over mechanical capture confirmed by femoral pulse). • Atropine 0.5 mg IV. • Consider epinephrine (2-10 mcg/min) or dopamine (2-20 mcg/kg/min) infusion. • Definitive (transvenous) pacing.

TABLE 1-1	Arrhythmias—Approach and Characteristics (*Continued*)		
PATHOLOGY	RHYTHM/CAUSE	CHARACTERISTICS	MANAGEMENT
Asystole/PEA	Various: Search for causes = 6 Hs and 5 Ts (see Table 1-3)	• ECG flat. No rhythm. (Or a rhythm but no pulse is able to be palpated.)	• CPR. • Do not defibrillate unless shockable rhythm (VF or VT). • Epinephrine 1 mg IV/IO q 3-5 min. • May give vasopressin 40 U IV/IO to replace first or second dose epinephrine. • May consider atropine 1 mg IV/IO q 3-5 min.
Metabolic/ drugs	Cocaine toxicity	• Tachycardia +/− ischemic changes	• Do not give beta-blocker.
	Hyperkalemia	• Peaked T waves, slurred/elongated QRS, loss of P wave	• Cardio-protection with calcium gluconate 10% 10 mg over 2 min (will normalize ECG). • Decrease potassium with insulin+dextrose, beta agonist (salbutamol), diuretic.
	Digoxin toxicity	• ST depression with inverted T waves (V_5-V_6) • Short QT segment	• Digoxin immune Fab (Digibind)
	*Opioid	• Cardiac/respiratory arrest (* *included in 2015 ACLS protocol*)	• Begin CPR. • Administer Naloxone 0.4 mg IM / 2 mg intranasal q 4 min.

Abbreviations: A fib, atrial fibrillation; PEA, pulseless electrical activity; SVT, supraventricular tachycardia; V Fib, ventricular fibrillation; V Tach, ventricular tachycardia.

TABLE 1-2	Heart Blocks	
RHYTHM	CHARACTERISTICS	TREATMENT
1st-degree AV block	Long PR interval (>200 ms)	No treatment
2nd-degree AV block Mobitz 1	Progressive increase in PR interval until a dropped beat, PR then resets	Stop offending drugs
2nd-degree AV block Mobitz 2	No change in PR with patterned dropped QRS beats (2:1 or 3:1)	Pacemaker
3rd-degree AV block	No relationship between P wave and QRS complex	Pacemaker

TABLE 1-3	6 Hs and 5 Ts (Underlying Causes for Bradycardic and Tachycardic Arrhythmias)	
Hypovolemia **H**ypoxia **H**ydrogen ion (acidosis) **H**ypo/Hyperkalemia **H**ypoglycemia **H**ypothermia	**T**oxins **T**amponade (cardiac) **T**ension pneumothorax **T**hrombosis (coronary or pulmonary) **T**rauma (hypovolemia, increased ICP)	

Bibliography

AHA. 2015 American Heart Association guidelines update for cardiopulmonary resuscitation and emergency cardiovascular care. *Circulation* 2015;18(2):132.

ASA. American Heart Association guidelines for cardiopulmonary resuscitation and emergency cardiovascular care. *Circulation* 2010:122.

Loss of Consciousness
Priority Topic 59

Definition

The occurrence of a loss of the ability to perceive and respond.

History

Must differentiate between **traumatic** LOC and **nontraumatic** LOC.

- SAMPLE history is important
  - **S**—signs and symptoms
  - **A**—allergies
  - **M**—medication
  - **P**—past medical history
  - **L**—last meal
  - **E**—event, the details of what happened
- History from witnesses is very important
- Seek information on:
  - Trauma
  - Medications (Rx, over-the-counter, and supplements)
  - Toxins (illicit drugs, poisons)
  - Seizure activity
  - Psychological history

Physical Examination

This is a critical care scenario! Switch into ACLS/ATLS/ICU mode. Do your ABCs. Do a thorough examination and **do not skip** any steps. Use collateral history via EMS, bystanders, and family.

- ABCDEs
  - Ensure a patent airway; intubate if necessary.
  - Ensure air is moving appropriately.
  - Attain a full set of accurate vitals including glucose, look for signs of shock.
  - Check pupils and calculate Glasgow Coma Scoring (GCS)—(see Table 1-4)
    - If GCS less than 8, intubate! (usually). Consider intubation for hypopnoea, pulmonary toilet, delay in transport or expected deterioration in clinical course.
  - Check for, and manage hypothermia via warmed fluids, warm blankets, increasing room temperature, etc.

TABLE 1-4	Glasgow Coma Scoring				
EYES		**VERBAL**		**MOTOR**	
4	Open spontaneously	5	Alert and oriented	6	Follows command
3	Open to speech	4	Disoriented	5	Localizes to pain
2	Open to pain	3	Inappropriate words	4	Withdraws from pain
1	No response	2	Moans	3	Decorticate (arm flexion)
		1	No response	2	Decerebrate (arm extension)
				1	No response

TABLE 1-5	Neurologic Signs	
UPPER MOTOR NEURON		**LOWER MOTOR NEURON**
Injury above anterior horn cell of spinal cord		Injury below anterior horn cell of spinal cord
Plantar reflex upgoing		Plantar reflex downgoing
Tone increased, secondary to unregulated spinal cord reflex arcs		Tone flaccid, secondary to lost muscle innervation
DTRs increased		DTRs decreased, normal, or absent Atrophy, fasciculations in long term

- Perform a **systematic** head to toe examination.
  - Look for signs of trauma.
  - Check for localizing neurologic signs (see Table 1-5).
  - Note smell of alcohol or ketones.
  - Look for asterixis, indicating renal or hepatic failure.
- Consider various causes of LOC (see Tables 1-6 and 1-7).

TABLE 1-6	Differential Diagnosis—Traumatic Head Injury			
	SAH	**EPIDURAL**	**SUBDURAL**	**TRAUMATIC BRAIN INJURY: CONCUSSION-DIFFUSE AXONAL INJURY SPECTRUM**
Definition	The presence of blood in the SA space, in the absence of trauma	The presence of blood between the dura and skull	The presence of blood between the dura and arachnoid membrane	Traumatic damage to white matter tracts
Presentation history	"Worst headache ever" "Thunderclap headache" Immediate onset Occasionally confusion Occasionally seizures Occasionally neck stiffness	Altered mental status, changing minutes to hours May have lucid interval-beware!	Mental status change over days to weeks May have hemiparesis	Ranging from the mild "fog" of a mild concussion to profound coma secondary to DAI Within minutes of head trauma: "Foggy" Headache Amnesia Transient LOC Coma DAI may declare itself in a delayed fashion on imaging, as majority of damage is biochemical
Physical examination	Decreased GCS Coma May have pupillary dilation if ICP is raised high enough to incite uncal herniation Meningismus	Decreased GCS Coma May have pupillary dilation if ICP is raised high enough to incite uncal herniation	Decreased GCS Coma May have pupillary dilation if ICP is raised high enough to incite uncal herniation	If mild symptoms, sideline concussion assessment and appropriate restriction of activity If comatose, begin critical care style assessment and treatment
Risk factors	Preexisting vascular malformations Trauma	Trauma, especially shearing and rotatory forces	Alcoholism Elderly (falls) Anticoagulation therapy	Trauma Contact sports
Investigation	CBC, renal panel, INR/PTT, serum glucose, ABG, serum EtOH, tox screen, U/A CT head Lumbar puncture if CT is negative	CBC, renal panel, INR/PTT, serum glucose, ABG, serum EtOH, tox screen, U/A CT head	CBC, renal panel, INR/PTT, serum glucose, ABG, serum EtOH, tox screen, U/A CT head	If conscious, perform SCAT 2 assessment If unconscious, perform CT
Treatment	Neurosurgery consultation	Neurosurgery consultation	Neurosurgery consultation	Concussion: activity restriction and graduated return to sport/activity DAI: supportive care in ICU to limit ongoing axonal injury

TABLE 1-7	Differential Diagnosis—Nontraumatic Head Injury
Definition	The occurrence of a loss of the ability to perceive and respond, in the absence of a traumatic event
Presentation	Stupor, confusion, unconscious
Physical examination	Recognize a sick patient, record vitals, perform focused, thorough head-to-toe examination as discussed earlier
Etiologies	"The 6 Hs and the 5 Ts" **H**ypovolemia **H**ypoxia **H**ydrogen ion (acidosis) **H**ypo/Hyper K$^+$ **H**ypoglycemia **H**ypothermia **T**oxins **T**amponade **T**ension pneumothorax **T**hrombosis **T**rauma
Investigation	CBC, renal panel, INR/PTT, serum glucose, ABG, serum EtOH, tox screen, U/A, CT head
Treatment	Appropriate recognition of a critically ill patient Supportive critical care management as needed • ABCDE • Warming • Fluid resuscitation Correction of biochemical abnormalities and coagulopathies

Intubation

Rapid sequence induction—"O BLAST HIM" to prepare prior to intubation.

The use of an Airway Checklist should be mandatory[3]

- O—O$_2$ available and working (use Apneic Oxygenation technique; NRB *plus* high-flow nasal at 15 L/min prior to intubation attempt to saturate with oxygen. For bag-valve-mask ventilation use two persons and a PEEP valve)
- B—Blade and bag (blade 2-3 for most adults)
- L—Laryngoscope available and working
- A—Airway (oropharyngeal/guedel airway—measure angle of mouth to angle of jaw to choose size. Consider nasopharyngeal airway as adjunct—measure nares to the lobe of the ear)
- S—Suction and stylet
- T—Tube; ET tube (size 7-8) or laryngeal mask airway (size 3-4)
- H—HELP (get some)/hinder (identify any signs of difficult airway)
- I—IV access
- M—Medications

Medications

Induction Options

- Ketamine 1 to 1.5 mg/kg is effective for induction with less risk of hypotension.
- Propofol 1.5 to 3 mg/kg as an induction bolus.[1] High risk of hypotension.
- Fentanyl 1 to 2 mcg/kg ideal body weight.[1]
  - bolus as above, followed by 10 mcg/kg/h
- Midazolam 0.05 to 0.1 mg/ kg (maximum 5 mg) for amnesia and induction[1,2]

Paralytic Options

1. Succinylcholine 1 to 1.5 mg/kg for paralysis
   - Intubate once fasciculations stop.
   - Contraindicated if state of high potassium (eg; burns, renal failure, polytrauma).
   - Expect succinylcholine to increase K by 1.0 mmol/L—beware in a renal failure patient.
   - Expect bradycardia!
2. Rocuronium 1 mg/kg for paralysis.

Management of Blood Pressure

TABLE 1-8	Management of Blood Pressure	
Phenylephrine	For hypotension Pure alpha (vasoconstrictive) effect	100-200 mcg/dose q 10-15 min PRN *Dosing is almost always bolus use.*
Norepinephrine	For hypotension Strong alpha (vasoconstriction) and weaker beta effects (chronotropy and inotropy)	Infusion 0.01-1 mcg/kg/min In practice, maximum dose usually 0.5 mcg/kg/min
Epinephrine	For hypotension and bradycardia Potent alpha and beta activity	Infusion 0.01-1 mcg/kg/min In practice, maximum dose usually 0.5 mcg/kg/min

RSI Cheat Sheet

1. Establish airway (chin lift, jaw thrust) +/− in-line C-spine stabilization.
2. Preoxygenate 100% high-flow O_2 for 2 to 3 minutes.
3. IV access and give fluids ** note: if able to, do your neuro examination prior to paralysis! **
4. Medications (example of possible options).
   - Midazolam 0.1 mg/kg (maximum 5 mg)
   - Fentanyl 2 mcg/kg
   - Succinylcholine 1 to 1.5 mg/kg
5. Expect bradycardia: have atropine 0.5 mg q3 to 5 min (maximum 3 mg).
   Expect hypotension: have phenylephrine 100 to 500 mcg ready to push.
6. WATCH for fasciculation to cease, indicating paralysis (roughly 45 seconds).
7. Laryngoscope w/ size 2 to 3 blade for most adults.
   - Head in the sniffing position
   - Observe lips and teeth carefully
   - THEN look into the blade and PUSH the tongue **forward** and **slightly up** until you see chords. **NEVER, EVER,** rotate your wrist, or leverage on the upper teeth.
   - Visualize the epiglottis.

** Choose an agent that you are familiar with, and is suited for the situation. Take an airway course! Taking control of an airway is lifesaving but high risk. You need to be comfortable with the skill or delegate to someone who is.

- Introduce ETT (+/− stylet or bougie).
- Inflate cuff with about 10cc of air and check for leak.
- To confirm appropriate tube placement, look for:
  a. multiple occurrences of mist in tube (the stomach can give you a puff or two of steam and CO_2),
  b. bilateral air entry with **no** breath sounds in epigastrium,
  c. end expiratory CO_2 on indicator strip or capnograph. Capnography is the standard of care.

Once tube placement is confirmed, care should be taken to match minute ventilation (rate and volume) of patient pre-intubation until an ABG can be obtained. Keep oxygen on high-flow with bag or 100% on ventilator until consultation is obtained.

Bibliography

AHS Critical Care MCGs. RSIP algorithm. https://www.ahsems.com/public/protocols/templates/desktop/#set/13/browse/3663/view/31311/Algorithm. Accessed Jan 18 2017.

ATLS Subcommittee. American College of Surgeons' Committee on trauma; International ATLS working group. Advanced trauma life support (ATLS®): the ninth edition. *J Trauma Acute Care Surg* 2013;74(5):1363-1366. doi: 10.1097/TA.0b013e31828b82f5.

Cardo D. Induction Agents for Rapid Sequence Intubation in Adults. In: Walls RM, Grayzel J, eds, *UpToDate; 2016.* Retrieved from http://www.uptodate.com/.

Hardy G, Horner D. BET 2: Should real resuscitationists use airway checklists? *Emerg Med J* 2016;33(6):439-441.

Strayer R, Weingart S, Andreus P, Arntfield R. Emergency Department intubation checklist, Mount Sinai School of Medicine, v13, updated 7/8/2012, accessed 10/11/2016. http://emupdates.com/2012/07/08/emergency-department-intubation-checklist-v13/.

Canadian Head CT Rules

- Ask yourself is a head CT indicated?
- Use mnemonic BEAN DASH. CT if any one of the following is present:
  - Basal skull fracture (hemotympanum, racoon eyes, CSF otorrhea/rhinorrhea, Battle sign)
  - Emesis ≥2
  - Age ≥65
  - Neuro symptoms (GCS <15 at 2 hours after injury)
  - Dangerous mechanism (pedestrian struck by a vehicle, occupant ejected from motor vehicle, fall from ≥3 feet, etc)
  - Amnesia (≥30 minutes prior)
  - Skull fracture suspected (open or depressed)

General Management

1. ABCDEs—These people may well have **very** serious associated injuries.
   - Manage critical care issues as needed
2. Supportive management—**prevention of further injury is all you can offer them**.
   - ICP management: Neutral head position; head of bed at 30 degrees.
   - Prevent hypoxemia.
   - Prevent hypotension (remember cerebral perfusion = ICP—mean arterial pressure). If possible aim for MAPs above 80 mm Hg.
   - Prevent hypothermia/hyperthermia.
   - Prevent seizure activity.
3. Begin correction of biochemical and coagulation abnormalities.
4. Critical care and neurosurgical consultations as needed for definitive management.

Bibliography

Stiell IG, Wells GA, Vandemheen K, et al for the CCC Study Group. The Canadian CT Head Rule for patients with minor head injury. *Lancet* 2001;357(9266):1391-1396.

All primary care providers should consider taking an ATLS course. ATLS provides everyone with a systematic way to bring calm to a chaotic scenario, optimize patient outcomes, and at times, save a life. For more information see: http://www.traumacanada.org.

Trauma

Priority Topic 92

Trauma is one of the leading causes of morbidity and mortality in young age groups.

OVERVIEW

- Be prepared. Know your facility and your team's capabilities.
- Review what is available, and ensure that necessary equipment is available.
  - Warmed IV fluids
  - Warm blankets
  - Chest tube tray
  - Intubation set
  - Cricothyroidotomy set
  - Appropriate drugs
  - A Broselow tape for peds
  - Fabric pelvic binders—not just a sheet if at all possible
  - Blood, if feasible
  - Appropriate monitoring

MANAGEMENT

- Be as prepared as possible
- Upon arrival:
  - Ensure C-spine immobilization.
  - Apply oxygen, monitors, and start two large bore IVs—defined as **16 g or larger**.
  - Attain a **complete** and **accurate** set of vitals.
    - HR
    - Respiratory rate
    - SaO_2
    - Blood pressure
    - Temperature
    - Glucose

PRIMARY SURVEY

- Airway—Is it patent? Will it remain patent? Is intubation required?
- Breathing—Is air moving in both lung fields?
- Circulation—Is there a pulse? What is the BP? Skin colour? Any active bleeding?
- Disability—Assess pupillary responses and calculate GCS (*see LOC section for GCS*).
- Exposure—Completely uncover the patient. Ensure you are warming them as much as possible—via warmed IV fluid and covering the patient with warm blankets as soon as possible.

Recheck your ABCDEs constantly. If there is a change in condition, immediately revert to "A."—"A" is your safe zone, your "happy place" if you will….

ADJUNCTS TO THE PRIMARY SURVEY

- Monitors
  - ECG, pulse oximeter, BP, ventilatory rate
- Urinary catheter
- Trauma labs
  - CBC, electrolytes, blood type and crossmatch, urinalysis, toxicology screen, serum EtOH, arterial blood gas
- X-rays
  - AP pelvis.
  - CXR.
  - In most cases a lateral C-spine view is not required. Leave patient in C-spine precautions if concerned.

SECONDARY SURVEY

- Does not begin until the primary survey is completed, resuscitative efforts are underway, and the normalization of vital functions has been demonstrated.
- Recheck ABCDEs.
- A thorough and systematic examination from head to toe (including log roll and rectal examination) is to be performed.
- This means a full history and physical examination.
- Attain AMPLE history from patient, family, or EMS.
  - A—allergies
  - M—medications
  - P—past medical history
  - L—last meal
  - E—events, what happened? Ask about the mechanism of injury

ADJUNCTS TO THE SECONDARY SURVEY

- NG or OG tubes—if you are certain there is no sign of basal skull fracture
  - No Battle sign, no otorhinorrhea
- Foley catheter—if you are certain there is no bladder or urethral trauma
  - No blood at meatus, normal rectal examination
- ECG if indicated—that is, if cardiac ischemia or contusion is suspected
- Additional imaging
  - X-rays of extremities, CT scan if indicated—**ONLY IF PATIENT IS STABLE**

DEFINITIVE MANAGEMENT

- Stabilize the patient to the best of your, and your facilities, ability.
- Seek help and advice early from a traumatologist.
- Discuss most appropriate mode of transfer—ground versus airplane versus helicopter.
- "Package up" the patient for transfer:
  - Intubation and placement of chest tubes in an ambulance is very unpleasant. It's also unpleasant on the side of a busy highway. It's almost impossible in a plane or helicopter. Anticipate what your patient might need before transferring.

- If transferring via air, remember that a pneumothorax will progress faster as altitude increases during flight. Also, remember that FiO_2 decreases with altitude. If a patient is not maintaining sats at ground level, this will be made worse during flight.

But......

- Do not take extra time with procedures or diagnostics (ie, CT scans) unless they contribute appropriately to the patient's stability in preparation for transfer. Do not undertake diagnostics that your facility is not equipped to act upon (ie, if you do not have surgical coverage, don't do a CT scan).
- Travel with the patient in the ambulance/plane/helicopter if there is ongoing hemodynamic instability. Early consultation with a transport service is important as soon as you recognize that the person will outstrip you facilities capabilities.

LIFE-THREATENING TRAUMA EMERGENCY SCENARIOS THAT FAMILY PHYSICIANS SHOULD KNOW

Tension Pneumothorax

- Signs/symptoms: Hemodynamic instability, respiratory distress, increased HR, asymmetrical chest wall motion, tracheal deviation, hyperresonance to percussion, unilateral absence of breath sounds.
- Rx: Needle thoracostomy at second intercostal space at mid-clavicular line. Do not delay for X-ray. Follow with chest tube at fifth intercostal space at anterior axillary line.

Cardiac Tamponade

- Signs/symptoms: Usually with penetrating chest wound. Beck triad (hypotension, distended neck veins, muffled heart sounds), pulsus paradoxus (abnormally large drop in SBP on inspiration), Kussmaul sign (rise in JVP on inspiration).
- Rx: Confirm with ECHO or bedside U/S if possible; pericardiocentesis (at xiphoid, aim needle at 45 degrees towards nipple).

Bibliography

American College of Surgeons Committee on Trauma. *Advanced Trauma Life Support for Doctors*. 9th ed. Chicago, IL: American College of Surgeons; 2012.

Chen YA, Tran C. *Toronto Notes–Comprehensive Medical Reference & Review for MCCQE I and USMLE II*. Toronto, Canada: Toronto Notes for Medical Students; 2013.

Tintinalli JE, Stapczynski JS, Cline DM, Ma OJ, Yealy DM, Meckler GD, eds. *Tintinalli's Emergency Medicine: A Comprehensive Study Guide*. 8th ed. New York, NY: McGraw-Hill; 2015.

Shock

Supplementary Topic

Definition

Inadequate end-organ perfusion resulting in loss of aerobic cellular function

The "end organs" are

- Brain (signs—altered consciousness, loss of consciousness)
- Kidneys (signs—decreased urine output)
- Skin (signs—cool, clammy, dusky, pale)
- Heart (signs—myocardial ischemia, decreased cardiac output, hypotension)

TYPES OF SHOCK

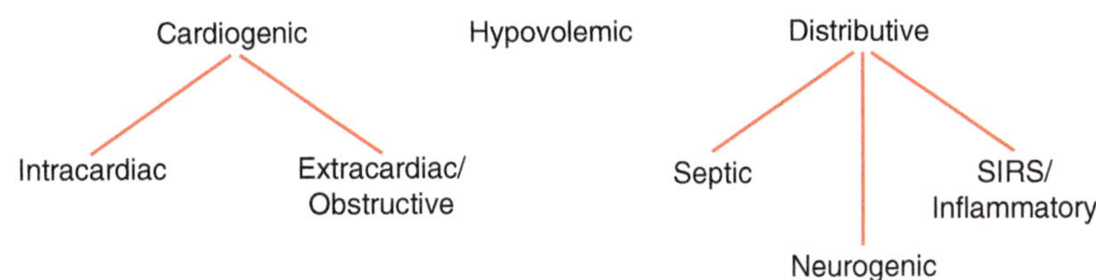

Hypovolemic Shock

Definition

Lack of effective circulating blood volume

- Beware:
  - Bleeding might not be external—meaning gastrointestinal (GI) bleed, ruptured ovarian cyst, femur fracture, pelvic fracture, etc.
  - "Blood" isn't just the red stuff. Large serum losses, such as in burn patients, nausea and vomiting, high output ileostomy, and pancreatitis can also lead to hypovolemia.

Signs

Tachycardia; peripheral vasoconstriction leading to cool, clammy skin; acidosis; tachypnea; altered mental status

Decreased urine output is the most sensitive, and simplest, method to monitor response to hypovolemic shock resuscitation.

Treatment

- Stop the bleeding!!!
- Simultaneously restore blood volume with crystalloid, transfusions.
- In patients with life-threatening hypotension, use vasopressors in addition to fluids to maintain target arterial pressure. Fill the tank, then optimize the pump and plumbing!!!

Cardiogenic Shock

Definition

- Decreased cardiac output and evidence of tissue hypoxia in the presence of adequate intravascular volume
- Occurs most often due to myocardial ischemia, but can also occur due to valve disease, cardiac trauma, massive pulmonary embolus, or cardiac tamponade

  Intracardiac:
  - Ischemia
  - Valve disease, involves endocarditis, chordae rupture, but is rare
  - Contusion

  Extracardiac—also referred to as obstructive
  - Cardiac tamponade
  - Massive pulmonary embolism

Signs

Distended jugular veins (increased JVP); arrhythmia and/or tachycardia, altered LOC, decreased urine output

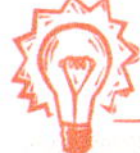

Cardiogenic shock—Think of this as a pump problem

Distributive shock—Think of this as a plumbing problem.

Treatment

- Treat ischemia if present.
- If ischemia not present, as evidenced by normal ECG and troponins, consider another possible diagnosis, valve issue, contusion, tamponade, or massive PE, and get help (you're gonna need it)!!!!
- Often there is a role for inotropic medications to temporize until definitive treatment can be reached.
- Early consultation with expert is recommended early for suspected massive PE.

Distributive Shock

Definition

- Loss of vascular tone, and in turn, poor venous return leading to poor cardiac function and output
- Distributive shock is of three types:
  1. Septic
  2. SIRS/inflammatory
  3. Neurogenic

1. Septic Shock

Definition

Acute circulatory failure characterized by persistent arterial hypotension despite adequate fluid resuscitation or by tissue hypoperfusion (as defined by a lactate concentration >4 mg/dL), and not explained by other causes.

Signs

Fever (not always), hypothermia (if severe sepsis), decreased LOC, decreased urine output

Treatment

Most important step is recognition of a patient as **very** sick, and that they are in need of the services of a facility that offers critical care services!!

- Attempt to identify a possible focus of infection
- If possible draw cultures **prior to** starting antibiotics
- Start empiric, broad-spectrum antibiotics ASAP based on suspected source and community susceptibility patterns
  - Time of first dose of antibiotics is directly linked to outcome
- Supportive care
  - Think ABCs
  - Oxygen by mask
  - Intubate if necessary
    - To improve oxygenation and/or
    - To reduce the work of breathing
    - Can reduce oxygen needs by up to 30%
  - Fluid resuscitation and monitoring via Foley and urometer. Most patients will require 20 to 40 mL/kg over the first 6 hours
  - Vasopressors have a definite role

2. Inflammatory Shock/SIRS

Definition

A combination of multiple, synergistically destructive, pathophysiologic processes that lead to endothelial dysfunction, fluid losses, and in turn, end-organ dysfunction

- Criteria:
  - Two or more of the following factors:
    - Body temperature <36°C or >38°C

- ○ Heart rate >90 beats/min
- ○ Tachypnea >20 breaths/min or arterial partial pressure of carbon dioxide <32 mm Hg
- ○ White count <4000 cells/mm³ (4×10^9 cells/L) or >12,000 cells/mm³ (12×10^9 cells/L) or the presence of >10% bands

Causes

- Anaphylaxis
- Pancreatitis
- Toxins, insect or snake bites
- Bowel ischemia or necrosis
- Burns
- Toxic shock syndrome
- Sepsis

"SIRS" is a bit of an odd classification for the nonintensivist, in that it encompasses some of the rarer causes of shock, but the main causes (hypovolemia, cardiogenic, septic, etc.) can cross over into SIRS.

Septic shock is simply SIRS with a known infection.

3. Neurogenic Shock

Definition

Hypotension caused by loss of vascular tone, secondary to loss of sympathetic outflow from the T1 to L2 sympathetic chain.

Common error is to confuse this with "spinal shock." **Spinal shock and neurogenic shock are completely different**. They are a terrible practical joke of medical nomenclature, sorry about that.

Spinal shock is a state of transient physiologic (vs anatomic) loss of cord function below the level of injury, with associated loss of all reflex and sensorimotor functions. This lasts somewhere from 1 to 24 hours. It has **nothing** to do with hemodynamics or end-organ function.

Classic Manifestations of Neurogenic Shock

- Hypotension **and** bradycardia (typically hypotension would be accompanied by **tachy**cardia)

Treatment

- Recognition of underlying spinal cord injury and transfer to appropriate specialist
  - Vasopressors play a definite role. Goal MAPs should be >80 mm Hg to perfuse the watershed area of the injury.

Beware of concomitant hypovolemia that often occurs along with spinal cord injuries. Car accidents with enough energy to crush a spinal cord often have enough energy to break a pelvis, a femur, or cause a hemothorax. Urine output is your best guide to ensuring proper end-organ perfusion.

Bibliography

Gaieski DF, Mikkelsen ME. Definition, classification, etiology, and pathophysiology of shock in adults. In: PE Parson, G Finlay eds, *UpToDate;* 2016. Retrieved from http://www.uptodate.com/.

Kearon C, Akl EA, Ornelas J, et al. Antithrombotic therapy for VTE disease: Chest Guideline and Expert Panel Report. *Chest* 2016;149(2):315-352.

ProCESS Investigators, Yealy DM, Kellum JA, Huang DT, et al. A randomized trial of protocol-based care for early septic shock. *N Engl J Med* 2014;370(18):1683-1693.

Tintinalli JE, Stapczynski JS, Cline DM, Ma OJ, Yealy DM, Meckler GD eds. *Tintinalli's Emergency Medicine: A Comprehensive Study Guide.* 8th ed. New York, NY: McGraw-Hill; 2015.

Approach to Poisoning

Priority Topic 74

INITIAL EVALUATION

ABCDEs

- Airway management
  - Give naloxone if considering opioid overdose (naloxone 0.4 mg IV or 2 mg intranasal q4min).

    Note: Naloxone is lifesaving but will immediately result in severe narcotic withdrawal. Naloxone has a shorter half-life than most ingested narcotics so repeat doses are required.
    - Respiratory rate <12 breaths/min is the best predictor of response to naloxone
- Breathing
  - Give 100% oxygen in carbon monoxide poisoning
- Circulation
  - ECG and cardiac monitor (arrhythmia, electrolyte abnormalities)
- Drugs
  - Universal antidotes; empiric treatment with naloxone, glucose, and thiamine should be considered as they are relatively cheap and safe treatments of three common causes of altered mental status (opioid overdose, hypoglycemia, and Wernicke encephalopathy).
- Decontamination
  - Ipecac syrup for inducing emesis should **not** be used as it has significant potential adverse effects.
  - Orogastric lavage is not recommended except in exceptional circumstance and under the direction of a trained toxicologist.
    - Airway protection is essential!
  - Activated charcoal
    - Indicated if within 1 to 2 hours post ingestion.
    - Complications include aspiration/vomiting/constipation and diarrhea.
    - Dosing: 10:1 (charcoal to drug) or 1 g charcoal/kg body weight, whichever is larger.
    - Drugs not bound by charcoal include; iron, lithium, lead, hydrocarbons, and toxic alcohols.
- Elimination
  - Urinary alkalinization
    - Enhances urinary elimination of certain drugs (salicylates, phenobarbital, methotrexate).
    - Achieved by IV sodium bicarbonate bolus or infusion (3 amps $NaHCO_3$ in 1 L D_5W at 1.5-2 × normal maintenance rate).
    - Most commonly used in moderate-to-severe ASA overdose.
    - Contraindicated in hypokalemia and renal insufficiency.
  - Hemodialysis
    - Used for removal of potentially life-threatening toxins that have either already been absorbed or do not bind to activated charcoal.
    - Common toxins include ASA, lithium, theophylline, toxic alcohols, and carbamazepine.

INDICATIONS FOR DIALYSIS:

A   Acidosis

E   Electrolytes (increased K)

I   Intoxication (ASA, methanol, ethylene glycol)

O   Overload (fluids)

U   Uremia

DRUGS THAT ARE NOT ABSORBED BY CHARCOAL:

P   Pesticides, potassium

H   Hydrocarbons

A   Alkali, acids, alcohols

I   Iron

L   Lithium, lead

S   Solvents

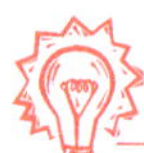

FORMULAS TO KNOW TO TREAT POISONED PATIENTS:

Anion gap = Measured − [Na^+ − (Cl^- + HCO_3^-)]

Normal <12

Osmolar gap = Measured − [$2Na^+$ + glucose + BUN + (1.25 × ETOH)]

Normal <10

Key Questions to Ask

- Who? (adult or pediatric)
- What was ingested? What else was consumed? (alcohol, acetaminophen, etc.)
- How much was ingested?
- How was it taken? (PO, IV, transdermal, mucous membranes, inhalational)
- When was the ingestion and how long was exposure?
- Collateral history from family, friends, paramedics, and police.

ANION GAP—CAUSES:

M	Methanol
U	Uremia
D	DKA
P	Paraldehyde
I	Iron, ibuprofen, isoniazid
L	Lactic acidosis
E	Ethylene glycol
S	Salicylates

TABLE 1-9　Common Toxidromes

TOXIDROME	CLINICAL PRESENTATION	TREATMENT
Alcohol (ethanol)	• Disinhibition, slurred speech, ataxia, aggression, hypoglycemia, retrograde amnesia, coma	• Thiamine (250-500 mg IM/IV BID × 3 days) • Folate (1-5 mg PO/IM/IV daily) • Treat hypoglycemia • Supportive treatments
Opioids	• Triad of miosis, CNS depression, and respiratory depression	• Ventilatory support • Naloxone (0.4 mg IV or 2 mg intranasal q4min)
Sympathomimetics (cocaine, amphetamines, alcohol withdrawal, decongestants)	• Agitation/excitation, hypertension, tachycardia, mydriasis, hyperthermia, diaphoresis, sudden death	• Cooling • Benzodiazepines for agitation and hypertension • Treat cocaine-induced MI as per ACS protocol • Avoid beta-blockers in cocaine OD
Anticholinergics (TCA, antihistamines, antipsychotics, gravol, benadryl, bladder medications)	• Hot as a hare-hyperthermia • Dry as a bone-dry skin and mucous membranes • Red as a beet-flushed skin • Blind as a bat-mydriasis • Mad as a hatter-altered mental status • Also dysrhythmias and seizure	• Benzodiazepines • Cooling • Physostigmine in certain situations
Cholinergics (organophosphates, pesticides)	**D**-diarrhea/diaphoresis **U**-urination **M**-miosis **B**-bradycardia/bronchorrhea **E**-emesis **L**-lacrimation **S**-salivation • Also muscle weakness and respiratory failure	• Airway and ventilatory support • Atropine (lots!) • Pralidoxime
TCA	**3Cs:** **C**ardiotoxicity (wide QRS and prolonged QT) **C**onvulsion/seizure **C**oma/sedation Other: ataxia, dry mouth, urinary retention	• Sodium bicarbonate (for wide QRS) • Circulatory support • Benzodiazepines for seizures
Sedatives (barbiturates, benzodiazepines)	• Decreased level of consciousness, slurred speech, ataxia, respiratory depression	• Supportive
Hallucinogens (phencyclidine hydrochloride [PCP], lysergic acid diethylamide [LSD])	• Psychosis, agitation, hallucination, hyperthermia, mydriasis, nausea	• Supportive • Benzodiazepines

ACETAMINOPHEN OVERDOSE

- The metabolite *N*-acetyl P-benzoquinone imine (NAPQI) causes hepatotoxicity.
- **Toxic dose = 150 mg/kg**.
- Have high clinical suspicion as it is often found in combination with other drug overdoses.
- Appropriate treatment with *N*-acetylcysteine (NAC) has a near 100% success rate if given <8 hours from ingestion.

Clinical Features

1.	<24 hours	Nausea, vomiting, and diaphoresis
2.	24 to 48 hours	Often asymptomatic or RUQ pain
		Minor increases in transaminases, bilirubin, and prothrombin time may be seen
3.	72 to 96 hours	Peak liver dysfunction, jaundice, pain, encephalopathy, GI symptoms
4.	4 days to 2 weeks	Spectrum ranges from full recovery to death or liver transplant

Treatment

- Initial evaluation and supportive treatment
- Decontamination
  - Consider activate charcoal if within 1 to 2 hours
- Consult poison control
- Serum NAPQI level at 4 hours post ingestion or as soon as possible → plot level on Rumack-Matthew nomogram
- Begin treatment with NAC if:
  - Time of ingestion is known and serum NAPQI level falls above the lower line on the nomogram.
  - Serum level not available until >8 hours post ingestion, first dose of NAC should be given.
    - NAC may be discontinued if acetaminophen level is subsequently found to be nontoxic.
    - Time since ingestion is not known or >24 hours.
    - Continue treatment after initial dose if serum acetaminophen >10 mcg/mL or elevated AST/ALT.

ASA OVERDOSE

- Mechanism/toxicity caused by direct stimulation of respiratory centre and chemoreceptor trigger zone, uncoupling of oxidative phosphorylation, increased fatty acid metabolism, ototoxicity.
- Chronic ingestion is associated with higher toxicity for a given salicylate level.

Clinical Features

- Nausea, vomiting, tinnitus, hearing loss, tachypnea/hyperventilation, altered mental status
- Mixed acid–base disturbance
  - **Metabolic acidosis**
    - ASA inhibits the Krebs cycle and oxidative phosphorylation leading to increased production of CO_2, heat, metabolic acids, and enhancing glycolysis and lipolysis.
    - Usually will have an elevated anion gap but in the case of co-ingestion it may be normal.

- **Respiratory alkalosis**
  - ◦ ASA causes direct stimulation of the medullary respiratory centre.

Diagnosis

- Salicylate levels—repeat Q2H until level falls and clinical improvement
- Blood gas—follow serially until metabolic acidosis resolves
- Electrolytes, liver function tests, CBC, urinalysis
- ECG
- Abdominal XR—concretions may appear on plain abdominal film

Treatment

- ABCs—significant volume depletion is common
- Decontamination—activated charcoal if within 2 hours
- Elimination
  - Urine alkalinization
    - ◦ For moderate-to-severe toxicity.
    - ◦ Bolus of 1 to 2 mEq/kg $NaHCO_3$ followed by an infusion (three ampules of $NaHCO_3$ added to 1 L of 5% dextrose in water).
    - ◦ Follow urine pH Q1H and titrate infusion to a pH >7.5.
    - ◦ Monitor for hypokalemia and replace as needed.
  - Hemodialysis
    - ◦ Indications include serum ASA >100 mg/dL, refractory acidosis, need for respiratory support, renal failure, altered mental status, and severe acid–base disorder.

Bibliography

Hall JB, Schmidt GA, Wood LDH, eds. *Principles of Critical Care*. 3rd ed. New York, NY: McGraw-Hill; 2005.

Longo DL, Fauci AS, Kasper DL, Hauser SL, Jameson JL, Loscalzo J, eds. *Harrison's Principles of Internal Medicine*. 18th ed. New York, NY: McGraw-Hill; 2012.

Tintinalli JE, Stapczynski JS, Cline DM, Ma OJ, Yealy DM, Meckler GD, eds. *Tintinalli's Emergency Medicine: A Comprehensive Study Guide*. 8th ed. New York, NY: McGraw-Hill; 2015.

CLASSIC ASA TOXICITY
Respiratory alkalosis
Increased anion-gap metabolic acidosis

Chest Pain

Priority Topic 13

Chest pain is one of the most common presenting complaints to the emergency department (ED). It is the responsibility of the clinician to identify those patients at high risk of life-threatening causes of chest pain and manage them accordingly.

Always start with ABCs and address life-threatening issues immediately.

If the patient has any of the following:

- Visceral-type chest pain (difficult to describe, radiates, imprecise location, *heaviness, discomfort, pressure, aching*)
- Abnormal vital signs
- Significant vascular disease risk factors
- Dyspnea

Place patient in treatment room, hook up a cardiac monitor, establish IV access, give O_2, and perform an ECG. Initiate ACLS protocols as appropriate.

History/Risk Factors

- HPI: Onset, duration, quality, severity, radiation, associated symptoms
- PMHx: DM, previous CV disease, dyslipidemia, HTN
- FHx: MI in first-degree relative (female <65, male <55)
- SHx: Obesity, smoking, EtOH, age

The HEART Score has been shown to reliably predict the risk of MACE (major adverse cardiac events).

TABLE 1-10   Chest Pain: Causes, Characteristics, and Management

ETIOLOGY	CLASSIC SIGNS/ SYMPTOMS	CHARACTERISTIC FINDINGS	APPROPRIATE WORKUP	TIMELY MANAGEMENT
Aortic dissection	Sudden, severe pain, described as "tearing," radiates to back	CXR-widened mediastinum, >20 mm Hg difference in BP on right vs left sides	TEE, MRI, or CT	ABCs, straight to OR if dissection otherwise admit to ICU Decrease contractility and arterial BP (BBs, CCBs, nitrates) Surgery if ascending aneurysm or if descending aneurysm >5 cm
Pulmonary embolism	Pleuritic CP, dyspnea, decreased O_2 saturation, anxiety, tachycardia	ECG (T-wave inversions in V_1-V_4, RBBB, S_1-Q_3-T_3 pattern) CXR-usually normal, 5% show Westermark sign or Hampton hump	D-dimer, ECG, CXR, Doppler U/S (to look for DVT), VQ scan, chest CT Use Wells or PERC score (see Table 1-12)	ABCs Heparin → oral anticoagulant
Pneumothorax	Pleuritic CP, dyspnea, tachycardia, tachypnea, hypoxia	Decreased/absent breath sounds on affected side Tension pneumothorax: Tracheal deviation away from affected side with mediastinal deviation on CXR CXR: Lung markings do not extend to periphery	CXR if patient stable	Tension pneumothorax: Needle decompression and/or chest tube If clinically significant: Chest tube/ Heimlich valve May consider watchful waiting if asymptomatic/small pneumothorax
Acute coronary syndromes (UA, NSTEMI, STEMI)	Retrosternal squeezing/ pressure, radiates to arm/shoulder/jaw/neck, dyspnea, n/v, syncope Remember: DM and women present nonspecifically	Unstable angina: No ST or biomarker elevation NSTEMI: No ST changes, biomarkers elevated STEMI: Biomarker and ST elevation	Troponin/CK-MB, ECG, CXR	ABCs Pain control (morphine), oxygen, ASA/clopidogrel, nitro Call cardio: PCI or thrombolysis
Pericarditis	Anterior, precordial CP, pleuritic, better with leaning forward	ECG: Diffuse ST elevation (saddle-shaped), PR interval depression Pericardial friction rub on auscultation	ECG Clinical diagnosis	Supportive treatment, fluids, NSAIDs, steroids
GERD/hiatal hernia/ esophageal perforation	Hx of frequent heartburn, dysphagia, relief with antacid If perforation: fever, dyspnea, subQ emphysema, tachycardia, hematemesis	CXR- rule out pneumomediastinum	Perf: CXR, CT, contrast swallow GERD/HH: Upper GI series, gastroscopy, or barium swallow	GERD/HH: trial of PPI, +/− gastroscopy, lifestyle modification Perf: ABCs, supportive, NPO, Abx, consult surgery
Peptic ulcer disease	Dyspepsia +/− UGI bleed, burning 1-3 h postprandial, improvement with food	*Helicobacter pylori*, stress Hx of NSAID or EtOH use	*Helicobacter pylori* serology, urea breath testing, gastroscopy	*Helicobacter pylori* eradication (PPI, Amox, Clarithro) Lifestyle modifications. D/C NSAID use, quit smoking, lose weight
Cardiac tamponade	Dyspnea, hypotension, tachycardia, CP	Elevated JVP, narrowed pulse pressure, muffled heart sounds	ECG, ECHO	ABCs, pericardiocentesis, surgery
Varicella zoster (shingles)	Tingling sensation → vesicular rash following a dermatome	Unilateral vesicular rash with dermatomal pattern Risks: immunocompromised (cancer, old, HIV+)	Clinical diagnosis, may do serology if unsure	Acyclovir (within 72 h of pain) Contagious until lesions crusted Post-herpetic neuralgia (NSAIDs, gabapentin, TCAs)
Esophageal spasm	Dysphagia (liquids and solids), CP		Barium swallow, manometry	Anticholinergics, nitrates, CCBs, botulinum toxin injection

TABLE 1-11 — The HEART Score for Chest Pain Patient in the ED

History	Highly suspicious	2 points
	Moderately suspicious	1 point
	Slight or non-suspicious	0 point
ECG	Significant ST-depression	2 points
	Nonspecific repolarization	1 point
	Normal	0 point
Age	≥65 years	2 points
	>45-64 years	1 point
	<45 years	0 point
Risk factors	≥3 risk factors or history of CAD	2 points
	1 or 2 risk factors	1 point
	No risk factors	0 point
Troponin	≥3 × normal limit	2 points
	>1 - < 3 × normal limit	1 point
	<normal limit	0 point

Risk factors: DM, current or recent smoker (< 1 month), HTN, hyperlipidemia, obesity, family history of CAD

Score 0-3: 2.5 % MACE over the next 6 weeks—Discharge home
Score 4-6: 20.3% MACE over the next 6 weeks—Admit for clinical observation
Score 7-10: 72.7% MACE over the next 6 weeks—Early invasive strategies

TABLE 1-12 — Wells Score for PE

FACTOR	POINTS
Suspected DVT	3
Alternative Dx less likely than PE	3
Tachycardia (HR >100 bpm)	1.5
Prior VTE	1.5
Immobilization/surgery within past 4 weeks	1.5
Active malignancy	1
Hemoptysis	1

Score <4 do D-dimer (sensitive, not specific, high NPV).
Score >4 do CT chest or VQ scan. (CT chest less sensitive than VQ scan)
Score >6 is high probability of PE (78.4%).
Score <2 is low probability of PE (3.4%).

Bibliography

Backus BE, Six AJ, Kelder JC, et al. A prospective validation of the HEART score for chest pain patients at the emergency department. *Int J Cardiol.* 2013;168(3):2153-2158. doi:10.1016/j.ijcard.2013.01.255. http://www.ncbi.nlm.nih.gov/pubmed/23465250.

Backus BE, Six AJ, Kelder JH, et al. Risk scores for patients with chest pain: evaluation in the emergency department. *Curr Cardiol Rev.* 2011;7(1):2-8. doi:10.2174/157340311795677662. http://www.ncbi.nlm.nih.gov/pubmed/22294968.

DynaMed. Chest Pain. Ipswich, MA: EBSCO Publishing; November 2016. Retrieved November 28, 2016 from http://search.ebscohost.com/login.aspx?direct=true&db=dme&AN=116633&site=dynamed-live&scope=site.

Green GB, Hill PM. Chest pain: cardiac or not. In: Tintinalli JE, Stapcznski JS, John Ma O, Cline DM, Cydulka RK, Meckler GD, eds. *Emergency Medicine: A Comprehensive Study Guide.* 8th ed. New York: McGraw-Hill; 2015.

Hollander JE, Dierks DB. Acute coronary syndromes: acute myocardial infarction and unstable angina. In: Tintinalli JE, Stapcznski JS, John Ma O, Cline DM, Cydulka RK, Meckler GD, eds. *Emergency Medicine: A Comprehensive Study Guide.* 8th ed. New York: McGraw-Hill; 2015.

Kline JA. Thromboembolism. In: Tintinalli JE, Stapcznski JS, John Ma O, Cline DM, Cydulka RK, Meckler GD, eds. *Emergency Medicine: A Comprehensive Study Guide.* 8th ed. New York: McGraw-Hill; 2015.

Six AJ, Backus BE, Kelder JC. Chest pain in the emergency room: value of the HEART score. *Neth Heart J.* 2008;16(6):191-196. http://www.ncbi.nlm.nih.gov/pubmed/18665203.

Wells PS, Anderson DR, Rodger M, et. al. Derivation of a simple clinical model to categorize patients probability of pulmonary embolism: increasing the models utility with the SimpliRED D-dimer. *Thromb Haemost.* 2000 Mar;83(3):416-20.

Atrial Fibrillation (AF)

Priority Topic 8

Definition

- A *regularly irregular* rhythm

Symptoms

- May be asymptomatic, especially with chronic AF
- Palpitations, SOB, lightheadedness/dizziness/presyncope, focal neurological deficit (with stroke)

Risk Factors

HTN	EtOH	Cardiomyopathy (ischemic/HF)
Thyrotoxicosis	Valvular heart disease	MI
PE	Pneumonia	Hypokalemia/hypomagnesemia
Hypoxia	Rheumatic heart disease	ASD
Pericardial disease	Sick sinus syndrome	Post-cardiac surgery
SVT	Familial/genetic	Obstructive sleep apnea
Obesity	COPD	Pulmonary HTN

Classification

Four categories:

1. New onset
2. Paroxysmal (short bursts with spontaneous conversion to sinus rhythm)
3. Persistent (lasts >7 days, requires pharmacological or electrical cardioversion)
4. Permanent (prolonged symptoms [>1 year] or refractory to cardioversion)

CHA_2DS_2-VASc Scoring

Used to determine appropriate anticoagulation treatment and to estimate stroke risk (Refer to Canadian Cardiovascular Society for detailed information on stroke prevention in AF)

C: CHF (1 pt)

H: HTN (1 pt)

A: age ≥75 (2 pt)

D: diabetes (1 pt)

S: stroke/TIA history (2 pts)

V: vascular disease (MI, PAD) (1 pt)

A: age 65 to 74 (1 pt)

S: sex = female (1 pt)

Score:

- 0: ASA 325 mg po daily
- 1: If female and <65—ASA 325 mg po daily
  Otherwise, may consider oral anticoagulant*—DOAC or warfarin (INR 2-3)
- 2+: Oral anticoagulant*—DOAC or warfarin (INR 2-3)

Management

- Always start with ABCs and address life-threatening issues first!
- Goal is to alleviate patient symptoms, improve quality of life, and decrease mortality/morbidity and not necessarily the elimination of atrial fibrillation.

Investigations

- CBC, INR/PTT, renal and liver panels, TSH (fasting glucose and lipids should also be done but as an outpatient, not in the ED).
- 12-lead ECG (rate, rhythm, conduction disturbances, signs of previous MI, ventricular hypertrophy, atrial enlargement).
- Echocardiogram (to document ventricular size, wall thickness, EF, left atrial size, **presence of valvular pathology**, or congenital heart disease)—does not need to be done in ED unless urgent cardioversion required (see electrical cardioversion section).

Treatment

For detailed guidelines refer to Canadian Cardiovascular Society (www.ccs.ca).

Rate and Rhythm Control

Goal is resting HR <100 bpm in persistent or permanent AF

A. Rate control:
   - Start with rate control, if symptoms continue then move on to rhythm control.
   - Initial rate control therapy
     - No history of MI or LV dysfunction—beta-blockers (eg, metoprolol) or nondihydropyridine calcium channel blockers (eg, diltiazem)
     - History of MI or LV dysfunction—beta-blockers

B. Rhythm control (maintenance of sinus rhythm): To be discussed with a cardiologist
   a. Nonstructural heart disease:
      i. Dronedarone, flecainide, propafenone, or sotalol
   b. Abnormal LV function but LVEF >35%:
      i. Dronedarone, sotalol, or amiodarone
   c. LVEF <35%:
      i. Amiodarone
   - Digoxin is not recommended as initial rhythm control therapy in an active patient. Reserve use for sedentary or LV systolic dysfunction patients (heart failure). Digoxin can be used as an adjunct to BBs and CCBs to achieve better rate control, but should not be used on its own.

C. Electric cardioversion
   - Initially use 120 to 200 J biphasic waveform
   - Indications
     - For unstable patients

---

*DOAC = direct oral anticoagulant; preferred over warfarin in nonvalvular AF.

- If AF <48 hours, or anticoagulation >3 weeks, and >4 weeks since previous cardioversion
- If AF >48 hour duration and not anticoagulated/subtherapeutic → need transesophageal echocardiogram to ensure no thrombosis in atria/ventricles prior to cardioversion

Anticoagulation

- Purpose: Prevention of thrombus/embolus
- Anticoagulate with ASA or oral anticoagulant as appropriate (see above for CHA_2DS_2-VASc scoring and anticoagulation determination)

Follow-Up

- Outpatient follow-up with cardiology and family physician.

Bibliography

Canadian Cardiovascular Society. *Atrial Fibrillation Guidelines*. 2016. Retrieved 28/11/2016, from http://www.ccs.ca/images/Guidelines/PocketGuides_EN/Pocket_Guides/AF_Pocket_Guide_2016.pdf

DynaMed. Atrial Fibrillation. Ipswich, MA: EBSCO Publishing; November 2016. Retrieved November 28, 2016, from http://search.ebscohost.com/login.aspx?direct=true&db=dme&AN=115288&site=dynamed-live&scope=site.

Piktel JS. Cardiac rhythm disturbances. In: Tintinalli JE, Stapcznski JS, John Ma O, Cline DM, Cydulka RK, Meckler GD, eds. *Emergency Medicine: A Comprehensive Study Guide.* 8th ed. New York: McGraw-Hill; 2015.

Seizures

Priority Topic 81

Definitions

- Seizure
  - An episode of abnormal neurologic function caused by the inappropriate electrical discharge of cerebral neurons
- Generalized seizure
  - Begins with **loss of consciousness** and is caused by nearly simultaneous activation of the entire cerebral cortex
  - May be generalized tonic-clonic (grand mal), absence (petit mal), or myoclonic
- Partial seizure (focal)
  - Electrical discharges begin in a localized region and may or may not spread to involve other regions or the entire cortex.
  - Consciousness not affected = **simple partial seizure**.
  - Consciousness affected = **complex partial seizure**.
- Status epilepticus
  - Seizure lasting 5 to 15 minutes or seizures that recur prior to the full return of consciousness.

History

- History of seizure disorder.
- Precipitating factors.
- Grand mal seizures will usually begin with the patient becoming very rigid with extremities extended and progress into the clonic phase of rhythmic jerking movements.
- Always attempt to determine if the movements were localized or generalized and symmetric.

- Duration typically 60 to 90 seconds. This is often overestimated by witnesses.
- Loss of bowel and bladder control, tongue biting.
- Apnea and cyanosis.
- Gradual return to consciousness and a postictal phase of confusion.

Physical Examination

- Vital signs, temperature, serum glucose
- Complete neurologic examination looking for any focal signs
- Examine for injuries that were sustained during the attack

Differential Diagnosis

- Syncope, migraine, narcolepsy, movement disorder, pseudoseizure, vagal episode

Treatment

- Protect airway, oxygen, and prepare for endotracheal intubation if unable to terminate seizure.
- IV access if possible.
- Bedside glucose.
- Terminate seizure.
  - First-line agents
    - Benzodiazepines—Lorazepam or diazepam
    - Diazepam may be given by rectal or endotracheal route and midazolam may be given IM if unable to secure IV access
  - Second-line agents
    - Phenytoin (15-20 mg/kg IV, max 50 mg/min)
    - Fosphenytoin—can be given faster (100-150 mg "phenytoin equivalents" per min IV or IM)
    - Consult neurology and consider ICU admission
- Investigations.
  - If known seizure disorder exists:
    - Serum anticonvulsant levels
  - If first time seizure:
    - CBC, glucose, renal panel, Ca, Mg, β-hCG, toxicology screen, head CT, EEG
- Neurology consult to determine need for long-term treatment.

Key Points

- Patient must be seizure free for 1 year before driving. Check provincial reporting laws.
- Warn patient about dangers related to swimming, living alone, operating heavy machinery, chewing gum, heights.
- Anticonvulsants are teratogenic; women should take 4 to 6 mg/day of folic acid during childbearing years and be on lowest-possible dose of anticonvulsant.
- Many antibiotics can interfere with anticonvulsant levels.
- Anticonvulsants can lead to osteoporosis, hematologic complications, liver dysfunction, GI upset, and fatigue.

Bibliography

Hall JB, Schmidt GA, Wood LDH, eds. *Principles of Critical Care*. 3rd ed. New York, NY: McGraw-Hill; 2005.

McPhee SJ, Papadakis MA, eds. *Current Medical Diagnosis & Treatment*. New York, NY: McGraw-Hill; 2012.

Tintinalli JE, Stapczynski JS, Cline DM, Ma OJ, Yealy DM, Meckler GD, eds. *Tintinalli's Emergency Medicine: A Comprehensive Study Guide*. 8th ed. New York, NY: McGraw-Hill; 2015.

FEBRILE SEIZURE

Criteria:
- Temperature >38°C
- Age <6 years
- No CNS infection/inflammation
- No metabolic abnormality
- No history of afebrile seizure

May be classified as benign (simple) if it lasts <15 minutes, there are no focal signs, and seizure does not recur in 24-hour period. Febrile seizures do not cause brain damage!

Lacerations

Priority Topic 56

History

Ascertain details surrounding the laceration.

- What is the cause of laceration?
- How clean are/were the surroundings (ie, dirty cut)?
- Was a bite involved? If yes, was it human, canine, feline, or other?
- How long ago did it occur?
- Is there any chance that a foreign body may remain deep in the wound?
- Is there a possibility that there is an underlying compound fracture?

  Must ask about tetanus immunization and booster status.

  Must ask about potential allergies to local anaesthetics and antibiotics that may be required.

Physical Examination

- Use appropriate sterile conditions and adequate lighting.
- Use appropriate analgesia (local or otherwise).
- Note the position of the wound, and what surrounding structures may be injured (nerves, vessels, tendons). Test for the function of the possibly injured structures distal to the injury.
- Document all findings.
- Under no circumstances should you blindly probe into a wound with an instrument. Do not snap or clamp bleeding vessels, use direct pressure for hemostasis.
- X-ray if foreign body or underlying fracture is suspected.

Management

- First classify a laceration as simple or complex, and seek specialist assistance (plastic surgery, orthopedic, general surgery, urology, ophthalmology) if complicating factors are present.
  - A wound is simple if it has following factors:
    - Small (under 10 cm)
    - Time to treatment of <6 hours
    - No neural compromise
    - No vascular compromise
    - No tendon involvement
    - Not involving complex facial anatomy (eyelids, lip margins, globe)
    - No foreign body present
- There are differing opinions on how long a wound can be left open and a safe primary closure can be performed. Factors that weigh in on this decision are:
  - Time from injury
  - Site of injury—face versus periphery—consider blood supply
  - Level and type of contamination of wound
  - Patient factors—diabetic, immunocompromised, trustworthiness
    - If you are concerned at all, always err on the side of safety. Irrigate and dress the wound **open**, start IV antibiotics, and perform a delayed primary closure in 48 hours. A gas-producing, necrotizing, anaerobic infection can definitely happen, and almost always results in a loss of limb, and sometimes a loss of life.

- If decision is made to close wound:
1. Ensure that appropriate tetanus prophylaxis and antibiotics are given, if required.
2. Ensure that appropriate analgesia is provided:
   - Lidocaine (xylocaine)
     - Without epinephrine
       - Duration 30 to 60 minutes
       - **Maximum dose 5 mg/kg,** not to exceed 300 mg
     - With epinephrine
       - Duration 2 to 6 hours
       - **Maximum dose 7 mg/kg**
   - Bupivacaine (marcaine)
     - Without epinephrine
       - Duration 30 to 60 minutes
       - Maximum dose 2 mg/kg, not to exceed 175 mg
     - With epinephrine
       - Duration 3 to 7 hours
       - Maximum dose 3 mg/kg, not to exceed 225 mg
3. Ensure that the wound has been irrigated and debrided appropriately. Use copious amounts of irrigation (ie, >1 L of NS for a 5-cm wound).
4. Close the wound accurately using a suture technique and material appropriate for the area to be closed.
   - Close in layers with absorbable suture (ie, Vicryl) if warranted.
   - Choice of skin closure based on cosmetic requirements (ie, small, nonabsorbable suture around the eyelid, eg, Prolene) or need for rapid closure (ie, stapler for an intoxicated or hemodynamically unstable patient), etc.
5. Dress wound appropriately and arrange for necessary follow-up.
   - Immobilize the area with a splint if needed to keep tension off the wound. Remember to use the position of safety if splinting a hand.
   - Consider more frequent follow-up for wounds at higher risk of infection. Use the criteria above to make this decision.

Always draw on the plunger of your syringe before injecting to ensure you do not inject local anaesthetic intravascularly.

TETANUS IMMUNIZATION

- Td (tetanus toxoid) and TIG (tetanus immunoglobulin) are safe in pregnancy.
- Provide booster if last tetanus update was >5 years ago.
- Only give TIG if unsure of immunization status (unknown if had childhood series) and high-risk wound. TIG is never required in nontetanus-prone wounds (see Table 1-13).

TABLE 1-13	Guidelines for the Treatment of Tetanus-Prone Wounds	
HISTORY	**TOXOID REQUIRED**	**TIG REQUIRED**
Dirty wound + Unknown baseline immunization status	Yes	Yes
Dirty wound + Booster >10 years	Yes	No
Dirty wound + Booster >5 years	Yes	No
Dirty wound + Booster <5 years	No	No

SPECIAL CONSIDERATIONS

1. Small puncture wounds over flexor tendon area and injection injuries (paint sprayers, sandblasters) often result in gross, deep contamination with minimal superficial evidence of this. Be very aware.
2. Bite wounds:
   a. Canine, feline, mammalian, or human in origin.
   b. Often infected with organisms that live in the mouth (*Pasteurella multocida*, *Staphylococcus aureus*, *Bacteroides*, *Streptococcus viridans*).
   c. Do not close and consider starting on prophylactic amoxicillin/clavulanate 500 mg TID. Duration of 3 to 5 days is commonly given.
   d. Consider possibility of HIV or hepatitis B/C transmission from human bites.
   e. Update tetanus.
3. Animal wounds can be at risk of transmitting rabies.
   a. Send animal to appropriate laboratory if available.
   b. Consider rabies vaccine and RIG treatment.

Generally, *do not* close cat or human bites. May close facial wounds (due to scar risk) with close follow-up.

80% of cat bites and 5% of dog bites become infected. Consider this when deciding if antibiotic is needed.

Bibliography

Anti-infective Review Panel. *Anti-infective Guidelines for Community-Acquired Infections.* Toronto: MUMS Guideline Clearinghouse; 2010:53.

Anti-infectives for common infections—overview. *Drug Comparison Charts*. 10th ed. Saskatoon, Canada: Rx Files; 2014:77.

deLemos D. Closure of minor skin wounds with sutures. In: Stack AM, Wolfson AB, Wiley JF, eds. *UpToDate; 2016*. Retrieved from http://www.uptodate.com/.

DynaMed. Mammalian bite. Ipswich, MA: EBSCO Publishing; September 2014. Retrieved September 18, 2016, from http://search.ebscohost.com.cyber.usask.ca/login.aspx?direct=true&db=dnh&AN=116837&site=dynamed-live&scope=site.

Yingming A, Tran C, eds. Wound closure. *Toronto Notes*. 27th ed. Toronto, ON: Toronto Notes for Medical Students; 2011: PL5-PL10.

Epistaxis

Priority Topic 36

Symptoms

- Bleeding from nose
- With or without associated symptoms such as hematemesis, pain, headache, rhinorrhea, itchy/watery eyes, lightheadedness/dizziness, nausea

Risk Factors

Risk factors include the following:

Nose picking	Chemical irritants
Trauma	Chronic nasal cannula O_2 use
Foreign bodies	Recent surgery
Dry environment	Hereditary hemorrhagic telangiectasia
Blood dyscrasias	Alcohol or cocaine abuse
Inflammatory neoplasm	URTI
Polyp	
Deviated septum	Nonsteroidal anti-inflammatory drugs (NSAIDs)/ASA/warfarin/heparin/DOACs
AV malformation	HTN (esp. for posterior bleeds)

Management

1. History

- History of present illness (HPI): Onset, duration, timeline, pattern, amount of bleeding, associated symptoms, event/trauma, prior/recurrent nosebleeds
- Personal or family history of bleeding/bruising/coagulopathy
- Medications: Specifically NSAID, warfarin, heparin, and ASA use; chemotherapy
- Alcohol or cocaine abuse
- History of HTN

2. Physical Examination

- ABCs/vitals.
- In "sniffing" position use a speculum to visualize bleeding source. Area of bleeding: most commonly involved are anterior nasal septum/Little's area/Kiesselbach plexus.
- Check whether there is any fracture or instability.

Note: In the ER, the diagnosis of a posterior bleeding source is probable when there has been failure to control an anterior bleeding source. Other features that suggest a posterior source include elderly patients with a coagulopathy, significant hemorrhage seen in posterior nasopharynx, bilateral hemorrhage, hematemesis/hemoptysis.

3. Laboratories/Investigations

- Only necessary if hemodynamically unstable, suspicion of bleeding diathesis, or use of anticoagulation
- CBC, coagulation, crossmatch
- X-ray if suspect fracture/trauma history

4. Treatment

- Address airway compromise if present
- Obtain IV access and cross-match if hemodynamic instability
- Reassure patient and address their fear or anxiety
  1. Apply direct nasal pressure by pinching nares for 10 to 15 minutes. Don't cheat on this timing.
  2. Topical cocaine, xylometazoline, lidocaine, and epinephrine can be used for vasoconstriction.
  3. Chemical cauterization with silver nitrate (may anesthetise nasal mucosa first). Electrocautery should be left to ENT due to risk of septal perforation.
  4. Thrombogenic foams/gels soaked in epinephrine or liquid cocaine (if available).
  5. Anterior nasal packing with layering of ribbon gauze, an anterior epistaxis balloon, or a nasal tampon/sponge.
  6. Posterior packing—use longer lengths of anterior packing materials or a commercially available posterior packing device and call ENT.

5. Follow-up

- In case of anterior epistaxis with hemodynamic stability and hemorrhage control for >1 hour, discharge home with clear instructions on what to do if nosebleed recurs, use of humidifier, and avoidance of nose blowing.
- Patients with therapeutic warfarin levels may continue their medication.
- D/C NSAIDs for 3 to 4 days. D/C ASA and antiplatelets for 5 to 7 days if possible. May need to review with cardiology if recent stents placed.
- If anterior packing is placed in both nostrils, give Rx for staphylococcus coverage (first dose in ER).
- Remove nonabsorbable packing in 2 to 3 days.

Bibliography

DynaMed. Nosebleed. Ipswich, MA: EBSCO Publishing; September 2014. Retrieved November 28, 2016, from http://search.ebscohost.com/login.aspx?direct=true&db=dme&AN=115407&site=dynamed-live&scope=site.

Summers SM, Bey T. Epistaxis, nasal fractures, and rhinosinusitis. In: Tintinalli JE, Stapcznski JS, John Ma O, Cline DM, Cydulka RK, Meckler GD, eds. *Emergency Medicine: A Comprehensive Study Guide.* 8th ed. New York, NY: McGraw-Hill; 2015.

MEMORY CUE

Allergic = Mucoid

Viral = Watery

Bacterial = Purulent

Chlamydia = Mucopurulent

Topical steroids should be avoided as treatment of red eye by family physicians.

Red Eye

Priority Topic 79

CONJUNCTIVITIS

- Most common cause of red eye (see Table 1-14)

TABLE 1-14	Red Eye: Causes and Management				
	BACTERIAL	**GONOCOCCAL AND CHLAMYDIAL**	**VIRAL**	**HERPES**	**ATOPIC/ ALLERGIC**
Clinical presentation	• Rapid onset • One or both eyes involved • Discharge is muco-purulent. "Eye glued shut in morning" • Can progress to peri-orbital cellulitis • Photophobia signals involvement of cornea	• Consider in neonates and sexually active persons • Rapid progression • Copious purulent discharge • Unilateral • Tender pre-auricular lymph nodes • May lead to corneal perforation	• Rapid onset • Usually becomes bilateral at 24-48 h • Often associated with a viral respiratory tract infection • Watery discharge • Itchy, foreign body sensation	• Red, irritated eye • Watery discharge • Vesicles on face and eyelid • May have corneal involvement	• Very itchy eyes • Tearing • Redness • Associated with other atopy symptoms • Bilateral • No exudate
Etiology	*Staphylococcus aureus, Streptococcus pneumoniae, Haemophilus. influenzae, Mycoplasma catarrhalis*	*Neisseria gonorrhoeae, Chlamydia trachomatis*	• Usually adenovirus • Coxsackie virus	Herpes simplex type 1 or 2	
Treatment	• Most often self-limited (day 2-5) • Topical antibiotics controversial • Contagious for 48-72 h *Use antibiotics if corneal involvement or contact lens user.	• Emergent referral • GO: Ceftriaxone 1 g IM×1 • CH: Azithromycin 1-2 g PO×1 • May add topical antibiotics *Treat for both GO and CH when initiating management.	• Resolves spontaneously without specific treatment • Cold compress for comfort • Very contagious so proper hand hygiene and avoidance of direct contact is important	• Refer to ophthalmology • Oral systemic antivirals (valacyclovir/ acyclovir) • Topical steroid drops	• Warm or cold compress • Antihistamines

GLAUCOMA

Definition

- Progressive optic neuropathy involving characteristic structural changes to optic nerve with associated visual field changes
  - Usually have increased intraocular pressure (IOP), but this is not required for diagnosis.
  - Loss of peripheral vision precedes central vision loss.

Causes, Presentation, and Management (see Table 1-15)

TABLE 1-15	Glaucoma: Causes, Presentation, and Management	
	PRIMARY OPEN ANGLE GLAUCOMA	**PRIMARY ANGLE-CLOSURE GLAUCOMA**
Risk factors	• Increasing age • African descent • Diabetes • Family history • Increased IOP	• Increasing age • Asian and Inuit descent • Female • Shallow anterior chamber of eye
Clinical features	• Gradual onset • Initially asymptomatic • *Painless* increase in IOP • Bilateral loss of peripheral vision • Optic disc cupping • No acute attacks	• Rapid onset • Fixed, mid-dilated pupil • *Painful*, red eye • Unilateral • Decreased vision, "halos around lights" • Nausea and vomiting • Usually IOP >50 mm Hg
Diagnosis	• Consistent and reproducible abnormalities in two of the following: • Optic disc, IOP, and visual field	• Clinical presentation and measurement of IOP
Treatment	• Topical prostaglandins, beta-blockers, cholinergics, osmotic diuretics • Prevention is important by screening high-risk patients • Laser trabeculotomy/trabeculoplasty	• Emergent ophthalmology consult • Medical and surgical treatments aimed at lowering IOP • Beta-blockers, cholinergics, osmotic diuretics • Laser iridotomy

ANTERIOR UVEITIS (IRITIS)

Definition

- Inflammation of the iris

Etiology

- Immunologic
  - Ankylosing spondylitis, Reiter syndrome, psoriasis, Crohn disease, ulcerative colitis, reactive arthritis
- Infectious
  - Syphilis, Lyme disease, tuberculosis, herpes simplex, herpes zoster, toxoplasmosis
- Other
  - Sarcoidosis, trauma

Clinical Features

- Photophobia, decreased visual acuity
- Pain
- Miosis

- Inflammatory cells seen within the anterior chamber
- Hypopyon (layer of white cells)

Treatment
- Urgent referral to ophthalmology
- Topical corticosteroids
- Mydriatics

TEMPORAL ARTERITIS (GIANT CELL ARTERITIS)

Definition
- A systemic inflammation of medium and large arteries which typically involves the temporal artery.

Risk Factors
- Female
- Age >60

Clinical Features
- Abrupt unilateral vision loss (Amaurosis Fugax—transient blindness)
- Pain over temporal artery
- Jaw claudication
- Scalp tenderness

Diagnosis
- Elevated ESR
- Temporal artery biopsy

Treatment
- Do not wait for biopsy to be performed before starting treatment.
- Immediate initiation of high-dose systemic steroids is required in all suspected cases.
  - Give prednisone 40 to 60 mg daily and begin tapering after 2 to 4 weeks.

AGE-RELATED MACULAR DEGENERATION

- Degenerative disease of the central retina resulting in loss of central vision.
- Many risk factors including age, smoking, family history, and cardiovascular disease.
- Patients have vision loss but are otherwise asymptomatic.
- Red eye is not a feature.
- Should be suspected and investigated for in patients who present with gradual blurring of vision in one or both eyes.
- Diagnosis is made clinically on slit lamp examination.

CATARACTS

- An opacity of the lens which is the leading cause of blindness in the world.
- Risk factors include age, smoking, alcohol use, sun exposure, DM, and poor lifestyle habits.
- Presentation is highly variable, but usually begins with an increase in near-sightedness (myopia) followed by problems with night driving and reading fine print.
- Vision loss is painless and red eye is not a feature.
- No preventative strategies have been proven effective.
- The only treatment includes surgical removal of the opacified lens.
- Delay of surgical intervention does not lead to worse outcomes.

Bibliography

Anti-infective Review Panel. *Anti-infective Guidelines for Community-Acquired Infections*. Toronto: MUMS Guideline Learninghouse; 2012.

Longo DL, Fauci AS, Kasper DL, Hauser SL, Jameson JL, Loscalzo J, eds. *Harrison's Principles of Internal Medicine*. 18th ed. New York, NY: McGraw-Hill; 2012.

McPhee SJ, Papadakis MA, eds. *Current Medical Diagnosis & Treatment*. New York, NY: McGraw-Hill; 2012.

Tintinalli JE, Stapczynski JS, Cline DM, Ma OJ, Yealy DM, Meckler GD, eds. *Tintinalli's Emergency Medicine: A Comprehensive Study Guide*. 8th ed. New York, NY: McGraw-Hill; 2015.

Allergy
Priority Topic 3

Definitions

Allergy: An exaggerated immune response mediated by histamine, leukotriene, C4, and prostaglandins (IgE).

Anaphylaxis: Severe life-threatening allergic syndrome involving multiple organs in a previously sensitized patient. Usually presents as respiratory insufficiency and hypotension.

History

- Must quickly recognize and treat the difference between the very serious anaphylaxis from simple allergy.
- Patient may be able to share with you a past history of severe allergy.
- Look for MedicAlert bracelet or necklace.

Physical Examination

- Dyspnea, stridor, wheeze, hoarseness.
- Erythema.
- Generalized urticaria.
- Edema.
- Pruritus, itchy eyes.
- Conjunctival injection.
- Tachycardia.
- Hypotension.
- Decreased LOC.
- Nausea, vomiting, diarrhea.
- Consider allergy in the differential diagnosis when patients present with recurrent respiratory symptoms otherwise unexplained.

Preventative Management and Education

- Always document allergies in chart, and update regularly.
- Clarify true allergy (angioedema, stridor, anaphylaxis, hives) versus intolerance (rash, GI upset, nausea).
- Educate all involved.
- Have patient acquire a MedicAlert bracelet.
- Advise patient to keep an EpiPen on their person, as well as an antihistamine (H_1 blocker +/– H_2 blocker), and prednisone (for delayed reaction) closeby.
- Be aware, and counsel appropriately, that many of today's young adults were kept in a very protected environment at home and school, and the world outside of these places may not be so allergen-free.
- Refer to allergist if reaction is significant and/or allergen unclear.

Acute Management of Anaphylaxis

- Remove causative agent if possible and known.
- ABCs—Secure airway; intubate if necessary. Loss of airway patency can occur quickly—err on the side of caution.
- **Epinephrine**
  - **Adult dose 0.3 to 0.5 mL 1:1000 IM (0.3-0.5 mg)**
  - **Pediatric dose: 0.01 mL/kg 1:1000 IM (0.01 mg/kg)**
- Diphenhydramine (Benadryl) 50 mg IM or IV.
- Ranitidine 50 mg IV (these offer an added benefit to H_1 blocker alone).
- Corticosteroid (methylprednisolone 50-100 mg IV if severe allergy), or concern over possible delayed or recurrent reaction.
- Salbutamol nebulizer 2.5 mg if airway reactivity concerns are present.
- Observe for 2 to 3 hours post-epinephrine to ensure no delayed or recurrent reaction.

Bibliography

Campbell RL, Kelson JM. Anaphylaxis—Emergency Treatment. In: Walls RM, Randolph AG, Feldweg AM, eds. *UpToDate 2016*. Retrieved from http://www.uptodate.com/.

Yingming A, Tran C, eds. *Toronto Notes*. 27th ed. Toronto, ON: Toronto Notes for Medical Students; 2011: ER30-ER32.

Deep Vein Thrombosis
Priority Topic 21

Definition

- A blood clot causing blood flow obstruction, usually in a deep vein of the leg.
- Distal: Thrombi are confined to deep calf veins, distal to knee.
- Proximal: Thrombi involve popliteal, femoral, or iliac veins, and are more likely to cause pulmonary embolus.
- Pathogenesis: Virchow triad, which consists of:
  - Endothelial damage (trauma, burns, surgery)
  - Stasis (travel, bed-bound, wheelchair)
  - Hypercoagulability (cancer, late pregnancy, factor V Leiden, protein C or S deficiency, etc)

Risk Factors

- Surgery, fractures, cancer, estrogen therapy, obesity, inflammatory bowel disease, oral corticosteroids, family history of deep vein thrombosis (DVT), pregnancy, trauma, sepsis, hematological disorders

Presentation

- Swelling, pain, and erythema of the involved limb—lower limb by far the most common.
- Consider massive DVT with buttock or groin pain, thigh swelling, or collateral superficial veins.

Physical Examination

- See Wells criteria (Table 1-16), as well as:
  - Homan sign: Pain during dorsiflexion of foot
  - Superficial venous distension with prominent superficial veins

TABLE 1-16	Wells Criteria for DVT (Used to Assess Pretest Probability)
CRITERIA	**SCORE**
Localized tenderness along the deep venous distribution	1
Entire leg swollen	1
Calf swelling ≥3 cm larger than on asymptomatic side (measure 10 cm below tibial tuberosity)	1
Pitting edema confined to symptomatic leg	1
Collateral non-varicose superficial veins	1
Paralysis, paresis, or recent plaster immobilization of the lower extremities	1
Recently bedridden for ≥3 days, or major surgery within the previous 12 weeks requiring general or regional anesthetic	1
Previously documented DVT	1
Malignancy-on treatment, treated in past 6 months or palliative	1
Alternate diagnosis is at least as likely as DVT	−2

Low risk <1, moderate risk 1-2, high risk >3. If both legs are symptomatic, score the more severe leg.

Diagnosis

Also see the diagnostic algorithm that follows.

Assess for pretest probability using the Wells criteria for DVT, and follow the steps in order below:

- In **low-risk** patients with Wells DVT score <1 and low clinical suspicion
  - D-dimer should be ordered
    - If negative—DVT excluded
    - If positive—order duplex ultrasound with compression
      - If the ultrasound is positive—DVT is confirmed and treatment should begin as given under the head level "Treatment (for DVT and PE)."
      - If the ultrasound is negative—DVT can be excluded.
- In **moderate/high-risk** patients with Wells DVT score of 1 or more
  - In the absence of contraindications, it is appropriate to start treatment immediately.
  - Duplex ultrasound should be ordered
    - If positive—DVT is confirmed, and treatment should continue as given under heading "Treatment (for DVT and PE)."
    - If negative—order D-dimer
      - If negative—DVT is excluded.
      - If positive—unable to rule out DVT; repeat duplex ultrasound in 3 to 7 days, *or* assess with CT venography (rarely done).
- Unprovoked DVTs should be referred to a hematologist, and consideration given to look for occult cause (eg, lung, GI, gyne malignancy).

Treatment

- See "Treatment" under the "Pulmonary Embolus" section, for further information

Pulmonary Embolus

Definition

- A mechanical obstruction of the pulmonary vasculature
- Usually due to thromboembolism from DVT

- Massive PE is an acute PE in the presence of:
  - Sustained hypotension with systolic BP <90, and not due to any other cause
  - Persistent profound bradycardia, HR <40
  - Pulselessness

<table>
<tr><td colspan="2">WELLS CRITERIA FOR PE (USED TO ASSESS PRETEST PROBABILITY)</td></tr>
<tr><td>CRITERIA</td><td>SCORE</td></tr>
<tr><td>Clinical signs of DVT</td><td>3</td></tr>
<tr><td>Alternate diagnosis is less likely than PE</td><td>3</td></tr>
<tr><td>Heart rate >100</td><td>1.5</td></tr>
<tr><td>Previous DVT/PE</td><td>1.5</td></tr>
<tr><td>Immobilization ≥3 days or surgery in past 4 weeks</td><td>1.5</td></tr>
<tr><td>Malignancy—on treatment, treated in past 6 months or palliative</td><td>1</td></tr>
<tr><td>Hemoptysis</td><td>1</td></tr>
<tr><td colspan="2">PE unlikely: score <4; PE likely: score >4.</td></tr>
</table>

PE RULE OUT CRITERIA (PERC SCORE)

- Age <50 years
- Heart rate <100
- Oxygen saturation ≥95%
- No unilateral leg swelling
- No hemoptysis
- No recent surgery or trauma requiring hospitalization in the past 4 weeks
- No previous DVT/PE
- No estrogen use
- *If all PERC criteria are met patient has a <2% chance of having a PE and requires no further investigation*

Carpenter CR, et al. Differentiating Low-Risk and No-Risk PE Patients: The PERC Score. *J Emerg Mgmt* 2009;36(3):317-322. Reprinted with permission of Elsevier.

Diagnosis

Also see the diagnostic algorithm that follows.

- Assess for pretest probability using the Wells criteria for PE, and follow the steps in order below
- In **low-risk** patients with **Wells PE score ≤4 and low clinical suspicion**
  - Assess using PERC
    - If all PERC criteria are met, then PE can be excluded and no further testing is required.
    - If any PERC criteria are positive, order a D-dimer.
      - If D-dimer negative, PE can be excluded
      - If D-dimer positive, order a V/Q or CTPA scan
        - If scan negative, can exclude PE.
        - If scan positive, then PE is confirmed and treatment should begin as given under the heading "Treatment (for DVT and PE)."
- In **high-risk** patients with **Wells PE score >4** and/or **high clinical suspicion**
  - Consider starting treatment immediately (recommended if Wells score ≥6)
  - Order CT—Pulmonary angiogram, or V/Q scan if renal concerns (see "Notes")
    - If scans are diagnostic, PE is confirmed and treatment should begin as given under the heading "Treatment (for DVT and PE)."
    - If scans are not diagnostic of PE, then duplex ultrasound with compression of bilateral legs should be performed.
      - If ultrasound negative, follow-up with repeat ultrasound in 3 to 5 days.
      - If ultrasound positive for DVT, treat for PE.
- Other tests:
  - Arterial blood gas: Not useful to diagnose or exclude PE
    - Typically show hypoxemia, hypocapnia, and respiratory alkalosis
  - ECG: Typically see nonspecific ST changes
    - The S1Q3T3 pattern with right ventricular strain and/or new incomplete RBBB are rarely seen in acute PE, but may be seen with massive PE and cor pulmonale.

- ◦ Poor prognosis in patients with atrial arrhythmias, RBBB, inferior Q waves, precordial T and ST changes.
  - CXR: Commonly see abnormalities (atelectasis, pleural effusion), but nothing diagnostic of PE
- ■ Notes on imaging and D-dimer
  - CT-PA
    - ◦ Contraindicated with renal failure or contrast allergy; high specificity, but reader expertise is required.
  - V/Q scan (ventilation/perfusion scan)
    - ◦ Consider for patients with contrast allergy or renal failure
    - ◦ Reported as: Normal, low probability, intermediate probability, or high probability
    - ◦ **Rules out** PE in the following situations:
      - ▫ Normal scan with any level of clinical probability
      - ▫ Low probability scan **and** low clinical probability
    - ◦ **Diagnostic of PE** if high probability scan **and** high clinical probability
    - ◦ For any other scan result/clinical probability combination, further testing with CT-PA, or duplex ultrasound should be done
  - Bilateral duplex ultrasound with compression
    - ◦ Presence of a proximal DVT in a patient with suspected DVT is sufficient to start treatment
    - ◦ Negative test insufficient to rule out PE
  - D-dimer (a degradation product of crosslinked fibrin)
    - ◦ Elevated postsurgery, with infection, malignancy, DIC
    - ◦ Good negative predictive value; can rule out PE with normal D-dimer and low clinical suspicion
    - ◦ Normal D-dimer levels are seen in only 40% to 68% of patients without PE; poor specificity

Treatment (for DVT and PE)

- ■ Certain patients will require inpatient management
  - Massive DVT, PE, bleeding risk, comorbidities
- ■ Anticoagulation
  - Start treatment immediately (ie, prior to investigation results) if there is a high index of suspicion of DVT or PE
    - ◦ Intermediate index of suspicion and results are likely to take >4 hours, treatment is recommended.
    - ◦ Low index of suspicion, it is reasonable not to start treatment if results are expected within 24 hours.
  - Bridge anticoagulation for at least 5 days and until INR ≥2 for 24 hours
    - ◦ Low molecular weight heparin (LMWH).
    - ◦ Unfractionated heparin (UFH); IV is preferred to subcutaneous.
    - ◦ In the absence of renal failure, LMWH is preferred.
  - Long-term anticoagulation
    - ◦ Long-term treatment is recommended for at least 3 months in patients with a transient risk factor (eg, surgery).
    - ◦ For patients with an unprovoked DVT or PE, evaluate risk/benefit of continuing therapy as these patients may benefit from a longer course of anticoagulation.
    - ◦ Warfarin (see "Notes")
      - ▫ Start dosing at the same time as initiating bridging of anticoagulation or diagnosis of DVT.

- ▫ Target INR is 2 to 3.
  - DOAC: Has been shown to be as effective as warfarin. In Canada, Rivaroxaban, and Apixaban are approved for treatment of DVT or PE. Do not need to follow INR levels.
  - LMWH: In patients with malignancy, long-term anticoagulation with LMWH is preferred to reduce recurrence risk, and duration is typically longer than 3 months.
- ■ Thrombolytics should be considered in patients with PE and hypotension where there is no increased bleeding risk.
- ■ Early ambulation is not harmful.
- ■ Elastic compression stockings may reduce risk of postthrombotic syndrome.
- ■ Inferior vena cava filters are only recommended for patients in whom anticoagulation is contraindicated or in cases of large emboli where a second event would be fatal.

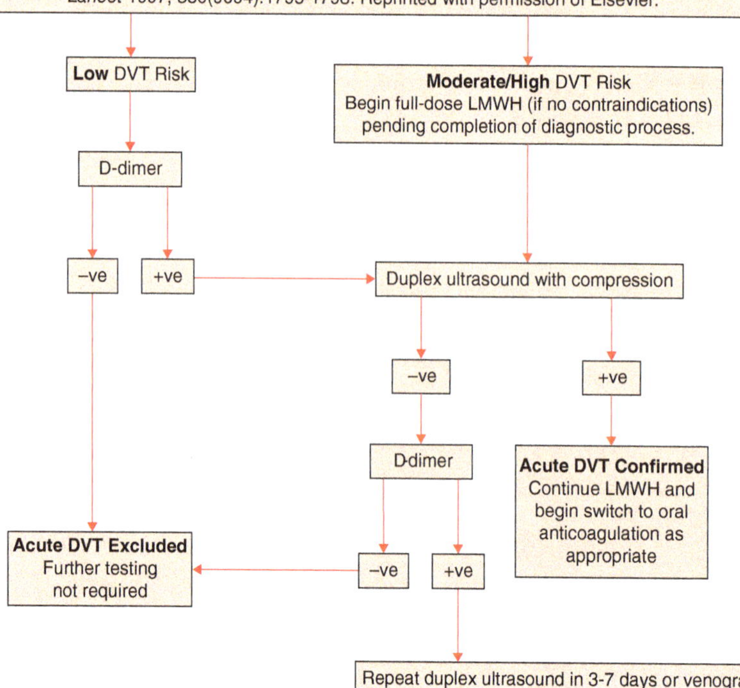

Clinical Signs and Symptoms of Lower Extremity DVT

Assess clinical pretest probability using Wells model	
Criteria	**Score**
Active cancer (on treatment for last 6 months or palliative)	1
Paralysis, paresis, or recent plaster immobilization of the lower extremities	1
Recently bedridden for 3 days or more, or major surgery within the previous 12 weeks requiring general or regional anaesthetic	1
Previously documented deep vein thrombosis	1
Localized tenderness along the distribution of the deep venous system	1
Entire leg swollen	1
Calf swelling at least 3 cm larger than that on the asymptomatic side (measured 10 cm below tibial tuberosity)	1
Pitting edema confined to the symptomatic leg	1
Collateral superficial veins (non-varicose)	1
Alternative diagnosis **at least as likely as** deep vein thrombosis	−2

SCORING: Low risk: <1; moderate risk: 1-2; high risk: >3
If both legs symptomatic, score the more severe leg.
Wells, PS, et al. Value of assessment of pretest probability of deep-vein thrombosis in clinical management. *Lancet* 1997; 350(9094):1795-1798. Reprinted with permission of Elsevier.

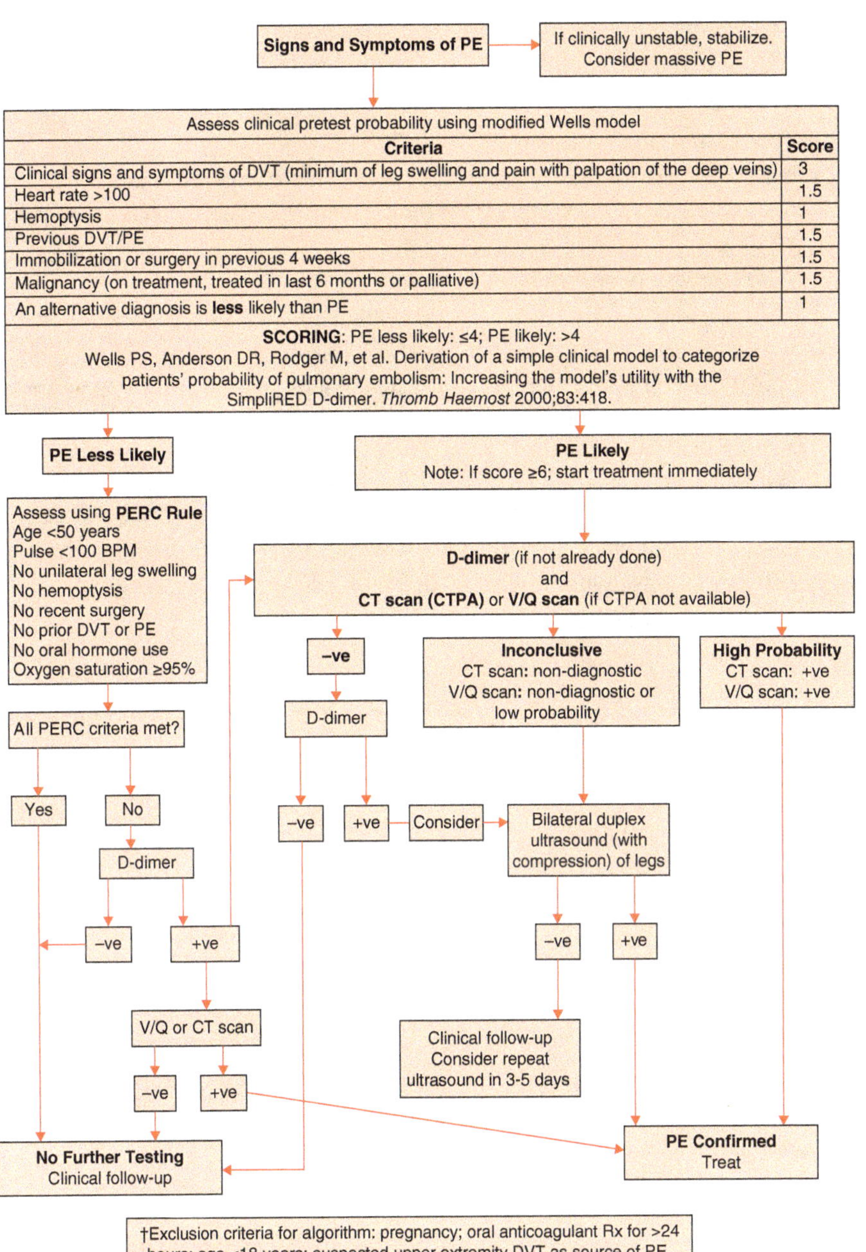

Warfarin Notes

- Target INR is 2 to 3 for most conditions, including DVT and PE (goal of 2.5).
- Target INR of 2.5 to 3.5 (goal of 3)
  - Indicated for: Recurrent VTE (venous thromboembolism) despite anticoagulation; mechanical aortic or mitral valve in the presence of Afib, some STEMIs, left atrial enlargement, low ejection fraction, hypercoagulable state, certain mechanical mitral valves, or older caged ball or caged disc valves.
- Risk factors for bleeding are as follows:
  - Elderly
  - Malnourished
  - Congestive heart failure
  - Liver disease
  - Recent surgery

- Alcohol use
- Previous GI bleed

■ Start warfarin
  - Typical starting dose is 5 mg.
  - Take an average of the doses over the previous 3 to 5 days in a patient with fluctuating doses to get a picture of the average daily dose that has produced an INR.
  - It is preferable to have same dosing every day to avoid confusion.

■ Medication interactions—increase INR monitoring with the following:
  - Increased warfarin response is caused by factors such as acetaminophen, NSAIDs, alcohol, amiodarone, allopurinol, fibrates, omeprazole, some statins, **many antibiotics**, thyroid hormone, some herbal preparations, for example, chamomile.
  - Decreased warfarin response is caused by factors such as antithyroid medications for hyperthyroidism (methimazole and propylthiouracil), barbiturates, carbamazepine, rifampin, phenytoin, St. John wort, increased vitamin K intake (Brussel sprouts, spinach, avocado, green tea, spinach, mayonnaise).

■ Perioperative warfarin management
  - Consider bridging anticoagulation (eg, LMWH)
    ◦ **High-risk** patients should receive bridging.
    ◦ For moderate-risk patients consider bridging.
  - Discontinue warfarin at least 5 days prior to procedures with intermediate/high risk of bleed.
  - Check INR 1 to 2 days prior to surgery.
    ◦ Give 1 to 2 mg of oral vitamin K if INR >1.5.
    ◦ Resume warfarin 12 to 24 hours after surgery if there is adequate postsurgical hemostasis.

■ Low-risk procedures not requiring discontinuation of warfarin are; diagnostic endoscopy, ERCP, cataract surgery, minor dermatological procedures, joint or soft tissue injections.

■ For dental procedures obtain INR prior to procedure. Need for discontinuation of warfarin is at the discretion of the dentist or dental surgeon performing the procedure.

■ Delay procedure if INR is supratherapeutic.

Bibliography

Bauer KA. Approach to the diagnosis and therapy of lower extremity deep vein thrombosis. In: Leung LK, Mandel J, Finlay G, eds. *UpToDate; 2016.* Retrieved from http://www.uptodate.com/.

DynaMed. Deep vein thrombosis (DVT). Ipswich, MA: EBSCO Publishing; 2016. Retrieved November 28, 2016 from http://search.ebscohost.com.cyber.usask.ca/login.aspx?direct=true&site=DynaMed&id=113862.

DynaMed. Periprocedural management of patients on long-term anticoagulation. Ipswich, MA: EBSCO Publishing; 2012. Retrieved November 28, 2016 from http://search.ebscohost.com.cyber.usask.ca/login.aspx?direct=true&site=DynaMed&id=113862.

DynaMed. Pulmonary embolism (PE). Ipswich, MA: EBSCO Publishing; 2016. Retrieved November 28, 2016 from http://search.ebscohost.com.cyber.usask.ca/login.aspx?direct=true&site=DynaMed&id=113862.

Jensen B, Downey L, Regier L. Oral antiplatelet and antithrombotic agents. *RxFiles Drug Comparison Charts.* 10th ed. Saskatoon, SK: Saskatoon Health Region; 2014:15-16.

Lip GY, Hull RD. Venous thromboembolism: Initiation of anticoagulation (first 10 days). In: Leung LK, Mandel J, Finlay G, eds. *UpToDate, 2016.* Retrieved from http://www.uptodate.com/.

Righini M, Le Gal G, Perrier A, et al. The challenge of diagnosing pulmonary embolism in elderly patients: influence of age on commonly used diagnostic tests and strategies. *J Am Geriatr Soc.* 2005;53(6):1039-1045.

Thompson BT, Karbhel C. Overview of acute pulmonary embolism in adults. In: Mandel J, Finlay G, eds. *UpToDate; 2016.* Retrieved from http://www.uptodate.com/.

CHAPTER 2

Internal Medicine

Headache

Priority Topic 44

RED FLAGS FOR HEADACHE—"SNOOP"

- **Systemic** symptoms or illness: Fever, vomiting, neck stiffness, pregnancy, immunocompromised, anticoagulated;
- **Neurologic** signs and symptoms: altered mental status, focal neurologic signs, papilledema, seizures;
- **Onset** is new (especially <40 years old) or sudden;
- **Other** associated conditions and circumstances: Trauma, awakens from sleep, early morning headache, worsened by Valsalva manoeuvres;
- **Prior** headache history is different than current episode.

DIFFERENTIAL DIAGNOSIS, AND WORKUP (SEE TABLE 2-1)

TABLE 2-1	Headache: Type and Workup
DIFFERENTIAL DIAGNOSIS	**WORKUP**
Temporal arteritis,[a] mass lesion	ESR, imaging, biopsy
SAH,[b] vascular malformation, hemorrhage, stroke	Imaging, lumbar puncture
Meningitis[c]	Imaging, lumbar puncture, serology
Collagen vascular disease	Antiphospholipid antibody
Trauma (epidural, subdural)	Imaging—brain, skull +/− C-spine

[a]**In temporal arteritis give steroids before diagnosis is confirmed.**
[b]**In suspected SAH if imaging is negative do lumbar puncture.**
[c]**In meningitis give antibiotics before diagnosis is confirmed.**
Content adapted from Toronto Notes 2017. torontonotes.ca.

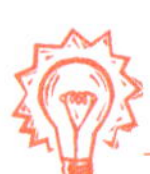

DIAGNOSIS OF MIGRAINE

1. ≥5 attacks fulfilling 2 to 4.
2. 4 to 72 hours duration
3. ≥2 of:
   Unilateral
   Pulsatile
   Worse with routine activity (eg, climbing stairs)
   Moderate-to-severe intensity
4. ≥1 of:
   Nausea/vomiting
   Phono/photophobia

SIGNS, SYMPTOMS, AND TREATMENT

TABLE 2-2   Headache—Signs/Symptoms and Treatments

	SIGNS/SYMPTOMS	ACUTE TREATMENT
Migraine (+/− aura)	2-72 h duration Unilateral Pulsatile Worse with activity Nausea/vomiting Phono/photophobia	See Table 2-3 NSAIDs Triptans Ergots Metoclopramide
Tension	Bilateral (frontal and occipital pain) Bandlike Exacerbated by stress, fatigue, noise Can be related to neck muscle pain	NSAIDs
Cluster	Unilateral and excruciating Peri-orbital 15 min to 3 h duration Conjunctival injection and lacrimation	High-flow O_2 Triptans Ergots
Medication overuse	Bilateral and bandlike Muscle contraction, tenderness Photosensitivity Occurs nearly every day	Discontinue analgesics Use triptan and ergots—during withdrawal

Content adapted from Toronto Notes 2017. torontonotes.ca.

TABLE 2-3   Step-Wise Approach to the Treatment of Migraines

Acute	Mild to moderate	NSAIDs or acetaminophen
	Moderate to severe	Triptans Ergots Metoclopramide/chlorpromazine (dopaminergic) Tylenol #3 if severe
Prophylaxis	If >3 per mo or decreased quality of life	β-blocker (propranolol) TCA (amitriptyline, nortriptyline) Anticonvulsant (divalproex, topiramate) Riboflavin Calcium channel blocker (verapamil)

Content adapted from Toronto Notes 2017. torontonotes.ca.

Bibliography

DynaMed. Migraine in adults. Accessed December 23, 2016.

Goadsby PJ, Raskin NH. Headache. In: Kasper DL, Fauci AS, Hauser SL, Longo DL, Jameson JL, Loscalzo J, eds. *Harrison's Principles of Internal Medicine*. 19th ed. New York, NY: McGraw-Hill Education; 2015: Chap. 21.

Goadsby PJ, Raskin NH. Migraine and other primary headache disorders. In: Kasper DL, Fauci AS, Hauser SL, Longo DL, Jameson JL, Loscalzo J, eds. *Harrison's Principles of Internal Medicine*. 19th ed. New York, NY: McGraw-Hill Education; 2015: Chap. 447.

Hall J, Premji A, eds. Toronto Notes 2015: A Comprehensive Medical Reference and Review for the Medical Council of Canada Qualifying Exam Part 1 and the United States Medical Licensing Exam Step 2. 31st ed. Toronto Notes for Medical Student Inc. Toronto; 2015.

Jensen B, Regier L, eds. *RxFiles Drug Comparison Charts*. 10th ed. Saskatoon, Sk: Saskatoon Health Region; 2014. Available from www.RxFiles.ca.

Anemia
Priority Topic 4

Definition
- Low hemoglobin (normal range: men 130-180 g/L; women 120-160 g/L)
- Categorized into microcytic, normocytic, and macrocytic based on MCV

TABLE 2-4	**Causes of Anemia**		
	MICROCYTIC	**NORMOCYTIC**	**MACROCYTIC**
MCV (fL):	<80	80-100	>100
Causes	Sideroblastic	Hemolytic	B_{12} deficiency
	Iron deficiency	Aplastic	Folate deficiency
	Thalassemia	Anemia of chronic disease	Alcohol
	Anemia of chronic disease	Renal failure	Hypothyroidism
		Pregnancy	Myelodysplasia
Key Test	Ferritin	Reticulocyte count	Blood smear

Content adapted from Toronto Notes 2017. torontonotes.ca.

Signs and Symptoms
- Fatigue
- Dyspnea
- Pallor (palms, nail beds, conjunctivae)
- Tachycardia
- Postural lightheadedness
- Worsening angina or CHF

Treatment
- Transfusion if symptomatic and Hb <70 g/L; at risk of decompensation (eg, hypovolemic, CHF, angina)
- If unstable vitals, consider fluids before blood transfusion

IRON DEFICIENCY ANEMIA

Symptoms
- Angular cheilitis
- Pica
- Atrophic glossitis
- Koilonychia
- Plummer–Vinson syndrome (esophageal web, atrophic glossitis, dysphagia)

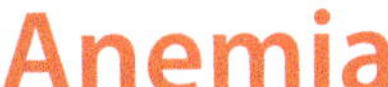

ANEMIA MNEMONICS
Microcytic TAILS (thalassemia, anemia of chronic disease, iron deficiency, lead poisoning, sideroblastic)
Normocytic HAARP (hemolytic, aplastic anemia, renal failure, pyridoxine deficiency (vit B_6), pernicious anemia (vit B_{12})

MEGALOBLASTIC ANEMIAS
B_{12} deficiency
Folate deficiency*

*After diagnosis, routine testing of folate levels not required

Diagnosis

TABLE 2-5	Diagnosis—Fe Deficiency vs Anemia of Chronic Disease						
LABS	MCV	RDW	FE	TIBC[a]	FERRITIN[b]	FE/TIBC	TRANSFERRIN
Fe deficiency	↓	↑	↓	↑	↓	<18%	↑
Anemia of chronic disease	↓or N	N	↓	↓	↑	>18%	N

[a] TIBC—only measure if ferritin is normal and clinically suspicious for iron deficiency or in kidney failure.
[b] Ferritin—best diagnostic test; iron deficient if <15 mcg/L.
Content adapted from Toronto Notes 2017. torontonotes.ca.

Etiologies

- Chronic blood loss (gastrointestinal [GI] loss, menorrhagia, frequent blood donation)
- Decreased absorption (Celiac disease, Crohn disease, GI surgery)
- Pregnancy
- Malignancy (note: low Hb +/− iron deficiency may be first sign of malignancy)

Treatment

- Target: Elemental Fe 180 to 200 mg PO OD.
  - A rise in Hb of 10 to 20 g/L in 2 to 4 weeks supports diagnosis.
  - Consider intravenous iron infusion in patients unable to tolerate oral iron, prior to GI surgery or on erythropoietin therapy.
- Anemia should be corrected in 2 to 4 months of treatment. However, treat for a total of 4 to 6 months to replenish iron stores.

VITAMIN B$_{12}$ DEFICIENCY ANEMIA

Symptoms

- Symmetric peripheral neuropathy
- Paresthesias
- Ataxia
- Glossitis
- CNS: Memory loss, personality changes, and dementia
- Late stage: Severe weakness, spasticity, clonus

Diagnosis

- Serum B$_{12}$ level and clinical picture
- Pernicious anemia tests: Anti-intrinsic factor antibody or Schilling test

Etiologies

- Malnutrition
- Fish tapeworm
- Drugs (eg, metformin, PPI, H$_2$ blocker)
- Bacteria overgrowth at terminal ileum
- GI tract abnormality
- Pernicious anemia—most common cause of vitamin B$_{12}$ deficiency

Treatment

- Vitamin B$_{12}$ (IM for pernicious anemia)
- High-dose oral vitamin B$_{12}$ (1000-2000 mcg/d) is also an option
- Follow levels of B$_{12}$ after starting

Symptoms

- Pallor
- Poor weight gain

Risk Factors

- Poverty
- Non–iron-fortified formula
- Ethnicity
- Whole cow's milk diet
- Exclusive breastfeeding after 6 months of age
- Poorly controlled maternal diabetes

Bibliography

Adamson JW. Iron deficiency and other hypoproliferative anemias. In: Kasper DL, Fauci AS, Hauser SL, Longo DL, Jameson JL, Loscalzo J, eds. *Harrison's Principles of Internal Medicine*. 19th ed. New York, NY: McGraw-Hill Education; 2015: Chap. 126.

DynaMed. Anemia differential diagnosis. Updated January 21, 2016. Accessed December 26, 2016.

DynaMed. Iron deficiency in children (infancy through adolescence). Updated November 21, 2016. Accessed December 23, 2016.

Hall J, Premji A, eds. Toronto Notes 2015: A Comprehensive Medical Reference and Review for the Medical Council of Canada Qualifying Exam Part 1 and the United States Medical Licensing Exam Step 2. 31st ed. Toronto Notes for Medical Student Inc. Toronto; 2015.

Jensen B, Regier L, eds. *RxFiles Drug Comparison Charts*. 10th ed. Saskatoon, Sk: Saskatoon Health Region; 2014. Available from www.RxFiles.ca.

Primack, BA, Mahaniah, KJ. Anemia. In: South-Paul JE, Matheny SC, Lewis EL, eds. *Current Diagnosis and Treatment: Family Medicine*. 4th ed. New York, NY: McGraw-Hill Education; 2015: Chap. 32.

Ray JC, Hemphill RR. Anemia. In: Tintinalli, JS Stapczynski, OJ Ma, DM Yealy, GD Meckler, DM Cline, eds. *Tintinalli's Emergency Medicine*. 8th ed. New York, NY: McGraw-Hill Education; 2016: Chap. 231.

Schrier, SL. Approach to the patient with anemia. In: Post TW, ed. *UpToDate*. Waltham, MA. Accessed December 26, 2016.

Stroke

Priority Topic 88

Definitions

Transient ischemic attack (TIA): Brief episode of neurological dysfunction without evidence of acute infarction. Returns to baseline in <24 hours.

- Signs/symptoms: Typically lasts <1 hour but by definition resolves in <24 hours; motor, sensory, speech/language, vision, or cerebellar dysfunction
- TIA is an important warning sign

Stroke: Sudden onset focal neurological dysfunction from infarction or hemorrhage in the brain lasting >24 hours.

- Signs/symptoms: Same as TIA but symptoms persist >24 hours

Signs/Symptoms

- Acute or abrupt onset
- Motor weakness
- Sensory deficits
- Decreased reflexes
- Mental status changes
- Hemiparesis
- Neglect
- Amaurosis fugax

ABCD2 SCORE—PREDICTION OF EARLY STROKE RISK AFTER TIA (AT DAY 2, 7, AND AFTER 90 DAYS)

	Score
A—Age ≥60	1
B—BP ≥140/90	1
C—Clinical features	
Unilateral weakness	2
Speech impaired only	1
D—Duration ≥60 min	2
10-59 min	1
D—Diabetes	1

Score: ≤3 = low risk; 4 to 5 = moderate; 6 to 7 = high

Score >3 needs admission to hospital.

RISK OF STROKE AFTER TIA
3%—in first 2 days
5%—in first 7 days
12%—in first 90 days

BELL PALSY
- Peripheral (lower motor neuron) CNVII palsy
- Abrupt onset: Unilateral facial paralysis
- **Includes** the forehead (central causes will spare the forehead)
- Treatment: Steroids within 3 days of onset (eg, prednisone 60-80 mg/d for 1 week) Antiviral therapy is no longer *routinely* recommended, but can be considered (eg, Valacyclovir 1000 mg TID for 1 week) in severe presentations

See http://www.acls.net/acls-suspected-stroke-algorithm.htm for ACLS stroke algorithm.

CONTRAINDICATIONS TO FIBRINOLYTICS
A—AVM/aneurysm
B—Bleeding: active internal or diathesis (INR >1.7; platelets <100,000/mm³)
C—Cancer (intracranial)
D—Dissection of aorta suspected
H—Hemorrhagic stroke/HTN uncontrolled
I—Ischemic stroke in past 3 months or large stroke on CT
S—Seizure at stroke onset/SAH suspected
T—Trauma (head) or stroke in past 3 months

- Slurred speech
- Inattention
- Impulsivity

Risk Factors
- HTN
- Diabetes
- Smoking
- Hyperlipidemia
- Prior TIA/stroke
- Obesity/sedentary lifestyle
- Cardiovascular disease
- Atrial fibrillation
- Excessive alcohol intake
- Coagulopathy
- Age (risk doubles with every 10 years after age 55)
- Aboriginal or black

Diagnosis
- **History and physical examination:** Look for the signs/symptoms listed earlier—may also help identify a hemorrhagic stroke
  - Increased likelihood of hemorrhage if blown pupil, history of trauma
- **Imaging**
  - Noncontrast CT—Useful to rule out hemorrhage; infarcts often do not show until 24 to 48 hours
  - MRI—Ischemic changes appear within hours
  - CT angiography
  - Ultrasound carotid Doppler—Useful for risk stratifying and identifying if surgical management possible
- **Laboratory investigations**
  - CBC, INR, PTT, glucose, Na$^+$, K$^+$, ECG

Differential Diagnosis
- Seizure
- Migraine
- Subdural hematoma
- Subarachnoid hemorrhage
- Mass effect
- Hypoglycemia (most common stroke mimic)
- CNS infection

Treatment
- ABCs.
- **Establish time of onset.**
- Rule out hemorrhage with CT scan.
  - In case of hemorrhage—consult neurosurgery
  - No hemorrhage—likely ischemic; **consider fibrinolytics if <3 to 4.5 hours from onset of symptoms**
- Contraindications to fibrinolytics (*Absolute* exclusion criteria).
  - Head trauma/stroke in previous 3 months
  - Clinical presentation of SAH
  - Arterial puncture at noncompressible site in previous 7 days
  - Hx of previous ICH

- BP ≥185/110
- Evidence of active bleeding on examination
- Bleeding diathesis including:
  - Platelets <100,000/mm^3
  - Heparin or warfarin—INR >1.7
- Blood glucose <2.7 mmol/L
- CT reveals multilobar infarction

■ If candidate for fibrinolytics—give rtPA, no anticoagulation for 24 hours. Consider mechanical thrombectomy if centre is capable.

■ If not a candidate for fibrinolytics—give ASA and clopidogrel.

Prevention

Primary Prevention

Please refer to www.ccpn.ca for more information on stroke prevention in AFib.

■ Determining the need for anticoagulation in AFib based on stroke risk: **CHADS$_2$ score**

■ Risk factor reduction

Secondary Prevention

■ ASA +/ − clopidogrel

■ Antihypertensives

■ Anticoagulation (eg, warfarin / DOAC)—if AFib or increased risk of cardiac source

■ Statin—not in first 48 hours, but long-term

■ Lifestyle modifications: Smoking cessation, regular exercise, diet control

■ Carotid Doppler and endarterectomy if >70% stenosis of ICA and >5 years life expectancy

- Carotid ultrasound: If carotid territory presentation of TIA/stroke assess for carotid blockage/source (Canadian 2006 Best Practice Standards state that TIAs need carotid imaging within 24 hour of a carotid distribution TIA).
- Echocardiogram/transesophageal echocardiogram (TEE)—Assess for cardio-embolic source

■ Early mobilization (<24 hours poststroke), swallowing assessment, nutritional support, and dedicated stroke unit leads to better outcomes

Medical Complications of Stroke

■ Cardiac—Common in the first 3 months post stroke

■ Depression—Occurs in approximately one-third of stroke patients

■ Dysphagia—Malnutrition/increased risk of aspiration

■ Ulcers

■ Venous thromboembolus (~25% of early death poststroke is from pulmonary embolism)—Consider heparin or leg compression stockings

■ Pain—Often associated with hemiplegia

CHADS2 SCORE: ANTICOAGULATION IN AFIB

- CHADS$_2$ Score
  - CHF — 1
  - Hypertension — 1
  - Age >75 — 1
  - Diabetes — 1
  - Stroke/TIA (prior) — 2
- Total score
  - 0 to 1 — ASA
  - 2 to 3 — Warfarin or ASA
  - >4 — Warfarin

Bibliography

ACLS training. Available from https://www.acls.net/acls-suspected-stroke-algorithm.htm.

Canadian Cardiovascular Society. Available from http://www.CCS.ca.

Coutts SB, Wein TH, Lindsay MP, et al. *Canadian Stroke Best Practice Recommendations: secondary prevention of stroke guidelines*. 5th ed. Updated December 2014. Available from http://www.strokebestpractices.ca/index.php/prevention-of-stroke/.

DynaMed. Prevention of stroke. Updated June 8, 2016. Accessed December 23, 2016.

DynaMed. Thromboembolic prophylaxis in atrial fibrillation. Updated July 15, 2016. Accessed December 23, 2016.

DynaMed. Transient ischemic attack. Updated October 28, 2016. Accessed December 23, 2016.

Go S, Worman DJ. Stroke syndromes. In: Tintinelli JE, Stepczynski JS, Ma OJ, Yealy DM, Meckler GD, Cline DM, eds. *Tintinelli's Emergency Medicine: A Comprehensive Study Guide*. 8th ed. New York, NY: McGraw-Hill Education; 2016: Chap. 167.

Insomnia

Priority Topic 53

Definition

Sleep disorder resulting in difficulty falling asleep, difficulty staying asleep, or early morning awakening despite adequate opportunity for sleep. This lack of sleep causes impairment in daily functioning.

History

- Ask people about their **sleep habits**:
  - Bedtime, time required to fall asleep, quality of sleep, number of awakenings
  - Distractions in the room: TV or computer in the bedroom
  - Activities before bed including exercise, caffeine, alcohol, medications, exposure late night to bright lights and to blue light spectrum
- Ask about recent stressors including travel, shift work.
- Assess impact on quality of life: fatigue, sleepiness, driving, concentration at work etc.
- Ask patients to complete a **sleep diary** including bedtime, sleep latency, total sleep time, awakenings, and quality of sleep.

Differential Diagnosis

The history will give clues to underlying sleep-related disorders that require further investigation and treatment:

- Psychiatric: Depression, anxiety, grief, PTSD
- Sleep apnea
- Restless leg syndrome
- CHF
- Pain
- Parasomnias: Sleep walking/talking
- Other: Central sleep apnea, hyperthyroidism, GERD, COPD, BPH

Advice for Good Sleep Hygiene

- Use an alarm clock to get up at the same time each day.
- **No** daytime naps.
- Use the bedroom for sleep and sex only.
- If not asleep in 20 minutes, get up and do something relaxing; return to bed only when tired.
- Relax before bed.
- Exercise during the day, not in the evening.
- Stop/limit caffeine and alcohol 6 hours before bed.
- No smoking for 1 to 2 hours before bed.

Treatment

Behaviour and cognitive strategies = foundation of treatment

1. Treat and manage any suspected medical or psychiatric cause.
2. Nonpharmacologic (see Sleep Hygiene discussed above).
3. Sleep restriction: Time in bed should match total hours slept.
4. Medication
   - Best if specific stressor identified: eg, travelling, divorce, returning military.
   - Use only if affecting daytime functioning.
   - Use for short-term only; after stopping expect two to three nights of poor sleep.
   - Avoid benzodiazepines and amitriptyline in elderly as the risk outweighs the benefit.

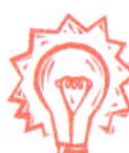

- Get a collateral history from the **sleep partner**.

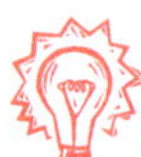

Depression and anxiety are the most common comorbidities in insomnia.

SUBSTANCES/MEDICATIONS THAT AFFECT SLEEP

Caffeine
Nicotine
Alcohol
Diuretics
Antihypertensives
Antidepressants
Bronchodilators
Decongestants
Steroids

INSOMNIA PHARMACOTHERAPY

1. Z-drugs: Zopiclone, zolpidem
2. Benzodiazepines: Lorazepam
3. Non-TCA antidepressants: Trazodone, mirtazapine
4. TCA antidepressants: Amitriptyline, doxepin
5. Antipsychotics: Quetiapine
6. Miscellaneous: Melatonin

5. If no improvement after 3 months:
   - Reassess for secondary causes.
   - Consider sleep study/polysomnography.
   - Consider referral for cognitive behavioural therapy.
6. Polysomnography suggested if:
   - High suspicion of sleep apnea or movement disorder
   - Initial diagnosis uncertain
   - Treatment failure
   - Violent or dangerous behaviour during sleep

Bibliography

DynaMed. Insomnia in adults. Updated October 31, 2016. Accessed December 23, 2016.

Jensen B, Regier L, eds. RxFiles *Drug Comparison Charts.* 10th ed. Saskatoon, Sk: Saskatoon Health Region; 2014. Available from www.RxFiles.ca.

Thyroid
Priority Topic 91

Screening for Thyroid Disease

- TSH considered the most sensitive screening test.
- Free T_4 should be done if TSH is abnormal.
- Free T_3 may be helpful if thyrotoxicosis is suspected.
- Test all symptomatic patients.
- Recommended for patients with nonspecific signs and symptoms of thyroid disease and risk factors.

Risk Factors for Thyroid Disease

- Woman >45 (female to male ratio is 5:1)
- Strong family history
- Pregnancy/postpartum
- Goitre
- Autoimmune disease (eg, DM Type I)
- Hx of neck radiation or thyroid sx/dx
- Hyperlipidemia
- Lithium and amiodarone use
- Down and Sjögren syndrome
- Psychiatric dx
- Infertility

HYPOTHYROIDISM

Definition

- Clinical syndrome caused by cellular responses to insufficient thyroid hormone production

MYXEDEMA COMA
- Decompensated hypothyroidism (rare)
- Decreased mental status
- Hypothermia
- ↓ BP and HR plus hypoventilation
- Rx: Hydrocortisone IV and LT_4 until stable—then LT_4 PO daily

Symptoms and Characteristics: "HIS FIRM CAP"

TABLE 2-6	Symptoms/Signs of Hypothyroidism
Fatigue, weakness	
Cold intolerance	
Bradycardia	
Dry skin, brittle hair, absent outer 1/3 of eyebrows	
Poor memory	
Dyspnea, hoarse voice	
Menorrhagia, later amenorrhea	
Constipation	
Weight gain with normal appetite	
Paresthesias, carpal tunnel syndrome, sluggish DTRs	
Anemia-normochromic normocytic	
Hyperlipidemia	
Puffy face, hands, feet	
Pretibial non pitting edema	
Effusions (pericardial, pleural, abdominal ascites)	

Content adapted from Toronto Notes 2017. torontonotes.ca.

COMMON ETIOLOGIES

- Hashimoto disease (most common)
- Iatrogenic
- Hypothyroid phase of thyroiditis

SICK EUTHYROID SYNDROME

Acute, reversible abnormalities in TSH/T_4/T_3 due to nonthyroid illness.

Occurs commonly after surgery, MI or with fasting, malnutrition, febrile illnesses, renal and cardiac failure, hepatic diseases, uncontrolled DM, CVD and malignancy

Does not require treatment, consider retesting!

Diagnosis: See Table 2-7

TABLE 2-7	Laboratory Tests to Assess Thyroid Function		
	TSH	FT_4	FT_3
Primary hypothyroidism	High	Low	Normal or low
Subclinical hypothyroidism	High	Normal	Normal
Abnormal hypothalamic-pituitary axis (insufficiency of pituitary TSH)	Normal or low	Normal or low	Normal or low

Content adapted from Toronto Notes 2017. torontonotes.ca.

Subclinical Hypothyroidism

- Prevalence 4% to 8% and every year 2% to 5% progress to overt hypothyroidism

Therefore treatment is recommended:

1. TSH >10 mU/L
2. TSH is above the upper reference interval limit but <10 mU/L and any of the following are present:
   a. Elevated thyroid peroxidase (TPO)
   b. Goitre
   c. Strong family history of autoimmune disorder

Treatment

Start low and go slow!

- L-thyroxine (dose range 0.05-0.2 mg PO OD)
- Elderly patients and those with CAD: Start at 0.025 mg daily and increase gradually

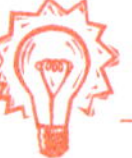

POTENTIAL BENEFITS OF TREATMENT

- Improves patient well-being
- Avoids patient from becoming symptomatic
- Protects fetus in pregnant woman
- Improves lipid profile

Monitoring TSH

- 6–8 weeks after initiating treatment and adjust dose until TSH returns to normal reference range. (TSH may remain abnormal for ~3 months. Free T_4 may be more reliable initially.)
- After a change of weight ≥10 lbs or clinical status.
- 4 to 6 weeks following a change in medication dose.
- Every 6 to 12 months once maintenance dose achieved.
- Thyroxine doses may increase by 25% to 50% during pregnancy, particularly in the first trimester, measure TSH in each trimester.

Key Points

- Remember your high-risk populations and who warrants screening.
- Screen with TSH. Check free T_4 only if TSH abnormal.
- For treatment—start low and go slow!
- Perform appropriate follow-up testing of TSH.

Bibliography

College of Family Physicians of Canada: Priority Topics and Key Features. Available from www.cfpc.ca/KeyFeatures/?p=72.

Cooper DS, Ladenson PN. The thyroid gland. In: Gardner DG, Shoback D, eds. *Greenspan's Basic and Clinical Endocrinology*. 9th ed. New York, NY: McGraw-Hill; 2011: Chap. 7.

DynaMed. Hypothyroidism in adults. Accessed December 23, 2016.

Hall J, Premji A, eds. Toronto Notes 2015: A Comprehensive Medical Reference and Review for the Medical Council of Canada Qualifying Exam Part 1 and the United States Medical Licensing Exam Step 2. 31st ed. Toronto Notes for Medical Student Inc. Toronto; 2015.

Jameson JL, Mandel SJ. Disorders of the thyroid gland. In: Kasper DL, Fauci AS, Hauser SL, Longo DL, Jameson JL, Loscalzo J, eds. *Harrison's Principles of Internal Medicine*. 19th ed. New York, NY: McGraw-Hill Education; 2015: Chap. 21.

Jensen B, Regier L, eds. *RxFiles Drug Comparison Charts*. 10th ed. Saskatoon, Sk: Saskatoon Health Region; 2014. Available from www.RxFiles.ca.

Ross, DS. Laboratory assessment of thyroid function. In: Post TW, ed. *UpToDate*. Waltham, MA. Accessed December 23, 2016.

HYPERTHYROIDISM

Definition

- Hyperthyroid: Excess production of thyroid hormone
- Thyrotoxicosis—Denotes the clinical, physiologic, and biochemical findings in response to elevated thyroid hormone

Symptoms/Characteristics: "THYROIDISM"

TABLE 2-8	Symptoms/Characteristics of Hyperthyroidism
T	Tremor
H	Heart rate up
Y	Yawning (fatigue)
R	Restlessness
O	Oligo/amenorrhea
I	Intolerance to heat
D	Diarrhea/decrease weight
I	Insomnia
S	Sweating
M	Muscle wasting/mood change

Content adapted from Toronto Notes 2017. torontonotes.ca.

May have hematological disturbances: Leukopenia, lymphocytosis, splenomegaly, lymphadenopathy (occasionally in Graves disease)

THYROID STORM
- Life-threatening!
- Decompensated thyrotoxicosis
- Fever, tachycardia, dehydration, delirium, coma, N/V diarrhea
- Causes: Trauma, surgery, RAI
- Rx: Beta-blockers, PTU, iodine, high-dose IV hydrocortisone

ELDERLY PRESENT ATYPICALLY
- Symptoms may be less obvious: Confusion, dementia, apathy, or depression
- May only have cardiovascular symptoms— Commonly new onset AFib, CHF

GRAVES DISEASE

- Goitre +/− thyroid bruit
- Ophthalmopathy: Proptosis/exophthalmos, lid lag/retraction, diplopia
- Acropachy: Clubbing and thickening of phalanges
- Dermopathy: Pretibial myxedema (nonpitting edema)

COMMON ETIOLOGIES

- Graves disease
- Thyroiditis
- Toxic nodular goitre
- Toxic nodule

GOITRE ETIOLOGY

Diffuse

- Graves disease
- Hashimoto disease
- Subacute thyroiditis (painful)

Nodular

- Multinodular goitre
- Adenoma
- Carcinoma

THYROID NODULES

- Benign tumours (eg, follicular adenoma)
- Malignancy (eg, thyroid carcinoma)
- Hyperplastic area in multinodular goitre
- Cyst

Physical Examination

Inspection:

- Scars, swellings (goitre, lump, nodule), or any other abnormalities.
- Ask patient to swallow—goitre will move.
- Ask patient to stick out tongue—thyroglossal cyst will move.

Palpation (from behind)

- Feel for isthmus (anterior to cricoid cartilage), retract SCM, and feel each lobe.
- Feel for nodules, tenderness, and consistency.
- Ask patient to swallow again—goitre will move.

Auscultate with bell for bruits.

Diagnosis: See Table 2-9

TABLE 2-9	**Causes of Hyperthyroidism with Investigations**				
PRIMARY CAUSES	**TSH**	**FT**$_{3/4}$	**RAIU 24-HOUR SCAN**	**ANTIBODIES**
Graves	Low	High $T_3 > T_4$	**Increased** homogenous pattern	TSI/TRAb/TBII
Thyroiditis	Low	High	Low	TPO
Toxic multinodular goitre	Low	High	**Increased** patchy/heterogenous pattern	None
Toxic adenoma (solitary hyperfunctioning nodule)	Low	High	Increased uptake in focal nodule with surrounding gland suppressed	None

Content adapted from Toronto Notes 2017. torontonotes.ca.

TSH may be suppressed as a normal finding in the first trimester, check Free T_4 for hyperthyroidism.

Imaging Goitres

- RAIU: Confirms Graves disease and exclude other causes (eg painless thyroiditis)
- Thyroid U/S: Assess size, nodules.
- Other investigations: Thyroid scan (Technicium 99)

Investigating Nodules

All patients require serum TSH and U/S.

- TSH to asses thyroid status and U/S to determine size, solid/cystic.
- Thyroid scan if TSH is low to determine if the nodule is hot (significant I 131 uptake into the nodule, which signifies very low malignant potential) or cold.
- FNA for all nodules >1 cm or 5 mm +/− suspicious features on U/S.

Treatment

- Graves disease
  - Thioamides: PTU or MMI.
  - Beta-blockers for symptomatic treatment.
  - Radioactive Iodine[131] if PTU or MMI does not produce disease remission.
  - Ophthalmopathy: High-dose prednisone in severe cases, orbital radiation, surgical decompression.
- Thyroiditis—Painful
  - High-dose anti-inflammatories (NSAIDs) and prednisone may be required for severe pain, fever, or malaise.
  - Beta-blockers for symptomatic treatment.

- Postpartum thyroiditis—Painless
  - Often self-limiting but monitor TSH every 6 to 8 weeks as at risk of hypothyroidism
- Toxic adenoma/toxic multinodular goitre
  - RAIU done over weeks.
  - Thioamides (eg, methimazole, or propylthiouracil) may be used initially to attain euthyroid state and avoid radiation thyroiditis.
  - Surgery may be used as first-line treatment.
  - Beta-blockers for symptomatic treatment prior to definitive therapy.

Monitoring TSH

- Check 4 to 6 weeks after initiating or changing treatment. TSH can be abnormal for months, free T_4 maybe more reliable.
- Check every 2 to 6 months once maintenance dose achieved.

Key Points

- Screen with TSH. Check free T_4 if abnormal and free T_3 if suspecting thyrotoxicosis.
- Have high index of suspicion in elderly who often present atypically.
- Examine the thyroid gland thoroughly for a goitre or nodules.
- Limit checking TSH testing to 4 to 6 weeks postinitiation or change in treatment and 6 to 12 months if stable, treated patient.

Bibliography

Cooper, DS, Ladenson, PN. The thyroid gland. In: Gardner DG, Shoback D, eds. *Greenspan's Basic and Clinical Endocrinology*. 9th ed. New York, NY: McGraw-Hill Companies; 2011: Chap. 7.

DynaMed. Hyperthyroidism and thyrotoxicosis. Updated March 21, 2016. Accessed December 23, 2016.

DynaMed. Thyroid nodule. Updated December 11, 2015. Accessed December 23, 2016.

Hall J, Premji A, eds. Toronto Notes 2015: A Comprehensive Medical Reference and Review for the Medical Council of Canada Qualifying Exam Part 1 and the United States Medical Licensing Exam Step 2. 31st ed. Toronto Notes for Medical Student Inc. Toronto; 2015.

Jensen B, Regier L, eds. *RxFiles Drug Comparison Charts*. 10th ed. Saskatoon, Sk: Saskatoon Health Region; 2014. Available from www.RxFiles.ca.

Ross DS. Diagnosis of hyperthyroidism. *UpToDate*. Waltham, MA. Accessed December 23, 2016.

Ross DS. Diagnostic approach to and treatment of thyroid nodules. *UpToDate*. Waltham, MA. Accessed December 23, 2016.

Ross, DS. Laboratory assessment of thyroid function. In: Post TW, ed. *UpToDate*. Waltham, MA. Accessed December 23, 2016.

Dizziness

Priority Topic 29

The term *dizziness* is a nonspecific term used to describe different sensations.

It is important to distinguish **(A) true vertigo from (B) nonvertiginous** *"dizziness,"* (presyncope, syncope, and disequilibrium).

Definitions

1. **Vertigo**—Illusion of motion: rotational, linear, or tilting movement of self or environment
2. **Disequilibrium**—Sense of imbalance, occurs primarily when walking, "unsteady on feet" (eg, peripheral neuropathy, cerebellar or posterior column disease, Parkinson disease)
3. **Presyncope**—Prodromal symptoms of fainting, "nearly fainted/blacked out"
4. **Syncope**—LOC and postural tone due to decrease in cerebral perfusion with spontaneous recovery

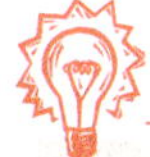

Vertigo *with* any CNS symptoms—assume a central cause!

Other key questions:
- Is there difficulty walking?
- Is the speech slurred?
- Are there visual disturbances (diplopia, poor vision, etc.)?

TRUE VERTIGO

There are two types:

1. Peripheral—Inner ear/vestibular nerve dysfunction (80%)
2. Central—Brain stem/cerebellum dysfunction

TABLE 2-10   True Vertigo—Signs and Symptoms

SYMPTOMS/SIGNS	PERIPHERAL VERTIGO	CENTRAL VERTIGO
Onset	Sudden	Sudden or gradual
Duration	Paroxysmal, intermittent	Constant
Severity	Severe	Less intense
Aggravated by movement	Yes	Variable
Position-dependent (typically head)	Yes	No
Associated nausea/vomiting	Yes	Variable
Associated fatigue	Yes	No
Hearing loss/tinnitus	May occur	No
Nystagmus: Direction Fatigable (with visual fixation)	Unidirectional, horizontal Yes	Bidirectional No
CNS signs (diplopia, dysphagia, dysarthria, ataxia)	No	Usually present
Gait: Postural instability/imbalance	Mild to moderate (leans in one direction)	Severe, falls when walking

Content adapted from Toronto Notes 2017. torontonotes.ca.

TABLE 2-11   Peripheral Vertigo—Causes, Symptoms, Diagnosis, and Treatment

CAUSES	VERTIGO	AUDITORY SYMPTOMS	NEUROLOGICAL SYMPTOMS	DIAGNOSIS	TREATMENT
BPPV Otolithic debris in semicircular canals	Sudden onset Change in head position results in symptoms (predictable) <30 seconds Intermittent: May recur for weeks/months	None	None	Dix–Hallpike test (negative test does not rule out condition)	Epley maneuver(canalith repositioning) Anticholinergics eg, SERC/Gravol
Vestibular neuronitis/ labryithitis Viral infection may precede attack Post-viral inflammatory disorder affecting the eighth CN	Sudden onset Worse with head movement in any direction Severe: Lasting hours to days Often resolves after 1 to 2 days	None	None	Rombergs test: Patient falls toward affected side	Steroids may hasten recovery Hydration Antihistamines eg, Benadryl

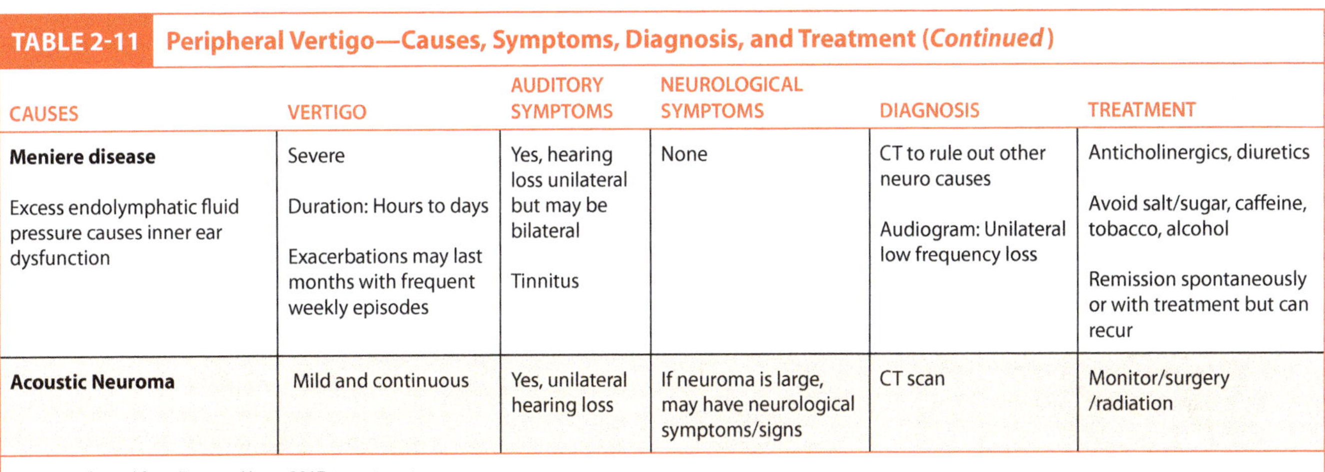

TABLE 2-11	**Peripheral Vertigo—Causes, Symptoms, Diagnosis, and Treatment (*Continued*)**				
CAUSES	VERTIGO	AUDITORY SYMPTOMS	NEUROLOGICAL SYMPTOMS	DIAGNOSIS	TREATMENT
Meniere disease Excess endolymphatic fluid pressure causes inner ear dysfunction	Severe Duration: Hours to days Exacerbations may last months with frequent weekly episodes	Yes, hearing loss unilateral but may be bilateral Tinnitus	None	CT to rule out other neuro causes Audiogram: Unilateral low frequency loss	Anticholinergics, diuretics Avoid salt/sugar, caffeine, tobacco, alcohol Remission spontaneously or with treatment but can recur
Acoustic Neuroma	Mild and continuous	Yes, unilateral hearing loss	If neuroma is large, may have neurological symptoms/signs	CT scan	Monitor/surgery /radiation

Content adapted from Toronto Notes 2017. torontonotes.ca.

TABLE 2-12	**Central Vertigo—Causes, Symptoms, and Diagnosis**			
CAUSES	VERTIGO	ASSOCIATED NEUROLOGIC SYMPTOMS	ASSOCIATED HISTORY	DIAGNOSIS
Vertebrobasilar insufficiency/TIA	Single to recurrent episodes—minutes to hours	Usually other brain stem symptoms Dysarthria/facial palsy/ataxia/uncoordinated limb movement	Older patient, vascular risk factors, cervical or carotid trauma	MRI may demonstrate vascular lesion
Cerebellar infarction or hemorrhage	Sudden onset, persistent symptoms for days to weeks	Severe gait impairment/falls when walking Headache, uncoordinated limb movements, dysphagia may occur	As above	Urgent MRI, CT will demonstrate lesion

Content adapted from Toronto Notes 2017. torontonotes.ca.

Key Points

- Divide vertigo into peripheral and central causes.
- Have a high index of suspicion for central causes in the elderly.
- Consult neurologist or neurosurgeon with central causes of vertigo or peripheral vertigo lasting >2 weeks.

CAUSES OF SYNCOPE

H	Hypoxia/hypoglycemia
E	Epilepsy
A	Anxiety/anemia
D	Drugs/dysfunctional brain stem
H	Heart attack
E	Embolism (PE)
A	Aortic dissection
R	Rhythm disturbance
T	Tachycardia/tamponade
V	Vasovagal (most common)
E	ENT
S	Situational
S	Subclavian steal syndrome
e	
L	Low systemic vascular resistance
S	Sensitive carotid sinus

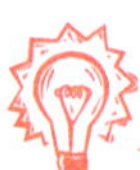

SAN FRANCISCO SYNCOPE RULE (QUINN)

The San Francisco Syncope Rule can predict patients at a high risk for serious outcome.

- **C**: History of congestive heart failure
- **H**: Hematocrit <30%
- **E**: Abnormal 12-lead electrocardiogram (eg, new changes or nonsinus rhythm)
- **S**: Shortness of breath
- **S**: Triage sBP <90 mm Hg

If positive for any one of the above critieria, 1/10 patients will have a serious outcome by day 7 & 1/250 will die by day 7.

Important to note: 1.4% of patients that do NOT meet any of the CHESS criteria will still have a 7-day serious outcome

NONVERTIGINOUS "DIZZINESS"—SYNCOPE/PRESYNCOPE

TABLE 2-13   Syncope/Presyncope: Causes, Signs/Symptoms, and Diagnostic Investigations

CAUSE/ORIGIN	SIGNS/SYMPTOMS/FEATURES	PMHX	DIAGNOSTIC INVESTIGATIONS
Cardiac	• No prodrome (heart block) • Palpitations/chest pain may precede (arrhythmia) • Syncope with exertion (aortic stenosis, HOCM) • Family hx (sudden cardiac death or cardiomyopathy)	Heart disease	ECG Echocardiography 24-h Holter monitor
Reflex 1. Vasovagal	• Young, healthy or elderly • Emotional stress or physical stress eg, prolonged standing, heat exertion • Prodrome: Sweaty, lightheaded, tinnitus, pallor, slow onset, nausea, blurry vision		Tilt-table testing Predominantly clinical diagnosis
2. Situational	Syncope immediately follows cough, sneeze, defecation, micturition		
3. Carotid sinus hypersensitivity	• Elderly (more common) • Often associated with head turning, tight shirt collars, taking of carotid pulse		Carotid massage (avoid if previous TIA/stroke/carotid bruits)

Orthostatic hypotension	• Prodrome: Postural change
	• Contributing factors:
	  ○ Volume depletion (diarrhea, vomiting, anemia, bleeding)
	  ○ Medications (vasodilators/antihypertensives, diuretics, antidepressants, alcohol)
	  ○ Autonomic failure
		Parkinson, DM, spinal cord injury	Postural BP (drop in systolic BP >20 mm Hg or diastolic >10 mm Hg with a postural change from supine/sitting to erect)

Content adapted from Toronto Notes 2017. torontonotes.ca.

Risk Factors

- Age >70
- CVD or previous TIA/CVA
- Low BMI
- DM
- Alcohol

Differential Diagnosis

- Vertigo, AAA, Stroke/TIA, DVT/PE, MI

Treatment

- Treat underlying cause.
- Educate avoiding triggers for orthostatic or situational syncope.
- Patients with recurrent syncope should avoid high-risk activities (driving).

Key Points

- All syncopal episodes warrant an ECG.
- Syncope is most often benign and self-limiting. Assess via a scoring matrix to risk stratify: example—San Francisco Syncope Rule (Quinn).
- Have high index of suspicion for a cardiac cause.
- Syncope is unlikely to have neurologic sequelae.

Bibliography

Benditt D. Syncope in adults. *UpToDate*. Accessed December 23, 2016.

Branch WT, Barton, JJS. Approach to the patient with dizziness. *UpToDate*. Accessed December 23, 2016.

DynaMed. Differential diagnosis. Updated November 28, 2016. Accessed December 23, 2016.

DynaMed. Orthostatic hypotension and orthostatic syncope. Updated November 1, 2016. Accessed December 23, 2016.

DynaMed. Syncope evaluation. Updated November 22, 2016. Accessed December 23, 2016.

Furman JM, Barton JJS. Evaluation of the patient with vertigo. *UpToDate*. Accessed December 23, 2016.

Hall J, Premji A, eds. Toronto Notes 2015: A Comprehensive Medical Reference and Review for the Medical Council of Canada Qualifying Exam Part 1 and the United States Medical Licensing Exam Step 2. 31st ed. Toronto Notes for Medical Student Inc. Toronto; 2015.

Quinn J, McDermott D, Stiell I, Kohn M, Wells G. Prospective validation of the San Francisco Syncope Rule to predict patients with serious outcomes. *Ann Emerg Med*. 2006;47(5):448-54.

Skin Disorders

Priority Topic 84

Key Points

- Evaluating a skin lesion:
  - Inspect **all areas of the skin** including scalp, nails, palms of the hands, soles of the feet, oral cavity, perineum.
  - Always consider a life-threatening condition such as melanoma, necrotizing fasciitis, Stevens–Johnson syndrome.
  - Use **biopsy or excision** to rule out serious pathology.
  - Use history, physical examination, and investigations to rule out a systemic disorder.
    - Autoimmune: SLE, ulcerative colitis
    - Endocrine: DM, thyroid disorders
    - Infectious: HIV, viral illness
    - Malignancy: Paget disease of the breast
    - Other: Liver or renal disease
  - Take a medication history and consider a drug reaction.
  - Determine the impact on the patient's life, including sleep in pruritic disorders.
  - In high-risk patients such as diabetics, bed- or chair-bound patients, peripheral vascular disease assess for skin lesions at every visit and treat minor lesions aggressively.
- Treating a skin lesion:
  - When the lesion is not responding to treatment:
    - Modify your treatment (eg, stepwise approach to acne)
    - Reconsider your diagnosis (dandruff vs psoriasis)
  - Optimize control of chronic diseases
  - Provide education and psychological support
    - Scars can be both physical and emotional.
    - Depression, anxiety, social isolation, and lack of self-confidence are not uncommon.
  - Provide information about support groups; for example, Psoriasis Society of Canada

COMMON SKIN DISORDERS

Acne Vulgaris

Definition

A common inflammatory pilosebaceous disease categorized with respect to severity.

MYTH BUSTER: ACNE

- Diet is not associated with acne.
- Not a disease of poor hygiene.
- Black tip of a comedone is oxidized sebum not dirt.

ECZEMA: TRIGGERS

- Irritants: Detergents, soaps, clothing (recommend wool, loose cotton)
- Contact and environmental allergens: Dust mites, pets
- Long, hot showers
- Sweating
- Stress

Eczema of the nipple: Suspect Paget disease of the breast!

ECZEMA CLASSIFICATIONS:

Atopic: Often associated with family history of atopy (eczema +/− asthma, allergic rhinitis)

Contact dermatitis: Precipitated by a particular irritant or allergen

Nummular: Often in elderly; annular, coin-shaped lesions

PSORIASIS: TRIGGERS

Trauma (Koebner phenomenon)

Infection

Alcohol

Stress

Drugs: Beta-blockers, NSAIDs, lithium

Clinical Categories

- Type I: Comedonal, sparse, no scarring
- Type II: Comedonal, papular, moderate +/− little scarring
- Type III: Comedonal, papular, and pustular with scarring
- Type IV: Nodulocystic acne, risk of severe scarring
- Predilection sites: Face, neck, upper chest, and back

Treatment

- Mild (type I and II)—topical treatment.
  - Appropriate skin hygiene
  - Benzoyl peroxide
  - Topical retinoid (tretinoin, adapalene)
  - Topical antibiotics
- Moderate (type III) or after topical treatments have failed.
  - Systemic antibiotics: Clindamycin or doxycycline × approx 3 months
  - Hormonal therapy (women): OCPs including Diane 35, Spironolactone
- Severe (type IV) or after above treatments have failed.
  - Isotretinoin (Accutane, Clarus, Epuris) for 4 to 6 months. Tx depends on optimal cumulative total dose (120-150 mg/kg/course). May extend the course (reduce the daily dose) if side effects are causing compliance issues. MUST counsel regarding teratogenic effects.

Eczema Dermatitis—The Itch That Rashes

Definition

An inflammatory, chronically relapsing, noncontagious, pruritic skin disorder.

Characteristics

- Xerosis and pruritus—"the itchy rash"

Physical Examination

- Skin findings:
  - Inflammation, erythema
  - Excoriation secondary to pruritus
  - Lichenification
  - Weeping, crusting—secondary bacterial infection
- Distribution varies according to age
  - Infants (2-6 months): Face, scalp, extensor surfaces
  - Childhood (>18 months): Flexural surfaces
  - Adult: Hands, feet, flexures, wrists, face, forehead, eyelids, neck

Treatment

I. Moisturize: Emollients restore the skin's protective barrier and maintain hydration (Vaseline>creams>gels). "The oilier the better!"

II. Avoid triggers! Consider antihistamines to break the itch-scratch cycle.

III. Steroids for flares: Topical corticosteroids (least potent dose that is effective). Advise about finger-tip unit, avoiding face and to use sparingly for 2 weeks at a time to avoid skin atrophy.

IV. Antibiotics for secondary bacterial infection: Topical fusidic acid (Fucidin), mupirocin, cephalexin, cloxacillin. Antivirals for superseding viral infections.

Psoriasis

Definition

A chronic, recurring inflammatory dermatosis of which a number of different presentations occur.

Plaque psoriasis (most common)

- Characterized by well-circumscribed erythematous papules/plaques with sliver-white scales
- May be mildly pruritic or painful
- Distribution: Scalp, extensor surfaces, trunk, intergluteal folds, pressure areas

Other manifestations include guttate, pustular, and erythrodermic psoriasis.

Treatment

Plaque psoriasis treatment is based on disease severity (CDA Guidance)[3]

- Mild: 5% of BSA
  - First line: Topical corticosteroids.
  - Other first-line options: Topical vitamin D analogues (calcipotriol) that can be used in combination with corticosteroids.
  - Second line: Topical retinoids (tazarotene), salicylic acid (removes scales), anthralin, and coal tar
  - Emollients can be used in combination with the above agents to help restore the barrier function of the skin.
- Moderate–severe: BSA >10% or significant affect on QOL, distribution of disease (face, hands, feet, or genitals), or uncontrolled pain +/− pruritus
  - Phototherapy
  - Systemic therapies (oral retinoids, cyclosporin, methotrexate, or biologics)

OTHER SKIN DISORDERS KEY POINTS

Lichen Planus

Characteristics

- Six Ps: Purple, pruritic, polygonal, peripheral, papules, penis
- Wickham striae: Greyish lines over surface
- Commonly presents on flexural surfaces, mucosa, and genitalia
- Associated with stress and hepatitis C virus infection

Treatment

- Spontaneously resolves over weeks or may persist for years
- Topical corticosteroids +/− intralesional steroid injections
- Chemo phototherapy for resistant cases

SKIN INFECTIONS

Dermatophytosis

- Fungal infection of the skin.
- Defined by infected location.
- Microscopic diagnosis: Skin scrapings prepared with KOH will demonstrate hyphae.
- Treat with topical antifungals. Use systemic antifungals for resistant cases or nail involvement.

Cellulitis

- Skin infection involving dermis and subcutaneous tissues
- Causative organism:
  - Common **beta-hemolytic** *Streptococcus* (group A more than group B, C, or G) or *Staphylococcus aureus*
  - Cat or dog bite: *Pasteurella multocida*
  - Saltwater exposure: *Vibrio vulnificus*

PSORIASIS: WHEN TO REFER?
- Confirmation of diagnosis required
- Inadequate response to appropriate, initial treatment
- Significant impact on patient's quality of life
- Clinician unfamiliar with other treatment options (PUVA, phototherapy, immunosuppressive meds).
- Widespread, severe disease
- Psoriatic arthritis (involve rheumatology)

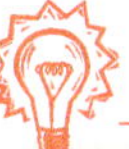

When treatment fails, consider an alternative diagnosis (eg, eczema could be a fungal infection).

DERMATOPHYTOSIS—DEFINED BY LOCATION OF INFECTION
Head: *Tinea capitis*
Body: *T. corporis*
Groin: *T. cruris*
Feet: *T. pedis*

TREATMENT
Abscesses require incision and drainage.

- Treatment
  - First-line treatment includes cephalexin PO or cefazolin IV (face, severe).
  - Consider risk factors for MRSA (hospital/LTC, incarcerated, immunosuppression, IVDU, implanted device, recent antibiotics)

Erysipelas

Type of superficial cellulitis presents as erythema with defined and elevated borders due to lymphatic involvement

Impetigo

- Infection of epidermis only.
- Often in children.
- **Honey-coloured** crusted lesions around mouth.
- Treat with topical antibiotics.

Necrotizing Fasciitis

- Severe, aggressive, and life-threatening form of skin infection.
- Most often polymicrobial.
- High fevers and severe systemic toxicity are seen.
- Treatment requires *urgent **surgical debridement*** +/– amputation and early broad-spectrum antibiotics (use bacteriostatic regimens).

Herpes Simplex Virus (HSV)

Consider abuse in preadolescents presenting with genital herpes.

- Affects more than one-third of the world's population.
- Presents with multiple *painful* orolabial or genital vesicles and ulcerations.
- Patients are the most sick with their first episode; many patients have fever, headache, malaise, and myalgias.
- Lifelong latent infection in sensory ganglia is standard.
- Subsequent recurrences are less severe. Prodrome of itching and burning often precedes the rash.
- Maternal-fetal transmission is associated with significant morbidity.
- Treatment:
  - Antivirals are needed early to be effective, for example, acyclovir, famciclovir, valacyclovir.
  - Chronic suppressive therapy is reserved for those with more than 4 to 6 outbreaks per year.

Dewdrops on a rose petal: Classic rash of VZV.

Varicella Zoster Virus (VZV)

- Manifests as varicella (chicken pox) and herpes zoster (shingles).
- Rash: Pruritic, papular changing to vesicular to pustular and finally to crusting.
- Vaccination is available (12 months and 4-6 years old) including vaccination for zoster for those over 60
- Chicken pox:
  - Disease of childhood, highly contagious
  - Incubation period of 14 to 21 days
  - Fever and malaise just before or with skin eruption

COMMON COMPLICATIONS
Second bacterial infection
Postherpetic neuralgia

- Herpes zoster:
  - More common in elderly and immunocompromised.
  - After primary infection, latent virus develops in spinal dorsal root ganglia.
  - Reactivation causes a rash along the dermatomal distribution.
  - *Pain precedes rash* and can be severe.

- Treatment:
  - Antivirals (acyclovir for 7 days).
  - Treat within 24 to 72 hours of rash appearing.
  - Prophylaxis: Treat household contacts.
- Herpes zoster ophthalmicus:
  - VZV infection of ophthalmic division of trigeminal nerve
  - Presents with lesions of nose, corner of eye
  - Risk of loss of vision, chronic ocular inflammation, and eye pain
  - Antivirals within 72 hours of rash help prevent ocular complications
  - Urgent referral of ophthalmologist if ocular involvement suspected
    - For example, conjunctivitis, keratitis, uveitis, ocular-motor nerve palsies

SKIN DISORDERS: SERIOUS DIAGNOSES NOT TO MISS!

Hypersensitivity Syndromes

- Erythema multiforme (EM)
  - Rapid onset of red macules to target-like papules with erythematous border and central sparring
  - Unlike urticaria, the lesions remain fixed 7 to 14 days
  - Rx: Stop causative drug, oral antihistamines
- Stevens–Johnson syndrome (SJS)/toxic epidermal necrolysis (TEN)
  - SJS: A severe expression of EM, though not as severe as TEN.
  - Severe cutaneous reaction often caused by drugs.
  - Presents as sick patient with fever >39°C, blisters on dusky macules, and **involvement of mucous membranes (mouth, eyes, genital lesions).**
  - Diagnosis is made based on the percentage of skin involved.
    - SJS <10%
    - TEN >30%
  - Mortality is due to fluid loss.
  - Treat aggressively. Hospitalize, stop causative drug, IV fluids, consider IVIG.

Skin Cancer

- Pay attention to sun-exposed areas: Face, lips, ears, scalp, and extremities.
- Always consider a life-threatening condition such as malignancy.
- Treatment generally involves excision +/− lymph node dissection for invasive disease.

Basal Cell Carcinoma (BCC)

- Eighty per cent of skin cancers are BCC.
- Spread locally and rarely metastasize.
- Nodular BCC (most common) presents as raised pearly white nodule with telangiectasia >6 mm.
- Superficial BCC presents as red scaling plaques with thready border.

Squamous Cell Carcinoma (SCC)

- Five per cent develop metastasis
- Tumour of keratinocytes
- Presents as persistent areas of ulceration, crusting, hyperkeratosis, or erythema
- Common in fair-skinned and organ-transplant patients
- Actinic keratosis = premalignant form
  - Presents as rough, scaly spots on sun-exposed skin
  - Often treated with cryotherapy; topical therapy includes: 5-fluorouracil, diclofenac, imiquimod

Rashes on the palms
- EM
- Rocky mountain spotted fever
- Drug eruption
- Secondary syphilis
- Scabies
- Hand, foot, and mouth disease

HSV—Herpes simplex virus is associated with EM in at least 60% of cases.

Use **biopsy or excision** to rule out serious pathology.

SKIN CANCER RISK FACTORS
Sun exposure
Age >50
Fair skin
Male gender
Family history
Multiple nevi (risk for melanoma)

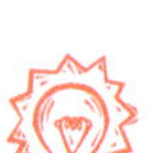

MELANOMA VS MOLE

A: Asymmetry
B: Border = irregular
C: Colour = varied
D: Diameter >6 mm
E: Evolving/elevation

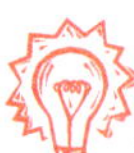

Think of pemphigus vulgaris when an oral ulceration lasts >1 month.

Malignant Melanoma

- Malignant neoplasm of pigment-forming cells
- ABCDE: To distinguish benign nevi versus malignant lesions (see sidebar)

Leukoplakia

- White lesion seen on oral mucosa which cannot be rubbed off
- Thought to be a premalignant lesion
- Associated with tobacco and alcohol use
- Requires biopsy and close follow-up +/− excision or cryotherapy

Cutaneous T-Cell Lymphoma (Mycosis Fungoides)

- Rare disease, more common in people of African descent.
- Malignant lymphoma of T-cells that usually remains confined to skin and lymph nodes.
- Diagnosis: Biopsy shows distinctive pathology.
- Ninety-five per cent are mycosis fungoides (limited superficial type)
  - Presents as erythematous, scaling patches or plaques that are often pruritic.
  - Hypo- and hyperpigmented lesions are common.
  - Lymphadenopathy is common.
- Five per cent of cases are Sézary syndrome (widespread systemic type).
- Treatment includes:
  - Topical: High-potency steroids, retinoids, or chemotherapy
  - Phototherapy: UVA/UVB

Pemphigus

- Rare but serious **autoimmune** disease—**refer to dermatologist!**
- **Bullous lesions** of skin and mucosa that quickly erode to **vesicles and ulcerations**.
- Most common form is pemphigus vulgaris.
- **Nikolsky sign:** Superficial detachment of the skin with lateral pressure.
- Treatment: Goal of treatment is initial remission.
  - Systemic steroids (prednisone 40-80 mg/d)
  - Nonsteroidal adjuvants: Azathioprine, mycophenolate, methotrexate, cyclophosphamide, rituximab, IVIG

Bibliography

Asai Y, Baibergenova A, Dutil M, et al. Management of acne: Canadian clinical practise guideline. *CMAJ*. 2016;188(2):118-126.

Corey L. Herpes simplex infection. In: Kasper DL, Fauci AS, Hauser SL, Longo DL, Jameson JL, Loscalzo J, eds. *Harrison's Principles of Internal Medicine*. 19th ed. New York, NY: McGraw-Hill Education; 2015: Chap. 216.

DynaMed. Atopic dermatitis. Revised December 21 2016. Accessed December 28, 2016.

DynaMed. Basal cell carcinoma. Updated December 28, 2016. Accessed December 28, 2016.

DynaMed. Cellulitis. Revised November 28, 2016. Accessed December 28, 2016.

DynaMed. Lichen planus. Updated April 7, 2016. Accessed December 28, 2016.

DynaMed. Pemphigus vulgaris. Updated November 12, 2014. Accessed December 28, 2016.

DynaMed. Psoriasis. Updated October 13, 2016. Accessed December 28, 2016.

Goldstein BG, Goldstein AO. Oral lesions. *UpToDate*. Updated December 2, 2015. Accessed December 28, 2016.

Hall J, Premji A, eds. Toronto Notes 2015: A Comprehensive Medical Reference and Review for the Medical Council of Canada Qualifying Exam Part 1 and the United States Medical Licensing Exam Step 2. 31st ed. Toronto Notes for Medical Student Inc. Toronto; 2015.

Hodak E, Amitay-Laish I. Variants of mycosis fungoides. *UpToDate*. Updated November 2, 2016. Accessed December 28, 2016.

Jensen B, Regier L, eds. *RxFiles Drug Comparison Charts*. 10th ed. Saskatoon, Sk: Saskatoon Health Region; 2014. Available from www.RxFiles.ca.

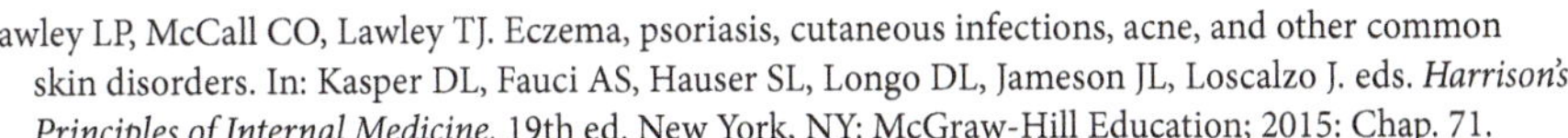

Lawley LP, McCall CO, Lawley TJ. Eczema, psoriasis, cutaneous infections, acne, and other common skin disorders. In: Kasper DL, Fauci AS, Hauser SL, Longo DL, Jameson JL, Loscalzo J. eds. *Harrison's Principles of Internal Medicine*. 19th ed. New York, NY: McGraw-Hill Education; 2015: Chap. 71.

Nirken MH, Whitney AH, Roujeau JC. Stevens-Johnson Syndrome and Toxic Epidermal Necrolysis. *UpToDate*. Accessed December 28, 2016.

Shinkai K, Fox LP. Dermatological disorders. In: Papadakis MA, McPhee SJ, Rabow MW, eds. *Current Medical Diagnosis and Treatment 2017*. 56th ed. New York, NY: McGraw-Hill Education: 2017: Chap. 6.

Whitley R. Varicella-zoster virus infections. In: Kasper DL, Fauci AS, Hauser SL, Longo DL, Jameson JL, Loscalzo J, eds. *Harrison's Principles of Internal Medicine*. 19th ed. New York, NY: McGraw-Hill Education; 2015: Chap. 217.

Cancer

Priority Topic 12

Use each visit as an opportunity to provide counselling regarding cancer prevention (eg, smoking cessation, practice safe sex).

Use the most up-to-date Canadian Cancer Screening Guidelines to screen all patients in your practice.

In patients who have been given a diagnosis of cancer:

- Provide emotional support and inquire about personal and social consequences of the illness.
- Provide close follow-up.
- Remain involved in the circle of care. Continue to stay involved in the specialist-driven treatment plan.
- Use each visit to ask about side effects of cancer treatments (eg, diarrhea, swelling, hair loss, paresthesias).
- Be realistic and honest when discussing prognosis with the patient.

In patients with a distant history of cancer, have a high index of suspicion for return/new cancer when presenting with new symptoms (eg, new shortness of breath, back pain) and investigate appropriately.

Bibliography

Canadian Cancer Society: Screening. Available from http://www.cancer.ca/en/prevention-and-screening/early-detection-and-screening/screening/?region=on

Canadian Taskforce on Preventative Healthcare. Available from http://canadiantaskforce.ca/guidelines/published-guidelines/

Loss of Weight

Priority Topic 60

- Unexplained, unintentional weight loss should be investigated through a thorough history, physical examination, and appropriate investigations as indicated.
- Patients' weights should be recorded on a regular basis (eg, annual basis for all patients but more frequently if weight loss is suspected). Persistent weight loss may indicate the need to work the patient up again for a possible cause.

Bibliography

The College of Family Physicians of Canada. Priority Topics and Key Features.

Evans AT, Gupta R. Approach to the patient with unintentional weight loss. *UpToDate*. Approach to the patient with unintentional weight loss. Updated March 14, 2016. Accessed December 26, 2016.

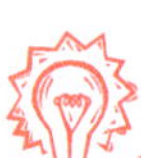

KEY PARKINSONIAN FEATURES: "TRAP"
Tremor
Rigidity
Akinesia/bradykinesia
Postural instability

Parkinsonism
Priority Topic 71

TABLE 2-14	Tremor of Parkinson's Disease
Upper extremity, often begins unilateral	
Four to six cycles per second	
At rest "pill rolling"	
Associated with: Rigidity Bradykinesia Postural Instability	
Increased with emotional stress Decreased with voluntary activity	
Content adapted from Toronto Notes 2017. torontonotes.ca.	

Symptoms/Characteristics

- Older age >60 years—number one risk factor
- Resting tremor—often unilateral
- Muscle rigidity/cogwheeling
  - Increase in resistance to passive movement
- Bradykinesia/akinesia
  - Slow movements
  - Difficulty initiating movements
- Gait
  - Small shuffling steps, decreased arm swinging, unsteady turning, and difficulty stopping
  - Flexed posture
- Postural instability—late feature
- Mask-like facial expression, infrequent blinking
- Seborrhea of face/scalp (dandruff)

Also look for:

- Changes in speech: Hypophonia (quiet voice/speech), monotonous speech, dysarthria (difficult articulation of speech), decreased spontaneous speech
- Micrographia: Small handwriting
- Sleep disturbances, personality changes, anxiety
- Falls

Etiology

- Idiopathic decrease in dopaminergic neurons in the pars compacta of the substantia nigra.

Diagnosis

- Classic 80%: Bradykinesia + unilateral asymmetric signs, pill rolling resting tremor, and good treatment response to levodopa.

Differential Diagnosis

When atypical features (below) are present → suspect secondary Parkinson or other syndromes

- Young age <60 years or Wilson disease
- Abrupt onset of symptoms
- Rapid progression

PEARL
Consider Parkinson disease in an elderly patient with functional status deterioration.

DRUGS THAT CAUSE PARKINSONISM
Amphotericin B
Calcium channel blockers
Chemotherapy
Cholinergics
Lithium
Metoclopramide
Neuroleptics
Prochlorperazine
SSRIs
Valproate

- Absent resting tremor
- Poor response to levodopa
- Ocular movement disorder: r/o supranuclear palsy
- Early autonomic dysfunction (eg, urinary incontinence, syncope): r/o multisystem atrophy parkinsonism
- Early dementia

Treatment

- General
  - Aim: Improve quality of life and functional status
  - Physical/occupational/speech therapy
    - For example, rails, large-handled cutlery, devices to amplify the voice.
    - Physiotherapy is helpful to prevent falls due to postural instability.
  - Early referral to neurology
  - Ongoing care
    - Assess functional status frequently.
    - Anticipate and monitor for medication side effects.
    - Recognize associated problems.
      - Depression, dementia, falls, and constipation
      - Urinary retention, sexual dysfunction, dysphagia (difficulty swallowing), sleep changes
- Medical
  - Dopamine precursor: First-line (eg, levodopa/carbidopa)
    - Carbidopa decreases the peripheral breakdown of dopamine.
  - Dopamine agonists: Best effect in early disease (eg, pramipexole)
  - Anticholinergics: Block acetylcholine in striatum (eg, benztropine)
  - NMDA-receptor antagonist: Blocks reuptake of dopamine (eg, amantadine)
  - MAOIs: Inhibits dopamine metabolism (eg, selegiline)
  - COMT inhibitor: Inhibits breakdown of dopamine (eg, tolcapone)
- Medication side effects:
  - Dopaminergic:
    - Dyskinesias (impairment in voluntary movement)
    - Brief duration of action—needs multidose regimen
    - Orthostatic hypotension/dizziness
    - Gastric upset
    - Depression/psychosis/hallucinations/disinhibition
  - MAOIs:
    - Arrhythmia
    - Hypertensive crisis with tyramine (cheese, wine)
- Surgical treatment options:
  - Deep brain stimulation
  - Reserved for unresponsive patients and late disease

Key Points

- Parkinson disease is the most common cause of bradykinesia.
- Distinguish idiopathic from atypical Parkinson disease (young age, drug-related).
- Use a team approach, by involving other health care professionals including early referral to neurology.
- In an elderly patient with functional status deterioration, consider parkinsonism.

WHEN TO REFER?
All patients should be referred to a neurologist.

Dyskinesia is the #1 side effect of levodopa.

Bibliography

Aminoff MJ, Douglas VC. Nervous system disorders. In: Papadakis MA, McPhee SJ, Rabow MW. eds. *Medical Diagnosis and Treatment 2017*. 56th ed. New York, NY: McGraw-Hill Education; 2017.

Chou KL. Clinical manifestations of Parkinson disease. Updated December 13, 2016. Accessed December 26, 2016.

College of Family Physicians of Canada. Priority Topics and Key Features. Available from http://www.cfpc.ca/ProjectAssets/Templates/KeyFeatures.aspx?id=5107&terms=priority+topics.

DynaMed. Parkinson disease. Updated November 14, 2016. Accessed December 26, 2016.

Hall J, Premji A, eds. Toronto Notes 2015: A Comprehensive Medical Reference and Review for the Medical Council of Canada Qualifying Exam Part 1 and the United States Medical Licensing Exam Step 2. 31st ed. Toronto Notes for Medical Student Inc. Toronto; 2015.

Jensen B, Regier L, eds. *Rx Files Drug Comparison Charts*. 10th ed. Saskatoon, Sk: Saskatoon Health Region; 2014. Available from www.RxFiles.ca.

Olanow CW, Schapira AHV, Obeso JA. Parkinson's disease and other movement disorders. In: Kasper DL, Fauci AS, Hauser SL, Longo DL, Jameson JL, Loscalzo J, eds. *Harrison's Principles of Internal Medicine*. 19th ed. New York, NY: McGraw-Hill Education; 2015: Chap. 449.

Restless Legs Syndrome

Supplementary Topic

Diagnostic Criteria

Must have all four criteria:

1. Urge to move the legs usually with accompanying uncomfortable sensations (eg, creeping).
2. Onset or exacerbation with rest.
3. Relief with movement.
4. Circadian pattern (worse in the evening and during the night).

   Supportive clinical features: Family history, response to dopaminergic therapy, periodic leg movements.

   No routine testing recommended, consider checking blood work (eg, iron deficiency, electrolytes) and for underlying medical conditions based on clinical judgment.

Causes

Idiopathic (primary) versus underlying medical condition (secondary)

1. DM/peripheral neuropathy
2. Iron deficiency
3. Pregnancy
4. Low magnesium
5. End-stage renal disease
6. Drug causes: Lithium, antidepressants (especially SSRIs and TCAs), antipsychotics, some CCBs, antiemetics (domperidone and ondansetron may have least effect)

Differential Diagnoses

1. Nocturnal leg cramps
2. Peripheral neuropathy
3. Varicose veins
4. Akathisia (inner restlessness and the urge to constantly move/inability to sit still)—occasional side effect of antipsychotic or antidepressant medications
5. Intermittent claudication
6. Periodic limb movements of sleep (PLMS)
7. Positional discomfort
8. Leg pain (eg, arthritis)
9. Fidgets or nervous leg shaking

Treatment

1. First-line treatment is nonpharmacologic.
   - Nutrition: Avoid caffeine, alcohol, chocolate, smoking/nicotine
   - Good sleep hygiene
   - Stretching/exercise
2. Treat any underlying causes.
3. Pharmacologic treatments
   - Dopamine agonists (eg, pramipexole, ropinirole)
   - Dopamine precursors (eg, levodopa)
   - Antiepileptics (eg, carbamazepine, gabapentin, pregabalin)
   - Opioids

Bibliography

DynaMed. Restless legs syndrome. Updated September 6, 2016. Accessed December 26, 2016.

Jensen B, Regier L, eds. *Rx Files Drug Comparison Charts*. 10th ed. Saskatoon, Sk: Saskatoon Health Region; 2014. Available fromwww.RxFiles.ca.

Restless Legs Syndrome Foundation. Available from www.rls.org.

Up to Date. Restless Legs Syndrome. Updated May 27, 2016. Accessed December 26, 2016.

CHAPTER 3

Infectious Diseases

Infections

Priority Topic 51

1. When investigating a patient with a possible infection:
   a. Use a selective approach in ordering cultures before initiating antibiotic therapy (eg, cultures usually not required for pneumonia, UTI, abscess, or uncomplicated cellulitis).
      - Use throat swabs according to guidelines in acute pharyngitis.
      - Perform a culture in patients with history of unusual or resistant organisms on previous culture.
      - Follow-up culture results to guide therapy when considering a broad infectious differential diagnosis (such as in immunocompromised patients).
   b. Use the correct techniques and protocols for cultures.
      - Selecting correct swabs and identification of appropriate culture and/or transport medium (eg, Diamond's medium for *Trichomonas vaginalis*).
      - Understanding and interpreting resistance and susceptibility patterns to influence choice of antimicrobial agent.
2. If considering treatment for an infection, antibiotic use should be:
   a. Judicious
      - Delayed treatment in otitis media (see Earache).
      - Antibiotics are not recommended in acute bronchitis, as etiology is primarily viral.
      - Avoiding screening for (or treating) asymptomatic bacteriuria in uncomplicated adult patients or those with indwelling catheters.
   b. Rational
      - Cost: Taking into account the direct cost of the antimicrobial, as well as dispensing fees, and degree of coverage by provincial or private drug plans.
      - Guidelines: Following Canadian guidelines where applicable, and recognizing situations in which guidelines will not directly apply.
      - Comorbidity: Adjusting dose amount, frequency of dosing, length of treatment or choice of antimicrobial agent based upon individual patient factors (eg, presence of renal disease, severity of illness, or history of immunocompromise).

- Local resistance patterns: Modifying antimicrobial selection and guidelines as needed.
- Ease of treatment: Considering the effect of dosing schedule and delivery route (eg, elixir vs tablet) on treatment adherence and outcomes.

3. Use empiric treatment when appropriate, for example:
   - Life-threatening sepsis without culture report or confirmed diagnosis.
   - Suspected meningitis.
   - Acute otitis media in children <6 months.
   - *Candida vaginitis* after antibiotic use.
   - Uncomplicated cellulitis, pneumonia, UTIs, or abscesses.

4. Consider infection as a possible cause of nonspecific signs and symptoms, such as:
   - Confusion in the elderly (eg, UTI, pneumonia)
   - Failure to thrive (eg, TB, HIV)
   - Unexplained pain (eg, necrotizing fasciitis, abdominal pain in children with pneumonia)
   - Fever of unknown origin (eg, endocarditis, intra-abdominal abscess)
   - Chronic diarrhea (eg, *Giardia lamblia*, *Entamoeba histolytica*)

5. When a patient is deteriorating or is not responding to treatment after an original diagnosis of a simple infection, consider the possibility of a more complex infection.
   - Look for a different type of organism (ie, viral vs fungal vs bacterial).
   - Consider a different dose, type, or route of antimicrobial.
   - Perform an appropriate culture or conduct further investigations if the etiology is unclear.
   - Reevaluate noninfectious causes (eg, neoplasm, autoimmune condition).

6. When using antibiotics to treat infections, employ other therapies as appropriate:
   - Fluid resuscitation in septic shock
   - Incision and drainage of abscesses
   - Tetanus booster as needed for lacerations and open wounds
   - Adequate analgesia

Bibliography

Working Group on the Certification Process. *Defining Competence for the Purposes of Certification by the College of Family Physicians of Canada: the evaluation objectives in Family Medicine.* The College of Family Physicians of Canada; 2010. http://www.cfpc.ca/uploadedFiles/Education/Certification_in_Family_Medicine_Examination/Definition%20of%20Competence%20Complete%20Document%20with%20skills%20and%20phases.pdf.

Antibiotics

Priority Topic 5

1. When antibiotics are required, agents should be selected based on multiple factors, including:
   - Differences among first-line therapies for a specific indication
     - Considering evidence-based effectiveness, cost, and minimization of side effects
   - Local resistance patterns
     - Tailoring treatment based on epidemiological reporting and clinical experience
   - Clinical context
     - Choosing antibiotics based on previous bacterial infections and treatments, known immunodeficiencies, and to minimize interactions with critical medications (eg, warfarin)

- Patient's context
  - Simplifying dose schedules to improve adherence, or ensuring that pre-scribed medications are covered by provincial or private drug plans.

2. Prescribe antibiotics only when the clinical presentation is likely to be caused by a bacterial infection, and when there is evidence for benefit from antibiotic treatment:
   - Avoiding antibiotics in nonsevere cases of acute otitis media for children >6 months of age (see Earache)
   - Relying on decision rules to minimize the use of antibiotics in cases of acute pharyngitis (see Upper Respiratory Tract Infections)
   - Prescribing antibiotics in sinusitis only if signs or symptoms of bacterial infection present (see Upper Respiratory Tract Infections)

3. Be vigilant when evaluating reported allergies and reactions to antibiotics, and differentiate these from nonallergic events, such as:
   - Intolerance to known side effects
   - Nonallergic exanthem
   - Concurrent symptoms not related to drug administration

4. Use bacterial cultures in specific instances in which the result is likely to alter your choice of antibiotic therapy:
   - Performing bacterial cultures to assess community resistance patterns, as well as for patients with systemic symptoms, history of unusual or resistant organ-isms, and for those who are immunocompromised.

5. Initiate antibiotics without delay before confirmation of the diagnosis in situa-tions in which:
   - The infection is life-threatening (eg, sepsis).
   - Patient factors increase the likelihood of deterioration (eg, febrile neutropenia).
   - The infection has the potential for a rapid clinical course (eg, meningitis).

Bibliography

Working Group on the Certification Process. *Defining Competence for the Purposes of Certification by the College of Family Physicians of Canada: the evaluation objectives in Family Medicine.* The College of Family Physicians of Canada; 2010. http://www.cfpc.ca/uploadedFiles/Education/Certification_in_ Family_Medicine_Examination/Definition%20of%20Competence%20Complete%20Document%20 with%20skills%20and%20phases.pdf.

Fever

Priority Topic 39

IN CHILDREN

Recognize the potential for occult bacteremia and other serious infections in young children

- For ages up to 3 months:
  - Fever defined as a rectal temperature ≥38.0°C.
  - Often a diagnostic challenge:
    - Usually caused by a self-limiting benign viral infection.
    - A cause may not be obvious despite a careful history and physical examination.
    - However, fever may be the only sign of a serious bacterial infection (eg, men-ingitis, pneumonia, UTI, bacteremia) or serious viral infection (eg, HSV) and should be further evaluated.
  - Investigate with CBC and differential, blood culture, CSF analysis and culture, and urine culture.

- Admit to hospital in most cases for empiric antibiotics, and consider chest radiograph and antiviral therapy (eg, acyclovir) based on clinical appearance as well as risk factors for serious infection (eg, prematurity, history of previous illness, prenatal complications, maternal history of HSV).
- For ages 3 months to 3 years:
  - Fever usually caused by a self-limiting viral infection, or a bacterial infection with a source identifiable on history and physical examination (eg, meningitis, UTI, pneumonia, skin infection, or osteomyelitis).
  - Consider urinalysis and urine culture.
  - If child appears toxic, or has risk factors for infection (based on medical or immunization history):
    - Investigate with CBC and differential.
    - Further workup might include blood culture, urine culture, CSF analysis and culture, and chest radiograph.

FEVER OF UNKNOWN ORIGIN

Definition

- Fever >38.3°C (oral)
  - Lasting >3 weeks
  - Or, diagnosis uncertain after 1 week of hospitalization or three outpatient visits

Symptoms

- Enquire about past medical history, travel history, immunizations, sick contacts, fever onset/duration/pattern, occupational activities, sexual activity, drug use, and animal contacts.
- Investigate symptoms of systemic illness suggesting less benign course such as weight loss or night sweats.
- Ask about potentially localizing symptoms, including cough, dyspnea, abdominal pain, back pain, diarrhea, dysuria, headaches, neck stiffness, arthritides, and rashes.

Physical Examination Findings

Complete examination, with particular attention paid to:

- Eyes: Redness, ulcers, retinal lesions
- Skin: Rashes, hemorrhagic/septic lesions, temporal artery tenderness
- Lymph nodes and spleen: Enlargement
- Heart: New murmurs or extra sounds
- Abdomen: Focal tenderness or masses
- Genitourinary: Genital lesions or discharge, rectal/prostate abnormalities
- Joints: Inflammation, swelling
- Neurological: Cranial nerve palsies, focal signs

Differential Diagnosis

- Infectious diseases (eventual diagnosis in 30%-40% of initial FUO cases), including meningitis, urinary tract infections, intra-abdominal abscess, hepatobiliary infection, endocarditis, osteomyelitis, or other systemic infections, such as:
  - Viruses (eg, HIV, HAV, HBV, EBV, CMV)
  - Bacteria (eg, TB, spirochetes, rickettsia)
  - Funguses or parasites (eg, malaria)
- Neoplasms (20%-30%) including lymphoma, leukemia, myelodysplastic syndromes, solid tumours
- Collagen-vascular diseases (10%-20%) including lupus, rheumatoid arthritis, giant cell arteritis, rheumatic fever

POSTOPERATIVE FEVER (5 Ws)
- Wind (atelectasis)
- Water (UTI)
- Walking (DVT, PE)
- Wound (infection)
- Wonder drugs (drug fever)

POSTPARTUM FEVER (TWO EXTRA Ws)
- Womb (endometrial infection)
- Weaning (mastitis)

- Other (15%-20%): Drug fever (eg, antibiotics, methyldopa, phenytoin), pulmonary embolism, Crohns disease
- Undiagnosed (5%-15%)

In special groups:
- Elderly: 30% of FUOs due to collagen-vascular diseases (eg, polymyalgia rheumatica, giant cell arteritis)
- HIV-positive: 75% due to infectious causes, 20% lymphoma, 5% HIV
- Patients with febrile neutropenia (temperature 38.3°C or >38°C for 1 hour, and ANC <500): High risk of infection

Investigations

Initial tests may include:
- CBC with differential
- Electrolytes and BUN/creatinine
- Urinalysis and urine culture
- Liver function tests
- ESR/CRP
- Chest x-ray
- Blood cultures

Additional tests to consider based on clinical scenario:
- Blood smear for parasites or spirochetes
- Cultures: CSF, sputum, and stool
- Infectious serological markers: HIV, EBV, CMV, HBV
- Other blood tests: TSH, ANA, RF, ACE
- Skin tests: PPD
- Biopsy: Lymph nodes or blood vessels
- Cytology: Urine

Imaging

- Abdominal ultrasound, CT, or endoscopy based on clinical signs and symptoms.
- MRI or bone scans for osteomyelitis.
- Ventilation-perfusion scans or CT pulmonary angiography for pulmonary embolus.
- PET scans for occult neoplasms.
- Echocardiography for endocarditis.

INFECTIOUS ENDOCARDITIS

- Infection of the heart endothelium.
- Risk factors: Prosthetic valves, previous endocarditis, congenital heart disease, intravenous drug use (IVDU).
- Common pathogens:
  - Native valve endocarditis or IVDU: *Streptococcus* or *Staphylococcus* spp.
  - Prosthetic valve endocarditis: *Staphylococcus epidermidis, Staphylococcus aureus, Enterococcus*
- Mitral valve is most commonly affected, while tricuspid valve involvement is most common with IVDU.
- Symptoms: Fever, chills, dyspnea, chest pain.
- Signs: Clubbing, new murmur, Osler nodes, Roth spots, petechiae, splinter hemorrhages, Janeway lesions.
- Immediate empiric IV antibiotics (vancomycin + gentamicin) after blood cultures are drawn but before diagnosis is confirmed for those who are unwell with continued IV treatment for 4 to 6 weeks, with duration counting from first day of negative blood cultures.

OTHER IMPORTANT POINTS

- When investigating a fever of unknown origin, stop all nonessential medications.
- Consider noninfectious causes of hyperthermia in a febrile patient.
- Provide immediate and adequate treatment for serious causes of fever before definitive confirmation of the diagnosis (eg, febrile neutropenia, infective endocarditis, meningitis, sepsis, drug fever, neuroleptic malignant syndrome, heat stroke).
- Elderly patients may not have a febrile response to an underlying infection.
- Do not give antibiotics for fever if the underlying infectious agent is likely viral.

Bibliography

Bleeker-Rovers, Chantal P, Jos W M van der Meer. Fever of unknown origin. In: Kasper DL, et al eds. *Harrison's Principles of Internal Medicine*. 19th ed. New York, NY: McGraw-Hill; 2015. http://access medicine.mhmedical.com.ezproxy.rqhealth.lib.sk.ca/content.aspx?bookid=1130&Sectionid=79724594.

Evans M. *Mosby's Family Practice Sourcebook*. 4th ed. Toronto: University of Toronto; 2006.

Karchmer, Adolf W. Infective endocarditis. In: Kasper DL, et al. eds. *Harrison's Principles of Internal Medicine*. 19th ed. New York, NY: McGraw-Hill; 2015, http://accessmedicine.mhmedical.com.ezproxy.rqhealth.lib.sk.ca/content.aspx?bookid=1130&Sectionid=79733720.

Roth AR, Basello GM. Approach to the adult patient with fever of unknown origin. *Am Fam Phy*. 2003;68(11):2223-2229.

Dysuria/Urinary Tract Infection

Priority Topics 32 and 95

Definitions

- Dysuria:
  - Pain, burning, or discomfort on urination
  - Differentiate:
    - "Internal": Pain felt inside the body → more likely to be a UTI
    - "External": Pain felt when urine passes over external genitalia → consider other diagnoses
- Uncomplicated UTI:
  - Otherwise healthy adult, premenopausal, nonpregnant women, without known urological abnormalities
- Complicated UTI:
  - Functional or anatomic abnormality of the urinary tract (eg, stones, strictures, reflux, neurogenic bladder)
  - History of urinary tract instrumentation (eg, catheters, ureteric stents, procedures, transplant)
  - Metabolic abnormalities (eg, renal failure)
  - Underlying disease (eg, poorly controlled diabetes, polycystic kidney disease, and immunosuppression)
  - Pregnancy
  - Most infections in men

Symptoms/Clinical Manifestations

- Cystitis: Dysuria, urinary urgency and frequency, suprapubic tenderness, cloudy urine, hematuria, absence of vaginal discharge or irritation, usually afebrile
- Pyelonephritis: Fever, chills, nausea, vomiting, back pain, +/− cystitis symptoms
- Populations who may present with nonspecific symptoms:
  - Children: Decreased appetite, irritability, fever, vomiting
  - Elderly: Delirium, functional decline, abdominal pain, falls, incontinence

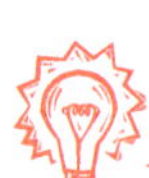

Recurrent infections: two or more UTIs within 6 months; or more than two positive urine cultures within 12 months

Reinfection: infection with a new organism >2 weeks after initial infection

Relapse: repeat or continued infection with the same organisms within 2 weeks of completing antibiotic course for a UTI

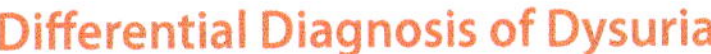

Differential Diagnosis of Dysuria

- Consider other diagnoses if external genital lesions, genital inflammation, or urethral discharge are present, or if the patient is experiencing scrotal, perineal, or rectal pain:
  - Infection (most common)
    - Includes cystitis, urethritis, prostatitis, epididymo-orchitis, and vulvovaginitis.
    - Common organisms causing urethritis include *Neisseria gonorrhea, Chlamydia trachomatis, T. vaginalis*, and HSV.
  - Mechanical or chemical urethral irritation (eg, sexual activity, sensitivity to topical products)
  - Hormonal (eg, endometriosis, hypoestrogenism)
  - Trauma (eg, catheterization)
  - Inflammatory disease (eg, Behçet syndrome, Reiter syndrome)
  - Neoplasms
  - Neurogenic and psychogenic conditions

UTI Risk Factors

- Previous UTIs
- Gender: Higher incidence in women than men
- Age: Higher rates among women aged 25 to 54; rates increase with increasing age in men
- Genitourinary tract abnormalities: BPH, strictures, renal cysts, diverticula, or bladder catheterization
- Other: Increased rates among women who are sexually active (postcoital voiding can be preventative)

Physical Examination Findings

- Perform in everyone:
  - Temperature (usually normal in cystitis)
  - Blood pressure and heart rate (hypotension and tachycardia may be present in pyelonephritis)
  - Assess for CVA tenderness (suggestive of pyelonephritis)
  - Abdominal examination for suprapubic tenderness
- If vaginal signs or symptoms → perform a speculum and bimanual examination
- In males, consider digital rectal examination

Urine Dipstick Testing

- Appropriate investigation in most scenarios when UTI considered.
- When to consider **not** performing:
  - Urine that is **not** cloudy: This alone has a 97% negative predictive value for a positive urine culture.
  - Catheterized patients (very low predictive value).
  - Note: There are no studies on the predictive value of dipstick testing in men.
- Nitrites: Positive test has high specificity for UTI.
- Leukocyte esterase: Positive test has reasonable sensitivity for UTI.
- If nitrites and leukocytes negative → UTI unlikely → explore other causes.
- Red blood cells → may be present in UTI, but persistent hematuria post-UTI requires follow-up.

Urine Cultures

- Do not wait for culture results before initiating treatment when UTI clinically suspected.

VALIDATED UTI SCORE FOR UNCOMPLICATED ACUTE CYSTITIS

- One point each for: (a) dysuria; (b) positive leukocytes on urine dip; and (c) positive nitrites on urine dip
- For a score of 0 to 1: consider urine culture or another diagnosis; empirical treatment only if symptoms are severe
- For a score of 2 to 3: empirical antibiotics +/– culture

- Consider cultures for:
  - All complicated UTIs (including all men)
  - Women >65 years
  - Pregnant women
  - Suspected pyelonephritis
  - Failed antibiotic treatment or persistent symptoms
  - Recurrent UTI (more likely to have a resistant strain)
- Culture **not** usually required
  - Symptomatic women <65 years (first episode).
  - Do not send cultures (or treat) asymptomatic bacteriuria in the elderly or those with indwelling catheters.

Further Investigations

- Anatomical and functional abnormalities should be ruled out (consider renal-bladder US +/− VCUG) for children in the following situations:
  - Diagnosis of pyelonephritis
  - Child with first UTI at <2 years
  - Child of any age with recurrent UTIs
  - Family/personal history of urologic or renal abnormalities
- In adults, renal ultrasound or CT (preferred) may be used to investigate the presence of a complicating anatomic or physiologic factors, especially if persistent clinical symptoms after 48 to 72 hours of appropriate antibiotic therapy (eg, severely ill pyelonephritis, history of renal colic or urolithiasis, poorly controlled diabetes, history of urological surgery, immunosuppression, repeated episodes of pyelonephritis, urosepsis).

Treatment

- Targeted at the most common organisms (*E. coli, S. saprophyticus, Proteus mirabilis, Enterococcus* spp., *Klebsiella* spp.) (see Table 3-1)

TABLE 3-1	**UTI Antibiotic Treatment Choices**	
	FIRST LINE	SECOND LINE
Uncomplicated UTI	TMP/SMX 1 DS tablet bid × 3 days Macrobid 100 mg bid × 5-7 days	Fosfomycin 3g PO × 1 dose Amoxicillin 500 mg tid × 7 days Cephalexin 250-500 qid × 7 days Ciprofloxacin 500 mg bid × 3 days
Complicated UTI	C and S Important! TMP/SMX 1 DS tablet bid × 10-14 days Macrobid 100 mg bid × 10-14 days	Amoxicillin/clavulanate 875 mg bid × 10-14 days Ciprofloxacin 500 mg bid × 5-14 days Levofloxacin 750 mg daily × 5-14 days
UTI in pregnancy	Amoxicillin 500 mg tid × 3-7 days Macrobid 100 mg bid × 5 days (do not use Macrobid at or near term) Fosfomycin 3 g PO × 1 dose	Cephalexin 250-500 qid × 7 days TMP/SMX 1 DS tablet bid × 3 days (Do not use TMP/SMX in the first trimester or the last 6 weeks of gestation)
UTI in children	TMP/SMX, dosed as 5-10 mg/kg/day TMP, divided bid × 7-10 days Nitrofurantoin 5-7 mg/kg/day divided q6h × 7-10 days	Amoxicillin 40 mg/kg/day divided tid × 7-10 days
Pyelonephritis	Ciprofloxacin 500 mg bid × 10-14 days	Amoxicillin/clavulanate 875 mg bid × 10-14 days TMP/SMX 1 DS tablet bid × 10-14 days (if no underlying structural or functional abnormalities or underlying disease)
	Outpatient treatment unless severe (eg, nausea/vomiting, hypotension)	

Key Points

- Query other diagnoses in addition to UTI when evaluating a patient with dysuria.
- Identify factors that may make the infection "complicated."

- Consider UTI as a diagnosis in elderly or young patients with nonspecific history.
- Use empiric antibiotic treatments before culture results are available in pregnant women, or in pyelonephritis or sepsis.

Bibliography

Anti-infective Review Panel. *Anti-infective Guidelines for Community-Acquired Infections*. Toronto: MUMS Guideline Clearinghouse; 2013.

Bremnor JD, Sadovsky R. Evaluation of dysuria in adults. *Am Fam Phys*. 2002;65(8):1589-1597.

Esherick JS, Clark DS, Slater ED. Disease Management. *CURRENT Practice Guidelines in Primary Care 2016*. New York, NY: McGraw-Hill; 2016. http://accessmedicine.mhmedical.com.ezproxy.rqhealth.lib.sk.ca/content.aspx?bookid=1701&Sectionid=110628313. Accessed December 27, 2016.

McIsaac WJ, Moineddin R, Ross S. Validation of a decision aid to assist physicians in reducing unnecessary antibiotic drug use for acute cystitis. *Arch Intern Med*. 2007;167(20):2201-2206.

Quick Reference Guide for Primary Care. http://www.hpa.org.uk/webc/HPAwebFile/HPAweb_C/1194947404720. Accessed April 4, 2012.

Robinson JL, Finlay JC, Lang ME, et al. Urinary tract infection in infants and children: Diagnosis and management. *Paediatr Child Health*. 2014;19(6):315-319. http://www.cps.ca/en/documents/position/urinary-tract-infections-in-children. Accessed December 27, 2016.

RxFiles: Urinary Tract Infections (UTIs). http://www.rxfiles.ca.ezproxy.rqhealth.lib.sk.ca/rxfiles/uploads/documents/members/CHT-UTI-Tx.pdf. RxFiles; May 2016. Accessed December 27, 2016.

Woodford HJ, George J. Diagnosis and management of urinary tract infection in hospitalized older people. *J Am Geriatr Soc*. 2009;57(1):107.

Earache

Priority Topic 33

ACUTE OTITIS MEDIA

Definition

- Acute signs and symptoms of illness with:
  - Evidence of middle ear inflammation
  - Fluid in the middle ear

Symptoms

- Acute onset of ear pain (though may be absent in up to 40% of those with otitis media)
- Fever, irritability, night-time awakening, decreased appetite, ear rubbing
- Usually presents with other symptoms of upper respiratory tract infection (eg, cough or rhinorrhea)

Risk Factors

- Age: Peaks between 6 and 18 months of age
- Exposure to cigarette smoke
- Attendance at large day care centres
- Family history
- First nations or Inuit ethnicity
- Formula feeding (especially supine bottle use)
- Use of a pacifier
- Household crowding
- Prematurity

Physical Examination Findings

- Note: The middle ear must be visualized for definitive diagnosis (ie, no wax occlusion).
- Not all red ears are infected: Mobility, appearance, and position of the tympanic membrane are more important.

Signs of Middle Ear Effusion

- Presence of liquid in the ear canal due to tympanic membrane rupture.
- Opacification of the tympanic membrane with loss of bony landmarks.
- Visible air-fluid level.
- Decreased tympanic membrane motility on pneumatic otoscopy.

Signs of Middle Ear Inflammation

- Bulging tympanic membrane with marked discoloration (ie, hemorrhagic, red, grey, yellow)
- No pain with pinna movement (unless coexisting otitis externa)

Differential Diagnosis of Ear Pain

- Eustachian tubule dysfunction
- Otitis externa
- Referred pain
- Cerumen impaction
- Foreign body
- Mastoiditis
- Basilar skull fracture
- Temporal arteritis
- Tumour
- Contact dermatitis
- Seborrheic dermatitis
- Herpes zoster oticus

Prevention

- Hand washing to minimize exposure to viral and bacterial agents (especially at day cares)
- Breastfeeding
- Minimize exposure to tobacco smoke
- Limit pacifier use
- Influenza vaccination

Management

- Immediate antibiotic therapy if:
  - <6 months of age.
  - Severe illness: Severe pain, toxic appearance, temperature >39°C orally before antipyretics, bilateral otitis media, or perforation with purulent discharge.
  - High-risk conditions: Immunodeficiency, chronic cardiac or lung disease, anatomic abnormalities of the head or neck (eg, cleft palate), history of complicated otitis media, or Down syndrome.
  - Uncertain follow-up: Patients or parents who have difficulty recognizing worsening illness or recontacting care if child is not improving.
- Watchful waiting (if >6 months of age) if mildly ill (fever <39°C) and symptoms for <48 hours:
  - Observe and provide analgesia, with reassessment at 24 to 48 hours for persistent or worsening illness.
    - Acetaminophen 10 to 15 mg/kg/day q4h, maximum of 75 mg/kg/day
    - Ibuprofen: 5 to 10 mg/kg/day q6 to 8h, maximum of 40 mg/kg/day
  - If symptoms do not improve after 1 to 2 days, verify the diagnosis and start antibiotics.

Antibiotics

- Ten-day course if <2 years, if associated perforated tympanic membrane or if frequent recurrent infections, 5-day course if >2 years and uncomplicated
- No tympanic membrane perforation (*Streptococcus pneumoniae, Moraxella catarrhalis, Haemophilus influenzae*):
  - Amoxicillin 75 to 90 mg/kg/day divided bid, up to 3 g/day maximum (capsules or susp) OR
  - Amoxicillin 45 to 60 mg/kg/day divided tid, up to 3 g/day maximum (capsules or susp)
  - Allergy to penicillin:
    - Nonanaphylactic:
      - Cefprozil 30 mg/kg/day divided bid
      - Cefuroxime axetil 30 mg/kg/day divided bid or tid
    - Anaphylactic:
      - Clarithromycin 15 mg/kg/day divided bid
      - Azithromycin 10 mg/kg once and 5 mg/kg daily for 4 days
- If Initial therapy fails (no symptomatic improvement after 2-3 days)
  - Amoxicillin-clavulanate (7:1 formulation of 400 mg/5 mL suspension) 45 mg to 60 mg/kg/day tid for 10 days OR 500 mg tid for children weighing >35 kg
  - Ceftriaxone 50 mg/kg IM or IV daily for 3 days
- Perforation or tubes in place (*Pseudomonas aeruginosa, S. aureus, S. viridans*)
  - Ciprofloxacin (Ciprodex) = 4 drops bid × 5 days

Follow-Up

- At 24 to 48 hours: If patient remains symptomatic, reassess for acute complications (eg, mastoiditis, meningitis), other diagnostic possibilities, and compliance with medications
- At 3 months: Assess for persistent otitis media with effusion (see later)
- If recurrent: Audiology and ENT referral if the patient has experienced >2 cases of acute otitis media in 6 months, or >3 cases in 12 months

Guideline Summary

- Immediate treatment for acute otitis media for those with severe illness and those <6 months of age.
- Consider watchful waiting approach for those >6 months of age with appropriate follow-up.
- Use amoxicillin as the first-line antibiotic, with second- and third-line agents if the patient has a penicillin allergy.

Key Points

- Always look for other causes of fever in a child presenting with fever and a red tympanic membrane.
- Provide parent/patient education that viruses are often the cause of acute otitis media, and are not amenable to antibiotics and that there is a high likelihood of resolution of acute otitis media without antibiotics in most cases.
- Address modifiable risk factors.
- Ensure appropriate follow-up.

OTITIS MEDIA WITH EFFUSION

- Definition: Fluid in the middle ear with ear discomfort, but without other signs or symptoms of infection, often following an episode of acute otitis media.
- Ninety per cent of effusions resolve spontaneously within 3 months of the acute infection.

- Antibiotics are not required.
- Refer for audiology and ENT assessment if the patient has or is at risk of speech, language, or learning problems, persistent hearing loss or abnormalities of the tympanic membrane at 3 months.

OTITIS EXTERNA

- Definition: Infection of the external ear (*P. aeruginosa, S. epidermidis, S. aureus*)
- Signs and symptoms:
  - Pain and tenderness of the tragus and on movement of the pinna
  - With or without pruritus, discharge, jaw pain, and hearing loss
  - Erythematous, edematous ear canal with pain on otoscopy
  - No fever, usually
- Treatment (duration typically for 7-10 days):
  - Adequate pain control with Tylenol and/or Advil
  - No perforation: Buro-Sol 2 to 3 drops tid-qid
  - Perforated TM: Ciprofloxacin (Ciprodex) 4 drops tid
- Necrotizing/malignant otitis externa (elderly diabetic patients, immunocompromised): Spread of *P. aeruginosa* infection to the bone, leading to deep ear pain, systemic signs and symptoms, fever, elevated ESR/CRP, and evidence of osteomyelitis on CT or MRI
  - Ciprofloxacin 750 mg po bid and ciprofloxacin (Ciprodex) 4 drops bid for 4 to 8 weeks

Bibliography

Alberta CPG Working Group for Antibiotics. Guideline for the diagnosis and management of acute otitis media in children; 2008. http://www.topalbertadoctors.org/download/366/AOM_guideline.pdf. Accessed November 2012.

Anti-infective Review Panel. *Anti-infective Guidelines for Community-acquired Infections*. Toronto: MUMS Guideline Clearinghouse; 2013.

Evans M. *Mosby's Family Practice Sourcebook*. 4th ed. Toronto: University of Toronto; 2006.

Forgie S, Zhanel G, Robinson J. Management of acute otitis media. *Paediatr Child Health*. 2009;14(7):457-460.

Hui CPS, Canadian Paediatric Society, Infectious Diseases, et al. Acute otitis externa. *Paediatr Child Health*. 2013;18(2):96-98. http://www.cps.ca/documents/position/acute-otitis-externa.

Le Saux N, Robinson JL, Canadian Paediatric Society, et al. Management of acute otitis media in children six months of age and older. *Paediatr Child Health*. 2016;21(1):39-44. http://www.cps.ca/documents/position/acute-otitis-media.

Cough

Priority Topic 17

ACUTE COUGH (<3 WEEKS DURATION)

Etiology:

- Virus—Most common cause
- Rhinitis (allergic)/postnasal drip—Watery/itchy eyes, sneezing, afebrile, seasonal
- Sinusitis—Fever, facial/tooth pain, purulent discharge
- Asthma—Worse with activity and at night; triggers; +/− wheeze, atopy, seasonal, family hx
- Aspiration
- Exclude serious causes: Pulmonary embolism (PE), pneumothorax, left heart failure, pneumonia, COPD exacerbation

Viral

- Low grade fever (<39°C); stable vitals; rhinorrhea; gradual onset; tend to get better over time

Bacterial

- High fever (>39°C); cough; more sudden onset; tend to get worse over time

PEDIATRIC PERSISTENT/RECURRENT COUGH (>8 WEEKS)

Differential Diagnosis

Infection, asthma, rhinitis, GERD, postnasal drip (PND), foreign body, pertussis

- Most common cause in infants: Infection, including otitis, bronchiolitis, bronchitis, *Bordetella pertussis*
- Most common cause in preschool child: Infection (otitis, sinusitis, bronchitis), asthma, foreign body
- Most common cause in school-age child: Asthma, infection, psychogenic

Treatment is based on suspected etiology. See specific sections for further details.

- **Do not** use cough suppressants and OTC medicines in children <6 years. Exceptions are drugs to treat fever (eg, ibuprofen, acetaminophen).
- Cough and cold medications are not recommended in the pediatric population.

ADULT PERSISTENT/CHRONIC COUGH (>8 WEEKS)

Three most common causes of chronic cough in adults: PND, asthma, GERD

- Other common causes: Rhinitis, smoking, COPD/chronic bronchitis, ACE inhibitors, congestive heart failure
- Less common causes: Think of restrictive (eg, pulmonary fibrosis) or obstructive lung diseases (eg, lung cancer), infections (eg, TB), and environmental factors (eg, workplace exposures)

History

- Onset, pattern/variations in cough, characteristics (eg, dry/productive, "barking," wheeze, nasal d/c), triggers and aggravating factors, occupation, smoking

Investigation

- CXR, CBC (WBC, Hgb), JVP, edema, $\%O_2$ saturation, pulmonary function testing
  - Note: Normal spirometry does **not** rule out cough-variant asthma
  - Assess for heart failure causing cough
  - Consider sinus imaging
  - Induced sputum after exclusion of common causes (cytology, infection, inflammatory cells)
  - Consider upper endoscopy after treatment failure (eg, query hiatal hernia)
  - Allergy testing if indicated by history
- Physical examination: Eye examination, ear, nasal, oropharynx, sinuses, mucosa, cardiovascular, respiratory, clubbing
- Diagnosis may be in combination with trial of treatment for presumed cause:
  - For example: Antibiotics, bronchodilation and evaluation with spirometry for possible asthma, H_2-blocker/PPI for possible GERD

Treatment

Depends on the presumed diagnosis, for example:

- Encourage smoking cessation; d/c ACE inhibitor
- Empiric treatment for PND, rhinosinus disease (including chronic sinusitis, allergic rhinitis) includes treatment with antihistamine/decongestant, nasal saline spray, intranasal steroids, and avoiding of allergens/triggers

- Empiric treatment for asthma (inhaled corticosteroid and bronchodilator)
- Empiric treatment for GERD with PPI or H_2-blocker, diet/lifestyle modifications
- Consider additional diagnostic testing if suboptimal response to treatment
- See relevant topic heading for more information about treating these conditions, for example, asthma and COPD sections, smoking cessation

CHRONIC COUGH IN SMOKERS

- Assess for COPD or chronic bronchitis
  - Chronic bronchitis = cough most days and increased sputum for 3 months in 2 consecutive years
  - COPD = spirometry = FEV_1/FVC <0.7 or FEV_1 <80% after bronchodilation
    - ◦ Dyspnea, decreased exercise tolerance, prolonged cough
  - Assess for lung cancer if suspected by history
    Canadian task force on lung cancer recommends screening *asymptomatic adults aged 55 to 74 with ≥30-pack year smoking history with low dose CT yearly for 3 years*. Therefore depending on history, a CT may be indicated over a CXR in a patient with significant smoking history.

Bibliography

Anti-infective Review Panel. *Anti-infective Guidelines for Community-Acquired Infections*. Toronto: MUMS Guideline Clearinghouse; 2013.

DynaMed. Chronic cough. Accessed Feb 2, 2012.

Gahbauer M, Keane P. Chronic cough: Stepwise application in primary care practice of the ACCP guidelines for diagnosis and management of cough. *J Am Acad Nurse Prac*. 2009;21(8):409-416.

Health Canada Releases Decision on the Labelling of Cough and Cold Products for Children. http://www.hc-sc.gc.ca/ahc-asc/media/advisories-avis/_2008/2008_184-eng.php. Accessed March 25, 2012.

Lewin G, Morissette K, Dickinson J, et al. Recommendations on screening for lung cancer. *Canadian Medical Association Journal*. 2016

Upper Respiratory Tract Infections
Priority Topic 94

LIFE-THREATENING URIs

- Epiglottitis
- Retropharyngeal abscess

BACTERIAL SINUSITIS

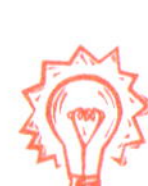

Two common features of bacterial sinusitis:

1. Persistent symptoms, >10 days
2. Severe symptoms (temperature >39°C and purulent nasal discharge)

Etiology

- Usually preceded by viral URTI
  - Most common acute: *S. pneumoniae, H. influenzae*
  - Chronic: *S. aureus, Pseudomonas, Enteribacteruaceae*
  - Children: *Moraxella catarrhalis*
  - Note: Infants are only born with ethmoid and maxillary sinus. By 5 years, they develop a sphenoid sinus; by 8 years a frontal sinus

Risk Factors

- Smoking, anatomy (eg, deviated septum, polyps), allergic rhinitis, asthma, medications (overuse of topical decongestants)

Signs/Symptoms

URI not improved in 7 to 10 days plus:

- Purulent nasal drainage
- Nasal congestion, hyposmia/anosmia
- Facial pain/pressure/fullness; pain can be increased by leaning forward, diffuse or localized headache
- PND
- Fever
- Cough
- Maxillary dental pain
- Ear fullness
- Poor response to nasal decongestants

Diagnosis

Clinical assessment more accurate than any single sign/symptom

- CDC (Centres for Disease Control and Prevention) criteria for clinical dx of acute bacterial rhinosinusitis:
  - Rhinosinusitis symptoms for ≥7 days (**7-10 days mark differentiates simple viral infection from bacterial sinusitis**) or with biphasic fever

PLUS ≥ 2 of the following:

  - Purulent nasal discharge/postnasal discharge
  - Maxillary tooth or facial (sinus) pain or tenderness (especially when unilateral)
  - Nasal obstruction
  - Smell disorder

Complications

- Orbital cellulitis, venous sinus thrombosis, bacterial meningitis, brain abscess, osteomyelitis, sepsis

Differential Diagnosis

Allergic/fungal sinusitis

Dental infection

- Rule out migraine—many patients with "sinus headache" may have migraine

Investigations

- Usually no tests, no evidence for culture
- Rule out allergic sinusitis with allergy testing if suspected
- CT only if suspect complications of infection

Treatment

Acute

- Most cases resolve without treatment.
- Symptomatic: Analgesics/antipyretics, intranasal corticosteroids, saline irrigation of nasal cavity
- **Mild-to-moderate**—Nasal steroids × 3 days, treat with antibiotics if not improving
  First-line —mild-to-moderate

  Amoxicillin—500 mg tid × 5 to 10 days (peds: 40-90 mg/kg bid)

  Second-line—mild to moderate, First-line for severe infection

  Amoxicillin/clavulanate—500 mg /day × 5 to 10 days (peds: 45 mg/kg/day × 10 days)

RED FLAGS FOR URGENT REFERRAL (BACTERIAL SINUSITIS)

- Systemic toxicity
- Altered mental status
- Severe headache
- Orbital swelling
- Change in vision

Penicillin allergic (5-10 days treatment duration):

>> Cefuroxime—250 to 500 mg od (peds: 30-40 mg/kg/day × 10 days)

>> Doxycycline—100 mg BID × 1 day, followed by 100 mg OD (peds: 4 mg/kg/day × 10 days)

Note: 5 days of antibiotic therapy in a healthy adult has the same benefit as longer course.

Successful treatment = improvement at 10 days but not complete resolution of symptoms

- **Severe**—Nasal steroids AND antibiotics (see above)
- **Chronic** (>2 weeks of inflammation, no response to treatment)
  - Repeated courses of antibiotics not recommended.
  - Refer to ENT if no resolution and continue/start intranasal steroids.
- Maintenance: Nasal steroids (modest benefit) and saline irrigation for symptom management

PHARYNGITIS/TONSILLITIS

Etiology

- Viruses—**cause 80% to 90% of pharyngitis cases in adults, 70% in children**
  - Adenovirus, Epstein-Barr, parainfluenza, influenza, rhinoviruses, and more
  - In presentation of pharyngitis, always consider EBV/mononucleosis
- Bacterial—group A beta-hemolytic streptococci, *Chlamydia trachomatis*
  - Fifty per cent of patients with GAS are 5 to 15 years old, uncommon before 3
  - *Chlamydia trachomatis* is rare, risk factors: Age 15 to 24, oral sex

History and Physical

- Abrupt onset of sore throat—may have fever/chills/headache/myalgias
- Tonsillar swelling and/or exudate
- Sore throat score for *Streptococcus pyogenes*, aka GABHS (group A beta-hemolytic streptococcus) (see Table 3-2)

TABLE 3-2   Sore Throat Score Card

The following SCORE CARD can assist health practitioners in the treatment (not diagnosis) of patients presenting with upper respiratory tract infection symptoms and a sore throat. Not to be used in epidemic situations; in populations in which rheumatic fever remains a problem; those individuals who have a history of rheumatic fever, valvular heart disease or immunosuppression.

Step 1
After a clinical assessment, where you conclude the patient has an uncomplicated upper respiratory tract infection with a sore throat, determine the patient's total sore throat score by assigning points according to the following criteria:

CRITERIA	POINTS
• Temperature > 38° C	1
• Absence of Cough	1
• Swollen, tender anterior cervical nodes	1
• Tonsillar swelling or exudate	1
• Age 3-14 yr	1
• Age 15-44 yr	0
• Age ≥ 45 yr	−1

TABLE 3-2	Sore Throat Score Card (*Continued*)

Step 2
Choose the appropriate management according to the sore throat score:

TOTAL SCORE RISK OF STREPTOCOCCAL	INFECTION (%)	SUGGESTED MANAGEMENT[1]
0 or less	1-2.5	No culture or antibiotic required.[1]
1	5-10	
2	11-17	Perform culture (or office Rapid antigen test).[2]
3	28-35	Treat only if test is positive for Group A Strep.
4 or more	51-53	Start antibiotic therapy on clinical grounds (patient has high fever or is clinically unwell and presents early in disease course). • If culture (or office Rapid antigen test)[2] is performed and result is negative then antibiotic should be discontinued.

[1] It is always appropriate to perform a throat culture if other clinical factors lead you to suspect Streptococcal infection (i.e., household contact with Streptococcal infection). Swab tonsils and peritonsillar pillars.

[2] If the antigen test is negative, then culture is still required for children. In adults, a negative antigen test alone is reasonable.

Adapted with permission from Anti-infective Review Panel. *Anti-infective Guidelines for Community-Acquired Infections.* Toronto: MUMS Guideline Clearinghouse; 2013. For updates see www.mumshealth.com.

Diagnosis

- **Clinical**: Repeat studies show it is not possible to differentiate between GAS and viral cause of pharyngitis by history and physical examination alone.
- Rapid streptococcus test (70% sensitive) or throat culture (90%-95% sensitive)

Differential Diagnosis

- Rule out mononucleosis/EBV pharyngitis.

Treatment for Streptococcal Pharyngitis (Table 3-3)

TABLE 3-3	Treatment for Streptococcal Pharyngitis	
	ADULTS	**CHILDREN**
Penicillin V (first line)	600 mg bid × 10 days	40 mg/kg/day
Erythromycin (penicillin allergy: Anaphylaxis)	250 mg qid × 10 days	40 mg/kg/day
Cephalexin (penicillin allergy: Rash/minor)	250 mg qid × 10 days	25-50 mg/kg/day

- **Primary purpose of treatment—prevent acute rheumatic fever (NNT 4000)**
  - Prevalence of rheumatic fever is 0.1 to 2 cases/100,000—in aboriginal communities is higher (Northern Ontario 8.33/100,000).
  - Antibiotics shorten duration of symptoms by **only 16 hours**.
  - Delay antibiotic treatment and await throat swab results*
- Antibiotic choices:
  - **GAS**: Penicillin is the drug of choice. No documented GAS resistance.
  - *Chlamydia Trachomatis*
    - Doxycycline 100 mg po BID × 7 days
    - Azithromycin 1 g × 1 dose

Note: If given beta-lactam antibiotics for suspected streptococcal pharyngitis, but the infection is actually caused by EBV, an urticarial and maculopapular rash will develop (morbilliform rash).

---

*Antibiotics started within 9 days of onset in GAS are shown to prevent rheumatic fever.

MONONUCLEOSIS/EBV PHARYNGITIS

Etiology

- Caused by Epstein-Barr virus; transmitted by infected saliva

Symptoms

- **Classic triad = generalized LAD, moderate-to-high fever, pharyngitis**
- Fatigue/malaise
- Headache

History and Physical

- Generalized lymphadenopathy typically involves inguinal, axillary, posterior auricular/cervical nodes
- Splenomegaly
- Tonsillar swelling (+/− greyish exudate)
- Vaginal ulcers may be present

Investigations

- Monospot test (+ heterophile Ab)
  - Negative result → order CBC with differential and EBV serology (anti-EBV titre)

Treatment

- **No antibiotics.** (Note: If given beta-lactam Abx, morbilliform rash will develop.)
- Avoid strenuous physical activity for 4 weeks, and avoid contact sports.
- Hydration and pain relief.
- Corticosteroids for acute airway obstruction or relief of sore throat; not for routine treatment.

Complications

- Splenic rupture
- Tonsil hyperplasia → airway obstruction

Prognosis

- Most patients recover to normal activities by 2 to 3 months

Bibliography

DynaMed [database online]. Acute sinusitis. EBSCO Publishing. http://web.ebscohost.com.cyber.usask .ca/dynamed/detail?vid=26&hid=9&sid=5fdbf4ec-bc94-440b-af64-b72b84140e48%40sessionmgr4& bdata=JnNpdGU9ZHluYW1lZC1saXZlJnNjb3BlPXNpdGU%3d#db=dme&AN=114974. Accessed December 5, 2012.

DynaMed [database online]. Infectious mononucleosis. EBSCO Publishing. http://web.ebscohost.com .cyber.usask.ca/dynamed/detail?vid=32&hid=9&sid=5fdbf4ec-bc94-440b-af64-b72b84140e48%40ses sionmgr4&bdata=JnNpdGU9ZHluYW1lZC1saXZlJnNjb3BlPXNpdGU%3d#db=dme&AN=114945. Accessed December 5, 2012.

DynaMed [database online]. Streptococcal pharyngitis. EBSCO Publishing. http://web.ebscohost.com .cyber.usask.ca/dynamed/detail?vid=30&hid=9&sid=5fdbf4ec-bc94-440b-af64-b72b84140e48%40ses sionmgr4&bdata=JnNpdGU9ZHluYW1lZC1saXZlJnNjb3BlPXNpdGU%3d#db=dme&AN=115782& anchor=anc-1428143566. Accessed December 5, 2012.

DynaMed [database online]. Upper respiratory infection. EBSCO Publishing. http://web.ebscohost.com .cyber.usask.ca/dynamed/detail?vid=28&hid=9&sid=5fdbf4ec-bc94-440b-af64-b72b84140e48%40ses sionmgr4&bdata=JnNpdGU9ZHluYW1lZC1saXZlJnNjb3BlPXNpdGU%3d#db=dme&AN=114537. Accessed December 5, 2012.

O'Toole D. Infectious disease: Family Medicine Notes: Preparing for the CCFP exam ED4. 2016:60-80.

Rx Files: Antibiotics and common infections: Stewardship, effectiveness, safety and clinical pearls. 2016:9.

Croup

Priority Topic 20

CROUP (LARYNGOTRACHEOBRONCHITIS [LTB])

Etiology

Parainfluenza virus is most common cause. Other causes: RSV, adeno/influenza/rhino-viruses, diphtheria, *Mycoplasma pneumoniae*

- Typically affects 6 month to 3-year olds during winter.
- Transmitted by respiratory droplets.
- Incubation period is 3 to 6 days.

Differential Diagnosis

- Rule out acute epiglottitis, anaphylaxis, foreign body, retropharyngeal abscess

Signs/Symptoms

Upper airway (laryngeal or tracheal) obstruction leading to acute clinical syndrome with

- Barking cough
- Inspiratory stridor (90% of kids with stridor have croup!)
- Hoarse voice
- URTI prodrome
- Worse at night
- Improves with cold air/mist
- Fluctuating disease course
- May have 2 to 5 day prodrome of mild fever, rhinorrhea, sore throat
- Nasal flaring = severe croup +/− coexisting pneumonia

Investigations

- Assess ABCs!
- Clinical diagnosis
  - —No viral studies required
  - —Imaging is typically not useful or indicated
- Frontal neck x-ray shows steeple sign = subglottic narrowing—do only if unsure of diagnosis

Complications

- Rare, but can get severe airway obstruction + respiratory failure.

Treatment

- PO dexamethasone 0.6 mg/kg (PO/IM) once (can repeat dose in 6-24 hours), improvement in 2 to 3 hours.
  - **Do not** undertreat mild-to-moderate croup (reduces rate of hospitalization, RTC, and duration of symptoms)
- Nebulized racemic epinephrine (for severe respiratory distress: Marked sternal wall retractions and agitation)
  - 0.5 mL of 2.25% solution diluted in 3 mL NS or sterile water via nebulizer. Can repeat back-to-back if severe respiratory distress. Observe for 2 to 3 hours post tx (the effect of epinephrine does not last >2 hours).
- Explain fluctuating disease course that usually lasts 4 to 7 days

It is a viral illness, antibiotics are *not* indicated, and will not change the disease course.

- Consider hospitalization if:
  - Severe croup: Cyanosis, decreased LOC, progressive/severe stridor, and retractions persisting 4 hours after corticosteroids, looks toxic
  - Dehydration
  - Relative indications for admission: Social factors (inability to monitor child as outpatient); distance from hospital

BACTERIAL TRACHEITIS

It is also known as "acute bacterial laryngo tracheobronchitis." An invasive, exudative bacterial infection of the soft tissues of the trachea. Usually occurs in setting of prior airway mucosal damage, for example, antecedent viral infection.

Etiology

- *Staphylococcus aureus* is most common cause. Other causes include *H. influenzae, S. pneumoniae, Moraxella catarrhalis, S. pyogenes.*

Epidemiology

- Rare, but is a pediatric airway emergency. Most occur in previously healthy children in setting of viral RTI. (Most common in 1-month to 6-year olds in fall/winter.)

Differential Diagnosis

- Epiglottitis, croup, peritonsillar or retropharyngeal abscess or cellulitis. Severe bacterial pneumonia, foreign body aspiration, diphtheria (rare if immunized), inflammatory bowel disease.

Presentation

- Prodromal signs/symptoms of viral RTI for 1 to 3 days before develop a *more severe illness with stridor and dyspnea.*
- Onset fulminant with progression to acute respiratory distress <24 hours.

Signs/Symptoms

- Stridor (inspiratory or expiratory)
- Cough (not painful; membranous exudates may be expectorated)
- Drooling—uncommon
- Preference to lie flat
- Fever may or may not be present
- Exudate can be minimal or extensive, sometimes forming pseudomembranes

Investigations

- Lateral neck or anteroposterior x-rays: Steeple sign (ragged edge or a membrane spanning the trachea).
- Pulmonary infiltrates common.
- Labs: CBC + inflammatory markers are *not* helpful and do not correlate with illness severity.
- Clinical diagnosis: Poor response with nebulized epinephrine or glucocorticoids can help differentiate from croup.
- Definitive diagnosis: Direct endoscopy visualization of inflamed, exudate-covered trachea, normal epiglottis (best done in OR or ICU).
- Gram stain and culture (aerobic and anaerobic) during endoscopy; or sputum specimen in older patients.

Treatment

- Admit to PICU.
- Maintenance of airway (most children require endotracheal intubation for airway obstruction related to purulent secretions).
- Supplement O_2, +/− fluid resuscitation.
- Endoscopy may be needed to remove pseudomembranous exudates.
- Trial of inhaled bronchodilators, but stop if no clinical response.
- Prevention:
  - Vaccination against pneumococci and virus (eg, measles, influenza) that can predispose to bacterial tracheitis
- Antibiotics—all intravenous administration (see below)
  - Initial therapy for most common pathogens:
    - Antistaphylococcal medicines (eg, vancomycin or clindamycin) + third-generation cephalosporin (eg, cefotaxime or ceftriaxone)

      or
    - antistaphylococcal medicines + ampicillin sulbactam
  - Ten-day course
  - If influenza etiology, use antiviral if symptoms present for <72 hours

BRONCHIOLITIS

Obstruction of the small airways caused by acute inflammation and edema of the cells lining the small airways, coupled with increased mucous production.

Etiology

RSV is the most common cause.

Others: Rhinovirus, parainfluenza, influenza, adenovirus.

- Typically affects 0 to 2-year olds (peak 2-6 months) from October to April
  - Most common LRTI in children <2
  - Leading cause of hospitalization in infants <1

Differential Diagnosis

- Viral-triggered asthma, pneumonia, foreign body, GERD, congenital heart disease/heart failure—*lack of preceding URT symptoms before onset of wheezing may help rule out bronchiolitis.*

Risk Factors for RSV

- Prematurity (<37 weeks GA), low birth weight, lung disease (eg, cystic fibrosis), congenital heart disease, congenital abnormalities of airway
- Environmental risk factors: Older siblings, First Nations, passive smoke, household crowding, day care

Signs/Symptoms

- Expiratory wheeze
- URTI prodrome (2-3 d) (eg, low grade fever, cough, nasal congestion/discharge, mild cough) peak symptoms 3 to 5 d.
- Respiratory distress (apnea/tachypnea, grunting, nasal flaring, tachycardia) ± hypoxemia
- Factors associated with increased severity: Toxic appearance, <95% O_2 saturation on room air, age <3 months, respiratory rate ≥70, atelectasis on CXR

Associated Findings

- Atelectasis and areas of hyperinflation on CXR (Note: Evidence does not support diagnostic imaging for typical cases.)
- Acute otitis media

- UTI
- Dehydration

Investigations

- Clinical diagnosis!
- CBC and CXR if <3 months with fever and signs of LRTI or if diagnosis unsure. May see hyperinflation, peribronchial thickening, and patchy atelectasis with volume loss from airway narrowing and mucus plugging on CXR.
- Pulse oximetry; ABG in severe cases
- NPS swab: Does not alter management
- Bacterial culture: Concomitant bacterial infection rare, consider in <2 mo infant

Treatment

- Patients generally recover without treatment in 2 to 4 days.
- Wheezing can last for >7 days in some cases.

Recommended

- O_2 if sats <90% (mainstay of treatment in hospital)
- Hydration

Equivocal Evidence

- Epinephrine nebulization
- Nasal suctioning
- 3% hypertonic saline nebulization

Not Recommended

- Trial of inhaled bronchodilators—Continue only if clinical response. The pathophysiology of bronchiolitis is airway obstruction, NOT constriction.
- Systemic corticosteroids should **not** be used routinely.
- Antibiotics.
- Antivirals—Ribavirin may be beneficial in high-risk patients.

Prevention

- Palivizumab prophylaxis if <24 months with chronic lung disease or history of prematurity <35 weeks gestational age or congenital heart disease

In bronchiolitis—bronchodilators have NOT been shown to improve O_2 saturations, or shorten the length of stay in hospital. The current CPS position statement does NOT recommend the use of bronchodilators in a clear diagnosis of bronchiolitis.

PERTUSSIS (AKA "WHOOPING COUGH")

- Defined as acute tracheobronchitis
- Cause—*B. pertussis* bacteria
- Transmitted by respiratory droplets—**highly contagious!**
- Most commonly affected are <6 months olds (too young to be immunized) and ~50% are adolescents/adults.
- Incubation period—7 to 10 days
- Most contagious during catarrhal period (first 1-2 weeks) and first 2 weeks of paroxysmal phase (increased repetitive coughing phase).

Risk Factors

- Lack of/incomplete vaccination, exposure to infected person (household contact is most common source of infection in <6 month infant).

Signs/Symptoms

- Prolonged illness, cough >2 weeks
- Inspiratory "whoop" (in kids)
- Paroxysmal coughing
- Posttussive vomiting

- Apnea (rather than cough)—young infants
- Low grade fever
- Stages of illness:
  - **Phase 1: Catarrhal phase** (1-2 weeks)
    - Nonspecific prodromal symptoms such as URTI: Coryza, rhinorrhea, mild cough, malaise, low grade fever
  - **Phase 2: Paroxysmal phase** (4-6 weeks in children, 2-3 months in adults)
    - Spasmodic cough during day/night with minimal symptoms between coughing episodes
    - Inspiratory "whoop" (more common in younger due to small trachea)
    - May have posttussive vomiting/syncope
  - **Phase 3: Convalescent phase** (1-2 weeks)
    - Gradual decrease in cough frequency and severity
- In adolescents/adults: most have been vaccinated or had previous infection; present late with persistent cough (>4 weeks of coughing); cough may be only at night

Investigations

- Nasal swab (PCR). Report suspected cases.
- Diagnostic criteria for confirmed pertussis (≥1 of following):
  - Acute cough with culture (+) for *B. pertussis.*
    - Culture from posterior nasopharynx is gold standard (not anterior nares or throat).
  - PCR (+) in patients meeting clinical diagnosis.
  - Clinical diagnosis is enough when patient is in contact with verified *B. pertussis.*

Treatment

- Supportive
- Erythromycin × 7 days (if child <1 month: Use azithromycin); (decreases infectivity, but does not alter disease course or cough severity!).
- Patient remains contagious for 5 days after starting antibiotics.
- Same antibiotic for close contacts and postexposure prophylaxis.
- Vaccination:
  - Part of routine childhood vaccination at 2, 4, 6, 18 months, 4 to 6 years, 14 to 16 years
  - Exposed close contacts
    - DTaP for incompletely immunized close contacts ≤7-years
    - Consider booster (Tdap) if immunized and age = 10 to 64 years
    - CDC recommendations for pregnant women and those having close contact with infant <12 months:
      - Tdap.
      - Tdap should be given to pregnant women with no previous dose after the 20th week gestational age (third trimester preferred) or immediately postpartum.
      - Pregnant women who have previously received Tdap and need tetanus or diphtheria vaccine should get Td vaccination WHILE pregnant.*

Tdap = **T**etanus toxoid, reduced **d**iphtheria toxoid, and **a**cellular **p**ertussis vaccine

Td = **T**etanus toxoid, reduced **d**iphtheria toxoid

DTaP = **D**iphtheria toxoid, **T**etanus toxoid, and **a**cellular **P**ertussis vaccine

EPIGLOTTITIS (MEDICAL EMERGENCY!)

High airway inflammation (and obstruction) due to rapid infection and edema of epiglottis

---

* The SOGC states: "Susceptible women to be vaccinated as per general guidelines for non-pregnant patients" and state there is no evidence of teratogenicity as diphtheria/tetanus is not a live virus.

Etiology

- *Haemophilus influenzae* type B, beta-haemolytic streptococci (groups A, B, C). Peaks at 2 to 8 years, and 35 to 39 years.

Signs/Symptoms

- Tripod position, stridor (late finding), hoarse/muffled voice, fever, sore throat, dysphagia, cervical adenopathy, drooling. Neck tenderness in adults.

Investigations

- Avoid inspection of airway and delay phlebotomy—can increase anxiety → complete obstruction!
- Lateral neck x-ray ("thumb sign," pencil-thin airway)
- Direct laryngoscopy—*done in OR! See "cherry-red" epiglottis
- Look for coexisting infections (otitis media, pneumonia, meningitis, cellulitis)
- CBC (increased neutrophils with left shift), blood culture

Treatment

- Intubation (in the OR is the best setting) and admit to ICU,
- IV corticosteroids
- IV ceftriaxone (drug of choice for *H. influenzae*) for 7 to 10 days until culture and sensitivity results
  - Alternative antibiotic: Ampicillin-sulbactam
- Supportive care: IV fluids, oxygen (Avoid racemic epinephrine.)

Prevention: Vaccinate!

RETROPHARYNGEAL ABSCESS

Deep neck space infection of the retropharyngeal space, potential for airway compromise

Epidemiology

- Seventy-five per cent of cases <5 years old. (Retropharyngeal lymph nodes regress by about 6 years)
- Unilateral presentation is more common in 15- to 30-years old.

Etiology

- GAS (50%) +/− aerobes/anaerobes of mouth flora.
- Extension of pharyngeal infection (45%).
- Foreign body (27%).
- In adults usually associated with local trauma, nontraumatic is rare (suspect immunocompromise in these cases).

Signs/Symptoms

- Prodrome of sore throat + fever (pain and fever in all cases)
- Odynophagia → decreased oral intake
- Torticollis
- Neck swelling/pain +/− mass, cervical lymphadenopathy

Investigations

- Aerobic and anaerobic culture and sensitivity of secretions/abscess
- Lateral neck x-ray*
  - Bulging posterior pharynx
  - Abnormal = >7 mm at C2, >14 mm at C6.

---

*Plain x-ray has limited use in evaluating deep neck space infections but can be helpful to detect retropharyngeal swelling or epiglottitis.

- U/S is tool for intraoperative aspiration and drainage; can distinguish between adenitis and abscess
- CT is **imaging of choice** for diagnosis of deep neck space infections
  - Shows fluid collection with central hypodensity
  - Fat stranding in early cellulitis phase

Treatment

- Secure airway
- Transoral approach for I&D (and to obtain aspirate culture, blood cultures are less accurate)
- Antibiotics: IV penicillin G × 10 days, with beta-lactamase inhibitor

PERITONSILLAR ABSCESS/QUINSY

- Polymicrobial infection with collection of pus behind tonsil(s).
- Can be life-threatening!
- Usually unilateral.

Etiology

- More common in 20- to 40-year olds.
- More common from November to December and April to May (highest incidence of streptococcal pharyngitis and exudative tonsillitis).
- Usually a complication of streptococcal pharyngitis or tonsillitis → cellulitis → abscess formation due to salivary duct blockage.

Risk Factors

- Oropharynx/dental infection, periodontal disease, smoking

Signs/Symptoms

- Sore throat/neck, dysphagia, odynophagia, fever, "hot potato" voice, trismus, otalgia
- Drooling, halitosis
- Deviation of uvula, asymmetry of soft palate, ipsilateral palatal edema

Diagnosis

- Clinical

Investigations to Consider

- Needle aspiration
- Neck CT or MRI. U/S can differentiate peritonsillar abscess versus cellulitis.

Treatment

- Aspiration or surgical drainage + antibiotics for 10 to 14 days
  - IV: Ampicillin sulbactam; or penicillin G + metronidazole
    - Alternative is clindamycin
  - Oral: Amox-clav or penicillin VK + metronidazole or clindamycin
- Hydration + pain control

Bibliography

CDC. http://www.cdc.gov/vaccines/pubs/vis/downloads/vis-td-tdap.pdf.

Chow AW, Calderwood SB, Thorner AR. Deep neck space infections. Up to Date.

DynaMed [database online]. Acute epiglottitis. EBSCO Publishing. http://web.ebscohost.com.cyber.usask.ca/dynamed/detail?vid=34&hid=9&sid=5fdbf4ec-bc94-440b-af64-b72b84140e48%40sessionmgr4&bdata=JnNpdGU9ZHluYW1lZC1saXZlJnNjb3BlPXNpdGU%3d#db=dme&AN=115468. Accessed January 7, 2017

DynaMed [database online]. Croup. EBSCO Publishing. http://web.ebscohost.com.cyber.usask.ca/dynamed/detail?vid=41&hid=9&sid=5fdbf4ec-bc94-440b-af64-b72b84140e48%40sessionmgr4&bdata=JnNpdGU9ZHluYW1lZC1saXZlJnNjb3BlPXNpdGU%3d#db=dme&AN=114811. Accessed February 2, 2012.

DynaMed [database online]. Peritonsillar abscess. EBSCO Publishing. http://web.ebscohost.com.cyber.usask .ca/dynamed/detail?vid=43&hid=9&sid=5fdbf4ec-bc94-440b-af64-b72b84140e48%40sessionmgr4&bdat a=JnNpdGU9ZHluYW1lZC1saXZlJnNjb3BlPXNpdGU%3d#db=dme&AN=115937. January 4, 2017.

DynaMed [database online]. Pertussis. EBSCO Publishing. http://web.ebscohost.com.cyber.usask.ca/ dynamed/detail?vid=45&hid=9&sid=5fdbf4ec-bc94-440b-af64-b72b84140e48%40sessionmgr4& bdata=JnNpdGU9ZHluYW1lZC1saXZlJnNjb3BlPXNpdGU%3d#db=dme&AN=114591. Accessed September 26, 2016.

DynaMed [database online]. Respiratory syncytial virus (RSV) infection in infants and children. EBSCO Publishing. http://web.ebscohost.com.cyber.usask.ca/dynamed/detail?vid=38&hid=9&sid=5fdbf4ec- bc94-440b-af64-b72b84140e48%40sessionmgr4&bdata=JnNpdGU9ZHluYW1lZC1saXZlJnNjb3 BlPXNpdGU%3d#db=dme&AN=115760. Accessed December 5, 2012.

DynaMed [database online]. Retropharyngeal abscess. EBSCO Publishing. http://web.ebscohost.com .cyber.usask.ca/dynamed/detail?vid=47&hid=9&sid=5fdbf4ec-bc94-440b-af64-b72b84140e48%40ses sionmgr4&bdata=JnNpdGU9ZHluYW1lZC1saXZlJnNjb3BlPXNpdGU%3d#db=dme&AN=115742. Accessed January 2, 2017.

Friedman J, Rieder M, Walton J, et al. Bronchiolitis: Recommendations for diagnosis, monitoring, and management of children one to 24 months of age. Practice position statement. Canadian pediatric society. http://www.cps.ca/en/documents/position/bronchiolitis1.

Guidelines for the diagnosis and management of croup. Towards Optimized Practice. 2008. http://www .topalbertadoctors.org/cpgs.php?sid=12&cpg_cats=35&cpg_info=7. Accessed March 25, 2012.

Ortiz-Alvarez, O. Acute management of croup in the emergency department. Practice position statement. Canadian Pediatric Society. http://www.cps.ca/en/documents/position/acutemanagemnt-of-croup.

O'Toole D. Infectious disease: Family Medicine Notes: Preparing for the CCFP exam ED4. 2016:60-80.

Rx Files: Antibiotics and Common Infections: Stewardship, Effectiveness, Safety and Clinical Pearls. 2016:3-14.

SOCG Clinical Practice Guideline. Immunization in pregnancy. 2008;220:1149-1154. http://www.sogc.org /guidelines/documents/gui220CPG0812.pdf.

Up to Date. Bacterial tracheitis in children: clinical features and diagnosis. Accessed January 3, 2017.

Up to Date. Bacterial tracheitis in children: treatment and prevention. Accessed January 3, 2017.

Up to Date. Bronchiolitis in infants and children: clinical features and diagnosis. Accessed January 7, 2017.

Up to Date. Bronchiolitis in infants and children: treatment; outcome; and prevention. Accessed February 12, 2012.

Pneumonia

Priority Topic 73

Definition

- Inflammatory condition of the lung affecting the alveoli (predominantly)
- Associated with fever, chest symptoms, and a decrease in air space (consolidation) on a chest x-ray
- Typically caused by an infection (bacteria, virus, fungi, or parasite)

ADULTS

1. Signs and symptoms
   - Dyspnea
   - Fever
   - Chest discomfort
   - Pleuritic pain
   - Productive cough
   - Increased heart rate and respiratory rate
   - Focal abnormal breath sounds
   - Atypical = Insidious onset of fever, nonproductive cough, constitutional symptoms
   - Keep pneumonia on differential diagnosis in points with deterioration, delirium, and abdominal pain

2. Comorbidity includes
   - Chronic heart/lung disease
   - Liver disease
   - Renal disease
   - Diabetes mellitus
   - Alcohol abuse
   - Malignancy
   - Asplenia
   - Immunosuppressed
   - Hospital admission in past 3 months
   - Nursing home resident
3. Investigations
   - WBC, ABG, CXR, sputum culture and sensitivity, electrolytes if needed.
   - The CURB-65 score can be used to assess severity and guides decision if patient should be hospitalized.
   - **CURB-65** score (see Table 3-4):

TABLE 3-4	CURB-65 Score for Pneumonia Severity
SCORE	SUGGESTED MANAGEMENT
0-1 points	Low severity (risk of death <3%). Outpatient therapy is usually appropriate.
2 points	Moderate severity (risk of death 9%). Consider hospitalization.
3-5 points	High severity (risk of death 15%-40%). Hospitalization indicated. Assess patient for possible ICU admission, especially if the CURB-65 score is 4 or 5.

   - **C**onfusion (based on specific mental test or new disorientation to person, place, or time)
   - **U**rea (BUN) >7 mmol/L (20 mg/dL)
   - **R**espiratory rate >30 breaths/minute
   - **B**lood pressure (systolic <90 mm Hg or diastolic <60 mm Hg)
   - Age >**65** years

CHILDREN

1. Kids <5 years and kids born at 24 to 28 weeks gestational age have increased risk of severe disease.
2. Signs and symptoms
   - Cough, tachypnea, dyspnea, fever, wheezing, lethargy, irritability, poor feeding, signs of dehydration, vomiting, diarrhea, abdominal pain, and headache
3. Social history
   - Daycare; exposure to second-hand smoke
4. Physical
   - Temperature, respiratory rate, O_2 saturation, laboured breathing, HEENT, chest, lungs, abdominal examination
5. Testing to consider
   - Pulse oximetry at triage to assess severity and then as needed
   - CXR, CBC, CRP/ESR
   - Bun/Cr, electrolytes
   - ABG if toxic
   - Blood culture
   - Nasopharyngeal specimen for rapid viral antigen testing for influenza and other viruses

Use ciprofloxacin if pseudomonas is a concern.

Consider empyema if patient is not improving on antibiotics.

PNEUMONIA IN ADULTS AND CHILDREN ETIOLOGY AND TREATMENT OVERVIEW

Etiology and Treatment (see Table 3-5)

- Fluoroquinolones—Reserved for treatment failures; recent antibiotic use; or allergy.
- Aspiration—Anaerobic coverage (amoxicillin-clavulanate or clindamycin).
- Duration of treatment: Generally 7 to 14 days. If considering shorter course, patients should be treated for minimum of 5 days and be afebrile for 48 to 72 hours.
- Children 1to 3 months → always admit and consult peds.

TABLE 3-5   Etiology and Treatment of Pneumonia

Age	PEDIATRICS				ADULTS		
	0-4 weeks	4 weeks-3 months	3 months-5 years	5-18 years	CAP	Elderly/nursing home/ comorbidities	HIV
Etiology	*E. coli* GBS *Listeria*	Viral GAS *E. coli* *S. pneumoniae*	Viral (RSV, adeno, others) *S. pneumoniae* *S. aureus* GAS	*Mycoplasma Chlamydia pneumoniae,* *S. pneumoniae* Viruses	*S. pneumoniae* *M. pneumoniae* *C. pneumoniae*	*Streptococcus Haemophilus influen-zae* Gram (–) rods *Staphylococcus Legionella*	PCP
Treatment	Ampicillin + gentamicin	Second-generation cephalosporin	Amoxicillin 40-90 mg/kg/day × 10 days or Macrolide *No antibiotic indicated if viral cause	Amoxicillin 40-90 mg/kg/day × 10 days Or macrolide Azithromycin 10 mg/kg × 1 day, 5 mg/kg × 7-10 days Clarithromycin 15 mg/kg/day × 10 days	First line: Doxycycline 200 mg po × 1, then 100 mg po bid × 5-7 days Amoxicillin 1 G po TID × 5-7 days (>50 years old) Concern of atypicals: Add a macrolide Clarithromycin 500 mg PO bid × 5-7 days	First line: Doxycycline 200 mg po × 1, then 100 mg po bid × 5-7 days Amox/clav 875 mg po bid × 5-7 days, add a macrolide for atypicals Note fluoroquinolones should be reserved: Treatment failures, comorbidities, recent antibiotics, or documented highly drug resistant infection. Remember to adjust dosing in patients with impaired renal dosing Levofloxacin 500-750 mg OD × 5 days Moxifloxacin 400 mg OD × 5 days	TMP-SMX

Further Management Considerations

- Look for decompensation (need to ventilate, CPAP, BiPAP) before it happens.
- Keep in mind to admit patients who may be at risk of complications.
- Vaccinate those with comorbidities with influenza and pneumococcal infections.
- Be aware of drug interactions (especially warfarin and antibiotics).
- Do contact tracing if needed.
- Follow-up is important.
- Always rule out aspiration, tuberculosis, and HIV before choosing antibiotics (or reassess the diagnosis if patient not improving).

Bibliography

Anti-infective Review Panel. *Anti-infective Guidelines for Community-Acquired Infections*. Toronto: MUMS Guideline Clearinghouse; 2013.

Bauer T, Ewig S, Marre R, et al. BRB-65 predicts death from community acquired pneumonia. *J Int Med*. 2006;260:93-101.

Chen AY, Tran C. Toronto Notes. Toronto, ON: Type & Graphics Inc; 2011.

CURB-65. http://www.mdcalc.com/curb-65-severity-score-community-acquired-pneumonia/. Accessed April 27, 2012.

O'Toole D. Infectious disease: Family Medicine Notes: Preparing for the CCFP exam ED4. 2016:60-80.

Rx Files. Anti-infectives—oral. *Drug Comparison Charts*. 8th ed. 2010:56-57.

Rx Files: Antibiotics and Common Infections: Stewardship, Effectiveness, Safety and Clinical Pearls. 2016:4-5.

Meningitis

Priority Topic 62

Definition

Inflammation of the meninges covering the brain and spinal cord.

Etiology

- Bacterial: *E. coli*, GBS, *H. influenzae*, *S. pneumoniae*, *Neisseria meningitides*, *Listeria monocytogenes*, *S. aureus*
- Viral: Enterovirus, HIV, HSV, West Nile
- Fungal: *Cryptococcus*, Coccidioidomycosis

Risk Factors

- Haematogenous spread (respiratory infection, bacterial endocarditis)
- Parameningeal focus (AOM, sinusitis)
- Head trauma (penetrating)
- Previous neurosurgery/shunts
- Immunocompromised/contact with infected person

TRIAD: Fever, altered mental status, nuchal rigidity

Physical Examination

- Fever, vomiting, lethargy, irritability, poor feeding, headache, confusion, neck stiffness, seizure, meningismus
- Brudzinski sign: Passive flexion of neck causes involuntary flexion of hip/knees
- Kernig sign: Resistance to knee extension when hip flexed to 90 degrees

Investigations

- Labs: Blood culture, WBC with differential, LP/CSF
- CSF: See Table 3-6

TABLE 3-6	CSF Profiles	
	BACTERIAL	**VIRAL**
Appearance	Normal or cloudy	Usually normal
Glucose	Low	Normal
Protein	High	Moderate increase
WBC count (cells/mm^3)	>1000	<1000
Predominant WBC	Neutrophils (PMNs) predominant	Lymphocytes and monocytes

Treatment

- See Table 3-7

TABLE 3-7   Treatment

	NEONATES (1-3 MONTHS)	INFANTS/KIDS	TEENS/ADULTS	ELDERLY	SHUNT
Bacterial	*E. coli*	*H. influenzae*	*S. pneumoniae*	*S. pneumoniae*	*S. aureus*
	GBS	*S. pneumoniae*	*N. meningitis*	*N. meningitis*	Gram (−)ve
	Listeria	*N. meningitis*		*Listeria*	
Treatment (empiric)	Ampicillin 200-300 mg/kg/day × at least 14 days + Cefotaxime 100-200 mg/kg/day × 21 days	Vancomycin 15 mg/kg q 6 hrs 10-21 days + Ceftriaxone 25-50 mg/kg/day 10-21 days	Vancomycin 15-20 mg/kg/dose q8 hrs × 10-14 days + Ceftriaxone 2 g q12 hrs × 10-14 days	Vancomycin 15-20 mg/kg/dose q8 hrs × 10-14 days + Ceftriaxone 2 g q12 hrs × 10-14 days + Ampicillin (for Listeria)	

Note: Chemoprophylaxis of close contacts needed for HiB and meningococcus. Add Acyclovir if HSV on differential diagnosis.

Prevention

See "Immunizations" for further details.

Bibliography

Agabegi S, Agabegi E. *Step-Up to Medicine*. 2nd ed. Philadelphia, PA: Lippincott & Williams & Wilkins; 2008.

Chen YA, Tran C. *Toronto Notes–Comprehensive Medical Reference & Review for MCCQE I and USMLE II.* Toronto, Canada: Toronto Notes for Medical Students, Inc; 2011.

Esherick JS, Clark DS, Slater ED. Disease Management. *CURRENT Practice Guidelines in Primary Care 2016*. New York, NY: McGraw-Hill; 2016. http://accessmedicine.mhmedical.com.ezproxy.rqhealth.lib.sk.ca/content.aspx?bookid=1701&Sectionid=110628313. Accessed December 27, 2016.

RxFiles: Urinary Tract Infections (UTIs). http://www.rxfiles.ca.ezproxy.rqhealth.lib.sk.ca/rxfiles/uploads/documents/members/CHT-UTI-Tx.pdf. RxFiles; May 2016. Accessed December 27, 2016.

CHAPTER 4

Surgery

Abdominal Pain

TABLE 4-1	Differential Diagnosis of Abdominal Pain by Quadrants	
Right hypochondrium • Gallbladder • Liver	**Epigastric** • Pancreatitis • Peptic ulcer	**Left hypochondrium** • Spleen • Cardiac or lung
Right lumbar • Kidney stone • Renal	**Umbilical** • AAA	**Left lumbar** • Kidney stone • Renal
Right iliac • Appendicitis • Ovarian/fallopian tube	**Hypogastric/suprapubic** • Urinary • Gynecological	**Left iliac** • Diverticulitis • Ovarian/fallopian tube

ABDOMINAL PAIN—GENERAL CONSIDERATIONS

- Acute abdominal pain
  - Consider life-threatening causes, resuscitate, and refer for definitive treatment
  - Signs of peritonitis include rebound tenderness, rigidity, guarding
    - DDX = perforation, appendicitis, cholecystitis/cholangitis, pancreatitis, diverticulitis
- Chronic abdominal pain
  - Ensure follow-up, manage symptoms with lifestyle modification and medication, consider malignancy
  - Consider extraintestinal manifestations of inflammatory bowel disease
- **Always consider pregnancy, pelvic examination, and rectal examination**

HEMORRHOIDS

- Arise from dilated vascular plexus in anal canal
- **Presentation**
  - Rectal bleeding, not typically mixed with stool, anal pruritus, prolapse, anemia if chronic
  - Painful if thrombosed (especially external hemorrhoids), painless if internal hemorrhoids

- **Risk factors**
  - Pregnancy, obesity, heavy lifting, portal hypertension, prolonged sitting, pelvic tumours, straining, advanced age, diarrhea, chronic constipation
- **Physical examination**
  - Location (above/below dentate line), +/− prolapse
  - External hemorrhoids arise from below dentate line
  - Classification of internal hemorrhoids:
    - Grade I—Bleeding but no prolapse from anal canal
    - Grade II—Prolapse with straining but reduce spontaneously
    - Grade III—Prolapse with straining requiring manual reduction
    - Grade IV—Permanently prolapsed, irreducible, may strangulate
- **Treatment**
  - Conservative management
    - Adequate fibre (25-30 g/day) and fluid intake (6-8 glasses water/day) is first-line treatment
    - Sitz baths, warm water sprays, avoid straining, weight loss, exercise
    - Steroid cream or suppository (short-term only)
  - Surgical management
    - Rubber band ligation
    - Sclerotherapy: Best for internal hemorrhoids. Injection of aluminium potassium sulphate and tannic acid (ALTA) or phenol
    - Surgical excision: Thrombosed external hemorrhoids or internal hemorrhoids unresponsive to conservative treatment

ANAL FISSURE

- Tear in the lining of the anal canal distal to the dentate line, resulting in spasm of sphincter muscle causing further tearing.
- **Presentation**
  - Very painful rectal bleeding, blood on paper not mixed in stool
- **Risk factors**
  - Local trauma (eg, passage of hard stool), Crohn's disease, tuberculosis, leukemia, tightening of anal canal due to nervousness or pain
- Physical examination: Gentle examination; may be too painful for DRE; posterior midline is most frequent location, second is anterior midline
- Treatment
  - Increase fibre: Bulking agents, for example, psyllium or polycarbophils, adequate fluid intake.
  - Sitz baths, avoid straining.
  - Topical nitroglycerin (increased local blood flow reduces pressure on sphincter to allow for healing).
  - Other: Botulinum toxin, calcium channel blocker (nifedipine, diltiazem) to reduce sphincter pressure.
  - Surgery if persistent and not responsive to above: lateral sphincterotomy.
  - Consider endoscopy if persistent/recurrent to assess for possible Crohn disease.

RECTAL ABSCESS AND FISTULA

- Bacterial infection of blocked anal gland
- **Presentation**
  - Painful, may have systemic symptoms/signs

- **Physical examination**
  - Look for signs of spreading infection, may feel mass on DRE
- **Treatment**
  - Timely incision and drainage, take swab for culture and sensitivity (C&S). If fistula, can milk into anal canal;
  - Antibiotics if evidence of cellulitis, or if immunosuppressed, diabetes, valvular heart disease.
- **Complications**
  - May develop chronic suppurative fistula which requires surgical treatment (except for patients with Crohn's disease)

APPENDICITIS

- Inflammation of appendiceal wall followed by localized ischemia, perforation, and generalized peritonitis +/− abscess formation
  - Appendiceal obstruction is primary cause; fecalith in adults and lymphoid in children
- **Presentation**
  - "Migratory pain": Pain starts periumbilical, then moves to **right lower quadrant** (RLQ).
    - McBurney's point: 1/3 Anterior Superior Iliac Spine (ASIS) to umbilicus
  - Atypical presentation may occur in children and elderly
- **Physical examination**
  - Rovsing sign: Palpation of left iliac fossa causes pain in right iliac fossa
    - Most common, indicates interior appendix
  - Psoas sign: Extension of right hip exacerbates pain
    - Indicates retrocecal appendix
  - Obturator sign: Rotation of flexed right hip exacerbates pain
    - Indicates pelvic appendix
- **Investigations**
  - Elevated WBC with left shift
  - Beta-HCG to rule out pregnancy
  - Urinalysis
- Imaging is unnecessary with high clinical suspicion and timely appendectomy, useful if appendicitis is suspected but unclear.
  - Ultrasound: Low sensitivity therefore can rule in but cannot rule out.
  - Contrast CT: Good sensitivity and specificity, and can provide alternate diagnosis.
- **Complications**
  - Perforated appendix (especially with symptoms >24 hours duration), abscess, phlegmon
- **Treatment**
  - NPO
  - IV fluids
  - Antibiotics
  - Surgery

INFLAMMATORY BOWEL DISEASE

- Crohn's disease; associated with HLA B27 + extraintestinal manifestations.
- Two major disorders: Ulcerative Colitis and Crohn disease (see Table 4-2).

TABLE 4-2	Ulcerative Colitis vs Crohn's Disease	
	ULCERATIVE COLITIS	**CROHN DISEASE**
Site of involvement	Only involves colon Rectum almost always involved	Any area of the gastrointestinal tract Rectum usually spared
Pattern of involvement	Continuous	Skip lesions
Diarrhea	Bloody	Usually non-bloody
Severe abdominal pain	Rare	Frequent
Perianal disease	No	In 30% of patients
Fistula	No	Yes
Endoscopic findings	Erythematous and friable Superficial ulceration	Aphthoid and deep ulcers Cobble stoning
Radiologic findings	Tubular appearance resulting from loss of haustral folds	String sign of terminal ileum, RLQ mass, fistulas, abscesses
Histologic features	Mucosa only	Transmural
	Crypt abscesses	Crypt abscesses, granulomas (<30%)
Smoking	Protective	Worsens course
Serology	p-ANCA more common	ASCA more common

Abbreviations: ASCA, anti-Saccharomyces cerevisiae antibodies; p-ANCA, perinuclear antineutrophil cytoplasmic antibody; RLQ, right lower quadrant.

CROHN'S DISEASE

- Chronic inflammatory multisystem disease affecting mainly the gastrointestinal (GI) tract.
- "Gum to Bum": Skip lesions affecting any part of GI tract from mouth to anus; cobble stoning
  - Transmural inflammation results in thickened, fibrotic, strictured gut.
  - Eighty per cent have small bowel involvement, usually in distal ileum.
  - Fifty per cent have ileocolitis.
  - Twenty per cent have colitis, and half of these will have rectal sparing.
  - Thirty per cent have perianal disease.
- **Presentation**
  - Fatigue, diarrhea, abdominal pain (may be severe), weight loss, fever, bleeding less common.
  - Gradual onset, chronic course with remission and relapses.
  - Bimodal age <30 and >60, male = female, higher risk in smokers and Ashkenazi Jews.
  - Smoking worsens course of disease.
- **Investigations**
  - Endoscopy with biopsies.
  - CBC, C-reactive protein (CRP), LFT, electrolytes, urea and creatinine.
  - Rule out infectious causes of diarrhea.
- **Complications**
  - Intestinal: Fistulas, strictures/stenosis, abscess, colon adenocarcinoma
  - Malabsorption: Anemia, gallstones, kidney stones, osteoporosis, vitamin B_{12} deficiency if terminal ileum affected

- **Extraintestinal manifestations**
  - Eye: Uveitis, iritis, episcleritis, sclera-conjunctivitis
  - Joints: Nondeforming arthritis, ankylosing spondylitis, sacroiliitis
  - Skin: Erythema nodosum, pyoderma gangrenosum
  - Other: Primary sclerosing cholangitis, venous thromboembolism (VTE), cancer (lymphoma, cervical dysplasia, lymphoma)
- **Treatment**
  - Acute therapy:
    - Mild-to-moderate: Oral steroids, 5-ASA, +/− antibiotics especially if perianal disease with fistula or abscess (metronidazole +/− ciprofloxacin)
    - Moderate-to-severe: Oral steroids, azathioprine or 6-MP, Anti-TNF (infliximab) or adalimumab
  - Maintenance therapy: Elemental diet, quit smoking
    - Mild-to-moderate: 5-ASA or no treatment
    - Moderate-to-severe: Azathioprine or 6-MP. Methotrexate, anti-TNF (infliximab) for resistant cases
    - Regular colonoscopy; 8 years from diagnosis then q8 to 10 years
  - Surgery: Not curative, usually reserved for complications

ULCERATIVE COLITIS

- Chronic inflammatory disease involving mostly the mucosal layer of the colon
- Typically affects rectum and extends proximally in a continuous fashion
- **Presentation**
  - Insidious or acute exacerbations and remissions
  - Abdominal pain, bloody diarrhea, urgency, tenesmus
- **Investigations**
  - Flexible sigmoidoscopy +/− colonoscopy with biopsy.
  - CBC, CRP, LFT, electrolytes, urea and creatinine.
  - Rule out infectious causes of diarrhea
- **Complications**
  - Colonic: Toxic megacolon, bowel perforation, colonic adenocarcinoma
- **Extraintestinal manifestations**
  - Joints: Arthritis, ankyloses spondylitis, sacroilitis
  - Eyes: Uveitis and episcleritis
  - Skin: Pyoderma gangrenosum, erythema nodosum, psoriasis
  - Other: Gallstones, kidney stones, VTE, cancer (lung cancer, lymphoma, prostate cancer)
- **Treatment**
  - Acute therapy: 5-ASA or sulfasalazine, oral or IV steroids for severe disease.
  - Maintenance therapy: 5-ASA, sulfasalazine, anti-TNF (infliximab), 6-MP, azathioprine.
  - Surgery can be curative but associated with multiple postoperative complications, and should be reserved for complications or patients unresponsive to medical treatment.

IRRITABLE BOWEL SYNDROME

- Chronic/recurrent abdominal discomfort with associated change in bowel habits, etiology unknown; female > male
- May be diarrhea- or constipation-predominant or mixed

- **Diagnosis**
  - Rome III symptom-based criteria:
    - Recurrent abdominal pain or discomfort at least 3 days/month over the past 3 months. Symptoms must be present for 6 months and include two or more of the following:
      - (1) Improved with defecation
      - (2) Associated with change in stool frequency
      - (3) Associated with change in stool consistency
- **Rule out alarm features**
  - Acute onset
    - Change in bowel habits in person >60 years
    - Fever
    - Nausea/vomiting
    - Unintentional weight loss >10 lb
    - Anemia, hematochezia, melena, positive fecal occult blood test
    - Family history of colon cancer or inflammatory bowel disease
    - Awakes from sleep
    - Rectal or abdominal mass
- **Investigations**
  - Bloodwork: Celiac antibodies, +/– CBC.
  - No other investigations necessary unless alarm features are present; do not overinvestigate.
- **Treatment**
  - Chronic course so patient–doctor relationship, patient education, and reassurance are important.
  - Diet: Slow eating, eat regular meals, adequate water intake, stool bulking (psyllium, polycarbophils), avoid triggers (insoluble fibre, lactose, caffeine, sorbitol, alcohol, carbonated beverages, menstruation with OCP, and stress).
  - Medications:
    - (1) Constipation-predominant: Psyllium, polycarbophil, MOM, PEG, lactulose, prucalopride, linaclotide (peptide agonist of guanylate cyclase 2C which aids increase intestinal fluid and accelerating transit)
    - (2) Diarrhea-predominant: Loperamide, rifaximin (2-week antibiotic course)
    - (3) Pain-predominant: Antispasmodics—peppermint oil, hyoscine, pinaverium
  - Probiotics: Bifidobacteria recommended, no evidence for lactobacillus, use minimum 4 weeks
  - Counselling, CBT, hypnotherapy, relaxation techniques
  - Consider antidepressants (SSRI or TCA) in refractory disease

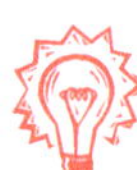

I GET SMASHED

Idiopathic

Gallstones (45%)

ETOH (35%)

Trauma

Steroids

Microbiology (mumps, TB, rubella, varicella, hepatitis, CMV, HIV)

Autoimmune (PAN, SLE, Crohn's)

Scorpion venom

Hyperlipidemia/hypercalcemia/hypothermia

ERCP/emboli

Drugs (diuretics, valproic acid, estrogen, azathioprine, didanosine)

PANCREATITIS

- Acute inflammation of pancreas
- Causes: **IGETSMASHED**
  - Gallstones and alcohol the most common
- **Presentation**
  - Rapid-onset upper abdominal pain (epigastric)
  - Constant, not colicky, band-like radiation to back, may improve with leaning forward
  - Associated with nausea and vomiting, +/– shock
  - Abdominal bruising: Cullen sign (umbilicus) and Grey Turner sign (flanks)

- **Diagnosis**
  - Typical history: tender epigastrium, elevated WBC, elevated lipase preferred over amylase (usually three times normal limit), abnormal LFTs (may be typical of gallstones or ETOH), lipids (TG >11.3), and calcium level
- **Imaging**
  - AXR: Sentinel loop and colon "cut off" sign
  - US: Diffusely enlarged pancreas and imaging of biliary tree to look for gallstones
  - CT is good for intra-abdominal complications (pseudocyst, pancreatic necrosis or hemorrhage, abscess formation)
- **Treatment**
  - IV fluids, analgesia, NPO, observation, investigation to treat cause
  - ICU may be required
- **Complications**
  - Abscess, pseudocyst, necrotizing pancreatitis (sterile or infected)
  - Pleural effusion, ARDS, pneumonia
  - Pericardial effusion, pericarditis

DIVERTICULITIS

- Inflammation of diverticula or pouch-like protrusions of the colon wall
  - Increased intraluminal pressure or stool can lead to erosion of the diverticular wall. This can lead to inflammation, followed by possible necrosis and perforation
- **Presentation**
  - Left lower quadrant pain, usually present for a few days prior to presentation
  - May have painless rectal bleeding
  - Alternating diarrhea and constipation, +/− nausea and vomiting, low grade fever, may have cramping, bloating, flatulence
- **Risk factors**
  - Age, lack of exercise, obesity, possibly low dietary fibre
- **Physical examination**
  - LLQ tenderness, distention, may palpate LLQ mass (abscess or phlegmon), may see signs of generalized peritonitis.
  - Asian population more likely to have right-sided disease so may see RLQ tenderness.
- **Diagnosis**
  - Based on history and examination; avoid colonoscopy or barium enema if acutely inflamed.
  - Other investigations are typically to rule out other causes of acute presentation.
  - CT scan with contrast will diagnose and assess for severity, can also assess for complications (perforation, abscess).
- **Treatment**
  - Uncomplicated
    - Bowel rest with clear fluids only for 2 to 3 days.
    - Antibiotics for 10 to 14 days, need to cover gram-negative rods and anaerobes.
    - High-fibre diet—no need to avoid seeds and nuts.
    - Admission decision based on comorbidities, ability to tolerate PO, severity of presentation.
  - Complicated: Resuscitation, broad-spectrum antibiotics, and surgical intervention may be required if obstruction, perforation, abscess, or fistula are present.

- **Follow-up**
  - Once acute episode has resolved, colonoscopy or barium enema and flexible sigmoidoscopy should be done to fully evaluate the colon.

ABDOMINAL AORTIC ANEURYSM

- Degeneration of aortic wall leads to dilation of the aorta.
  - Normal diameter approx. 2 cm
  - Aneurysmal ≥3 cm
- **Presentation**
  - Asymptomatic: Found incidentally on abdominal examination or US/CT/MRI for other reason
  - Symptomatic: Pain, may be abdominal, back, flank, groin; often mimics other disease presentations
    - May be described as ripping/tearing sensation
    - Pain unaffected by position or movement
  - Ruptured AAA
  - Life-threatening cause of acute abdominal pain
    - Triad is pathognomonic: Pain, pulsatile abdominal mass, hypotension
- **Risk factors**
  - Increased age, male gender (four to six times increased risk), smoking, atherosclerosis, hypertension, hypercholesterolemia, coronary artery disease, cerebrovascular disease, family history, Caucasian race, connective tissue disease (Marfan or Ehler's Danlos)
- **Physical examination**
  - Abdominal palpation: Widened pulse/pulsatile abdominal mass
    - More common if located between xiphoid and umbilicus (infrarenal and above inferior mesenteric arteries)
    - Increased sensitivity with increasing aorta diameter
  - Peripheral vascular examination
- **Diagnosis**
  - Abdominal US is investigation of choice.
  - CT can be used for monitoring of AAA size; however, higher radiation doses and contrast are required.
- **Treatment**
  - Serial monitoring:
    - Unlikely to rupture if <5 cm
    - Aneurysm 4.0 to 5.5 cm: US or CT every 6 to 12 months
    - Aneurysm 3.0 to 4.0 cm: US every 2 to 3 years
  - Medical treatment:
    - Risk factor reduction: Quit smoking, statin, ACEi are all recommended.
    - Antibiotic therapy for infectious or "mycotic" aneurysm typically caused by *Staphylococcus*, *Salmonella*, or fungal.
  - Surgical repair
  - Immediate if symptomatic or rapid rate of expansion (>0.5 cm in 6 months)
  - Elective if asymptomatic and ≥5.5 cm or growth >1 cm/year

ACUTE MESENTERIC ISCHEMIA

- Potentially fatal intestinal hypoperfusion due to an occlusive or nonocclusive obstruction affecting venous or arterial circulation.

- **Four major causes**
  1. Superior mesenteric artery embolism—50%
  2. Superior mesenteric artery thrombosis—15% to 25%
  3. Mesenteric venous thrombosis—5%
  4. Nonocclusive ischemia—20% to 30%
- **Risk factors**
  - Females and people >60 years
  - Coagulopathy, vasculitis, congestive heart failure, atrial fibrillation, peripheral vascular disease, aortic insufficiency, sepsis, cardiac arrhythmias, diuretics (reduce intestinal perfusion), digoxin, alpha-adrenergic agonists, history or family history of embolic events
- **Presentation**
  - One per cent of patients with acute abdominal pain and up to 10% in patients >70 years
  - Rapid onset of severe periumbilical pain +/− nausea, vomiting, diarrhea, distension
  - Hallmark is **pain out of proportion to physical findings (ischemic pain).**
- **Physical examination**
  - Abdominal examination may be normal; minimal tenderness until transmural bowel involvement
  - May see abdominal distention, signs of peripheral vasculopathy.
- **Investigation**
  - No serological marker is sensitive/specific to diagnose or rule out mesenteric ischemia; normal lab values do not exclude mesenteric ischemia
  - Abnormalities may be seen such as hemoconcentration, elevated WBC, increased anion gap, and lactic acidosis
  - Initial lab work may include CBC, electrolytes, urea, creatinine, LFTs, amylase, blood cultures, lactate, and blood gas
  - Imaging:
    - Contrast CT if no peritoneal signs on examination.
    - Mesenteric angiography if peritoneal signs present on examination.
- **Diagnosis**
  - Clinical suspicion plus radiological evidence on CT or mesenteric angiography
- **Treatment**
  - Depends on imaging findings of embolus, thrombosis, or vasoconstriction, but may involve: anticoagulation, thrombolytics, surgical intervention

CONSTIPATION

- Rome III criteria for constipation require the following criteria for 3 months, with symptoms present for at least 6 months:
  - Must include two or more of the following:
    - Straining during at least 25% of defecations
    - Lumpy or hard stools in at least 25% of defecations
    - Sensation of incomplete evacuation for at least 25% of defecations
    - Sensation of anorectal obstruction/blockage for at least 25% of defecations
    - Manual manoeuvres to facilitate at least 25% of defecations (eg, digital evacuation, support of the pelvic floor)
    - Fewer than three defecations per week
  - Loose stools are rarely present without the use of laxatives.
  - Insufficient criteria for IBS.

- **Types**
  - Primary (or idiopathic)
    - Functional, delayed (or slow) transit, and outlet obstructive (or mechanical)
  - Secondary (most common)
    - Diet, lifestyle, pregnancy, medications, or medical conditions
- **History**
  - Comorbidities or medications, diet, exercise (secondary causes)
  - Rule out alarm symptoms; acute change, intentional weight loss, family history of colon cancer or IBD, anemia, or melena/hematochezia
  - Specific populations: End-of-life care, Parkinson patients, and patients taking opioids
- **Physical examination**
  - Rectal examination to assess for presence of mass, pathology causing pain during defecation, abnormal tone
  - Abdominal examination
- **Diagnosis**
  - In the absence of alarm symptoms in patients <50 years, the diagnosis is clinical.
  - In the presence of alarm symptoms, further investigations are required.
- **Investigations**
  - None recommended routinely, investigation should be prompted by age and history/examination findings
  - If secondary cause suspected, or ≥50, consider:
    - CBC, electrolytes, calcium, blood sugar, thyroid
  - If alarm symptoms are present:
    - Fecal occult blood test and colon inspection (colonoscopy or flexible sigmoidoscopy with barium enema)
  - If refractory to treatment: Further investigations of colon transit time and anorectal physiology are required, and specialist referral should be made.
- **Treatment**
  - Lifestyle/prevention: Diet + physical activity (fluids, fruit, and fibre)
  - Bulk-forming laxative: Increases stool fluid content
    - Ex: Psyllium, inulin, guar gum, calcium polycarbophil
    - Avoid in dehydrated patients or patients with low fluid intake (ie, palliative)
  - Osmotic laxative: Draw fluid into intestinal lumen and stimulate peristalsis
    - Ex: PEG 3350, lactulose, sorbitol, glycerine, magnesium hydroxide
  - Lubricant: Aids in stool passage and slows reabsorption of water from GI tract
    - Ex: Mineral oil (avoid chronic use and not for infants)
  - Stimulants: Increase fluids, alter electrolytes, stimulate myenteric plexus, and induce peristalsis
    - Ex: Bisacodyl, sennosides
  - Stool softener: Reduces stool surface tension thereby increases fluid penetration into stool
    - Ex: Docusate sodium and docusate calcium
  - Prokinetic:
    - Ex: Metoclopramide, prucalopride (5HT-4 agonist)
  - Prosecretory: Used for IBS; constipation-predominant
    - Linaclotide, lubiprostone
  - Methylnaltrexone: Mu-opioid antagonist for opioid-induced constipation
  - Surgery is rarely indicated

CONSTIPATION ALARM FEATURES

Acute onset, fever, nausea/vomiting, unintentional weight loss >10 lb, anemia, hematochezia, melena, positive fecal occult blood test, change in bowel habits, symptoms refractory to current therapy, family history of colon cancer, or inflammatory bowel disease.

- Pediatric consideration:
  - Lifestyle instruction is very important (limit cow's milk to <24 oz/day, schedule routine toilet sitting, prop feet up with stool, use positive reinforcement.
  - Glycerin suppository, lactulose or PEG 3350 are preferred treatments.
  - Avoid mineral oil (due to risk of aspiration leading to lipid pneumonia) and manual disimpaction.

SMALL BOWEL OBSTRUCTION

- Obstruction is most often caused by mechanical obstruction of small bowel, but considers large bowel obstruction (usually due to malignancy) or nonmechanical obstruction secondary to ileus (see Table 4-3).
  - Low grade—partial obstruction
  - High grade—complete obstruction

TABLE 4-3	Obstruction: Type and Signs/Symptoms		
	SMALL BOWEL OBSTRUCTION	**LARGE BOWEL OBSTRUCTION**	**PARALYTIC ILEUS**
Nausea and vomiting	Early finding, may be bilious	Late finding, may be feculent	Present
Abdominal pain	Colicky	Colicky	Absent
Abdominal distention	+++	++	+
Bowel sounds	Normal or increased, may hear high-pitched BS	Normal or increased, may hear high-pitched BS	Decreased or absent
Abdominal x-ray findings	Air/fluid levels	Air/fluid levels	Air throughout colon

Adapted with permission from *Toronto Notes*.

- **Causes**
  - **H**ernia, **a**dhesions (60%), **n**eoplasm, **g**allstone ileus, **i**ntussusception, **v**olvulus
  - Also: Trauma, radiation, inflammatory bowel disease, foreign body
- **Presentation**
  - Crampy abdominal pain, abdominal distention, vomiting, inability to pass flatus
- **History**
  - Hematochezia, previous abdominal surgery, inflammatory bowel disease, history or family history of cancer, radiation
- **Physical examination**
  - Examine for abdominal masses, hernias, and signs of complications such as peritonitis or shock
- **Diagnosis**
  - Typically diagnosed based on history and examination, with x-ray to confirm.
  - Abdominal x-ray, three views: Air/fluid levels, dilated bowel loops.
  - WBC, pregnancy test, urea, creatinine, and blood gas to assess for metabolic acidosis.
  - CT with contrast may be considered for further information, for example, to identify a discrete transition point, or if x-ray is inconclusive.
    - Useful for patients with a history of malignancy, those with no history of abdominal surgery or risk factors for SBO, or postsurgery.

SMALL BOWEL OBSTRUCTION (SBO) CAUSES: HANG IV
- Hernia
- Adhesions
- Neoplasm
- Gallstone ileus
- Intussusception
- Volvulus

- **Complications**
  - Peritonitis, bowel necrosis, bowel perforation, sepsis
- **Treatment**
  - Conservative management if no signs of peritonitis, tachycardia, fever, elevated WBC, metabolic acidosis
    - ◦ More likely to be successful with partial SBO.
    - ◦ NG tube on suction, IV fluids, strict bowel rest, serial abdominal examinations, Foley catheter to monitor fluid status.
    - ◦ If no improvement within 12 to 24 hours, consider contrast imaging studies and/or surgery.

BILIARY TRACT AND CHOLELITHIASIS

- Cholelithiasis is the presence of stones (aka calculi) in the gallbladder.
  - Stone composition: Cholesterol, pigmented
- **Risk factors**
  - 4Fs: Fat, female, fertile, forty.
  - Also: Pregnancy, multiparity, OCP use, cyclical weight loss, rapid weight loss, postmenopausal estrogen, ceftriaxone.
- Gallstones are typically asymptomatic.
- Can precipitate biliary colic, acute cholecystitis, ascending cholangitis, acute pancreatitis.
- **Diagnosis**
  - Abdominal ultrasound
  - May see elevated bilirubin, LFT abnormalities (elevated ALP)
- **Complications**
  - Choledocholithiasis, biliary colic, cholecystitis, cholangitis, pancreatitis
- **Treatment**
  - No treatment required for asymptomatic cholelithiasis

BILIARY COLIC

- This occurs when the gallbladder contracts, often due to a fatty meal, resulting in hormonal or neural stimulation
  - Contraction forces a stone or sludge into the cystic duct opening, leading to increased pressure within the gallbladder, and resulting in pressure and pain.
  - As the gallbladder relaxes, the pain subsides, usually lasting <8 hours.
- **Presentation**
  - RUQ abdominal pain which is dull, intense, and constant (the term "colicky" is a misnomer)
  - May occur 1 to 2 hours following a fatty meal but often unrelated to meals
  - Pain lasts <8 hours (if >8 hours, consider other diagnosis/complications)
  - May be associated with nausea, vomiting, chest pain, diaphoresis
- **Diagnosis**
  - Known gallstones on abdominal ultrasound, typical history, normal WBC and no fevers, clinically stable, pain settles with time
- **Treatment**
  - Analgesia
  - Elective cholecystectomy or conservative management depending on frequency of attacks

CHOLEDOCHOLITHIASIS

- Stones are present in the common bile duct.
- Ductal stones can form in the absence of a gallbladder, but are usually formed in the gallbladder.
- **Complications**
  - Ascending cholangitis, obstructive jaundice, secondary biliary cirrhosis
- **Presentation**
  - RUQ pain, may radiate to back, associated with fever/chills, jaundice, pale stool, dark urine
- **Diagnosis**
  - **Elevated ALP, GGT, and total bilirubin**
  - Abdominal ultrasound, MRCP, ERCP (diagnostic and therapeutic)
- **Treatment**
  - Risk is stratified by visualization of CBD stone on abdominal US.
    - "Very strong" predictors—treatment of choice is ERCP
      - CBD stone on transabdominal ultrasound
      - Clinical ascending cholangitis
      - Serum bilirubin >68 μmol/L
    - "Strong" predictors—treatment is (1) laparoscopic cholecystectomy with intraoperative cholangiography, *or* (2) further imaging (MRCP/EUS) and reassessment
      - A dilated CBD on ultrasound (>6 mm)
      - Serum bilirubin 31 to 68 μmol/L
    - "Moderate" predictors—treatment is laparoscopic cholecystectomy or look for alternate diagnosis
      - Abnormal liver biochemical test other than bilirubin
      - Age >55 years
      - Clinical gallstone pancreatitis

ACUTE CHOLECYSTITIS

- Acute inflammation of the gallbladder with obstruction leading to gallbladder wall thickening and secondary infection
  - Calculous (>90%): obstruction of the cystic duct with a stone or sludge
  - Acalculous: no stones or sludge, difficult to diagnose, and high mortality rate
- **Common organisms**
  - *Escherichia coli* (40%), *Enterococcus* (12%), *Klebsiella* (11%), and *Enterobacter* (9%)
- **Risk factors**
  - Cholelithiasis, helminthic infection by ascariasis (common in Asia, Africa, Latin America)
- **Presentation**
  - Classic presentation is syndrome of fever, RUQ pain, and elevated WBC
  - Also anorexia, nausea and vomiting, change in mental status (especially in elderly)
- **Diagnosis and physical examination**
  - Clinical diagnosis requires at least one local sign/symptom and at least one systemic sign/symptom.
  - Local: Murphy sign, RUQ tenderness or mass.

- Systemic: Fever, elevated WBC, elevated CRP.
- Confirm acute cholecystitis with US or HIDA scan.
- Ultrasound findings: Distended gallbladder, pericholecystic fluid +/− stone in cystic duct. Thickened gallbladder wall >5 mm + Murphy sign when gallbladder compressed;
- Hepatobiliary scintigraphy: Absence of gallbladder filling within 60 minutes

■ **Treatment**

- NPO, IV fluids, IV antibiotics.
- Early cholecystectomy; if inflammation is severe, surgery may need to be delayed and gallbladder can be drained percutaneously in the interim

ACUTE CHOLANGITIS

■ Clinical syndrome where stasis of common bile duct causes biliary sepsis

■ **Risk factors**

- Biliary obstruction, stasis (often due to calculus or stricture)

■ **Presentation**

- Charcot triad occurs in 50% to 70%: Fever, RUQ pain, and jaundice
- Raynaud pentad: Fever, RUQ pain, jaundice, hypotension/shock, and confusion

■ **Diagnosis**

- WBC, LFT with transaminases transient and may be elevated at first and blood cultures.
- Elevated ALP, GGT, bilirubin more specific to cholestasis.
  ◦ May see transaminase around 1000 IU/L with abscess formation
- Abdominal ultrasound.

■ **Treatment**

- Antibiotics and biliary drainage/sphincterotomy
- ERCP or surgical cholecystectomy

CHARCOT TRIAD*

Fever

RUQ pain

Jaundice

RAYNAUD PENTAD*

Fever

RUQ pain

Jaundice

Hypotension

Confusion

*Suggests acute obstructive suppurative cholangitis

TABLE 4-4	**Pediatric Abdominal Pain**		
	DUODENAL ATRESIA	**PYLORIC STENOSIS**	**INTUSSUSCEPTION**
Definition	• Congenital defect of the duodenum • Leads to obstruction or complete atresia	• Thickened pylorus leads to gastric out-flow obstruction	• Telescoping of proximal bowel segment into distal segment
Presentation	• Bile-stained vomit • Feed intolerance	• Nonbilious projectile vomiting post feeds • Good appetite • May present with dehydration or weight loss	• Triad: Abdominal pain, sausage-shaped mass in RUQ, red-currant jelly stools • Sudden onset of severe paroxysms of pain • Pain-free intervals
Physical examination	• No abdominal distention	• Palpable olive-shaped pylorus muscle • Visible peristalsis	• RUQ sausage-shaped mass
Risk factors	• Down syndrome	• 3-8 weeks of age • Males	• Cystic fibrosis • 3 months-3 years old
Investigation	• Abdominal x-ray shows "double bubble" secondary to dilated stomach and duodenum • Consider upper GI series to rule out malrotation	• Abdominal ultrasound: pyloric muscle thickness >3 mm	• Abdominal x-ray with air or contrast enema • Abdominal ultrasound • Frequently at ileocecal junction
Treatment	• NPO and NG tube • Surgical correction	• Surgical pyloromyotomy	• Abdominal x-ray with air or contrast enema • Surgery for failed enema reduction

Bibliography

Afdhal NH. Acute cholangitis. In: Basow DS, ed. *UpToDate*. Waltham, MA; 2012. Retrieved from
http://www.uptodate.com/. Accessed March 23, 2012.

Black CE, Martin RF. Acute appendicitis in adults: Clinical manifestations and diagnosis. In: Basow DS, ed.
UpToDate. Waltham, MA; 2012. Retrieved from http://www.uptodate.com/. Accessed March 23, 2012.

Bleday R, Breen E. Overview of hemorrhoids. In: Basow DS, ed. *UpToDate*. Waltham, MA; 2012.
Retrieved from http://www.uptodate.com/. Accessed March 23, 2012.

Bleday R, Breen E. Treatment of hemorrhoids. In: Basow DS, ed. *UpToDate*. Waltham, MA; 2012.
Retrieved from http://www.uptodate.com/. Accessed March 23, 2012.

Breen E, Bleday R. Anal abscesses and fistulas. In: Basow DS, ed. *UpToDate,* Waltham, MA; 2012.
Retrieved from http://www.uptodate.com/. Accessed March 23, 2012.

Breen E, Bleday R. Anal fissures. In: Basow DS, ed. *UpToDate*. Waltham, MA; 2012. Retrieved from
http://www.uptodate.com/. Accessed March 23, 2012.

DynaMed. *Acute Cholecystitis*. Ipswich, MA: EBSCO Publishing; 2016. Retrieved from http://search
.ebscohost.com.cyber.usask.ca/login.aspx?direct=true&site=DynaMed&id=113862.

DynaMed. *Cholangitis*. Ipswich, MA: EBSCO Publishing; 2016. Retrieved from http://search.ebscohost
.com.cyber.usask.ca/login.aspx?direct=true&site=DynaMed&id=113862.

DynaMed. *Choledocholithiasis*. Ipswich, MA: EBSCO Publishing; 2016. Retrieved from http://search
.ebscohost.com.cyber.usask.ca/login.aspx?direct=true&site=DynaMed&id=113862.

DynaMed. *Constipation in Adults*. Ipswich, MA: EBSCO Publishing; 2016. Retrieved from http://search
.ebscohost.com.cyber.usask.ca/login.aspx?direct=true&site=DynaMed&id=113862.

DynaMed. *Duodenal Atresia or Stenosis*. Ipswich, MA: EBSCO Publishing; 2012. Retrieved from
http://search.ebscohost.com.cyber.usask.ca/login.aspx?direct=true&site=DynaMed&id=113862.

DynaMed. *Gallstones*. Ipswich, MA: EBSCO Publishing; 2016. Retrieved from http://search.ebscohost
.com.cyber.usask.ca/login.aspx?direct=true&site=DynaMed&id=113862.

DynaMed. *Hemorrhoids*. Ipswich, MA: EBSCO Publishing 2016. Retrieved from http://web.ebscohost
.com/dynamed/detail?vid=2&sid=bea65e50-18a3-4557-a8d1-4d48a7098753%40sessionmgr4007&hid=
4201&bdata=JnNpdGU9ZHluYW1lZC1saXZlJnNjb3BlPXNpdGU%3d#AN=116475&db=dme.

DynaMed. *Intussusception*. Ipswich, MA: EBSCO Publishing; 2010. Retrieved from http://search
.ebscohost.com.cyber.usask.ca/login.aspx?direct=true&site=DynaMed&id=113862.

Dynamed. *Irritable Bowel Syndrome (IBS)*. Ipswich, MA: EBSCO Publishing; 2016. Retrieved from
http://search.ebscohost.com.cyber.usask.ca/login.aspx?direct=true&site=DynaMed&id=113862.

DynaMed. *Pyloric Stenosis*. Ipswich, MA: EBSCO Publishing; 2012. Retrieved from http://search
.ebscohost.com.cyber.usask.ca/login.aspx?direct=true&site=DynaMed&id=113862.

DynaMed. *Small Bowel Obstruction*. Ipswich, MA: EBSCO Publishing; 2016. Retrieved from
http://search.ebscohost.com.cyber.usask.ca/login.aspx?direct=true&site=DynaMed&id=113862.

Farrell RJ, Peppercorn MA. Overview of the medical management of mild to moderate Crohn disease in
adults. In: Basow DS, ed. *UpToDate*. Waltham, MA; 2012. Retrieved from http://www.uptodate.com/.
Accessed March 23, 2012.

Freeman ML, Arain MA. Approach to the patient with suspected choledocholithiasis. In: Basow DS, ed.
UpToDate. Waltham, MA; 2012. Retrieved from http://www.uptodate.com/. Accessed March 23, 2012.

Heppell J. Surgical management of inflammatory bowel disease. In: Basow DS, ed. *UpToDate*. Waltham,
MA; 2012. Retrieved from http://www.uptodate.com/. Accessed March 23, 2012.

Hodin RA, Bordeianou L. Small bowel obstruction: Causes and management. In: Basow DS, ed.
UpToDate. Waltham, MA; 2012. Retrieved from http://www.uptodate.com/. Accessed March 23, 2012.

Hodin RA, Bordeianou L. Small bowel obstruction: Clinical manifestations and diagnosis. In: Basow DS, ed.
UpToDate. Waltham, MA; 2012. Retrieved from http://www.uptodate.com/. Accessed March 23, 2012.

Jim J, Thompson RW. Clinical evaluation of abdominal aortic aneurysm. In: Basow DS, ed. *UpToDate*.
Waltham, MA; 2012. Retrieved from http://www.uptodate.com/. Accessed March 23, 2012.

Kolodziejak L, Schuster B, Regier L, Jensen B. Constipation. *RxFiles Drug Comparison Charts*. 10th ed.
Saskatoon, SK: Saskatoon Health Region; 2014:57-59.

Kolodziejak L, Schuster B, Regier L, Jensen B. Inflammatory Bowel Disease *RxFiles Drug Comparison
Charts*. 10th ed. Saskatoon, SK: Saskatoon Health Region; 2014:60.

Kolodziejak L, Schuster B, Regier L, Jensen B. Irritable bowel syndrome (IBS). *RxFiles Drug Comparison
Charts*. 10th ed. Saskatoon, SK: Saskatoon Health Region; 2014:66.

Peppercorn MA. Clinical manifestations, diagnosis and prognosis of Crohn's disease in adults. In:
Basow DS, ed. *UpToDate*. Waltham, MA; 2012. Retrieved from http://www.uptodate.com/. Accessed
March 23, 2012.

Peppercorn MA. Clinical manifestations, diagnosis, and prognosis of ulcerative colitis in adults. In: Basow DS, ed. *UpToDate*. Waltham, MA; 2012. Retrieved from http://www.uptodate.com/. Accessed March 23, 2012.

Peppercorn MA, Ferrell RJ. Medical management of ulcerative colitis. In: Basow DS, ed. *UpToDate*. Waltham, MA; 2012. Retrieved from http://www.uptodate.com/. Accessed March 23, 2012.

Smink D, Soybel DI. Acute appendicitis in adults: Management. In: Basow DS, ed. *UpToDate*. Waltham, MA; 2012. Retrieved from http://www.uptodate.com/. Accessed March 23, 2012.

Tendler DA, LaMont JT. Acute mesenteric ischemia. In: Basow DS, ed. *UpToDate*. Waltham, MA; 2012. Retrieved from http://www.uptodate.com/. Accessed March 23, 2012.

Vege SS. Clinical manifestations and diagnosis of acute pancreatitis. In: Basow DS, ed. *UpToDate*. Waltham, MA; 2012. Retrieved from http://www.uptodate.com/. Accessed March 23, 2012.

Vege SS. Etiology and pathogenesis of chronic pancreatitis in adults. In: Basow DS, ed. *UpToDate*. Waltham, MA; 2012. Retrieved from http://www.uptodate.com/. Accessed March 23, 2012.

Vege SS. Etiology of acute pancreatitis. In: Basow DS, ed. *UpToDate*. Waltham, MA; 2012. Retrieved from http://www.uptodate.com/. Accessed March 23, 2012.

Vege SS. Treatment of acute pancreatitis. In: Basow DS, ed. *UpToDate*, Waltham, MA; 2012. Retrieved from http://www.uptodate.com/. Accessed March 23, 2012.

Wald A. Clinical manifestations and diagnosis of irritable bowel syndrome. In: Basow DS, ed. *UpToDate*. Waltham, MA; 2012. Retrieved from http://www.uptodate.com/. Accessed March 23, 2012.

Wald A. Etiology and evaluation of chronic constipation in adults. In: Basow DS, ed. *UpToDate*. Waltham, MA; 2012. Retrieved from http://www.uptodate.com/. Accessed March 23, 2012.

Wald A. Treatment of irritable bowel syndrome. In: Basow DS, ed. *UpToDate*. Waltham, MA; 2012. Retrieved from http://www.uptodate.com/. Accessed March 23, 2012.

Young-Fadok T, Pemberton JH. Clinical manifestations and diagnosis of colonic diverticular disease. In: Basow DS, ed. *UpToDate*. Waltham, MA; 2012. Retrieved from http://www.uptodate.com/. Accessed March 23, 2012.

Young-Fadok T, Pemberton JH. Epidemiology and pathophysiology of colonic diverticular disease. In: Basow DS, ed. *UpToDate*. Waltham, MA; 2012. Retrieved from http://www.uptodate.com/. Accessed March 23, 2012.

Young-Fadok T, Pemberton JH. Treatment of acute diverticulitis. In: Basow DS, ed. *UpToDate*. Waltham, MA; 2012. Retrieved from http://www.uptodate.com/. Accessed March 23, 2012.

Zakko SF, et al. Treatment of acute cholecystitis. In: Basow DS, ed. *UpToDate*. Waltham, MA: 2012. Retrieved from http://www.uptodate.com/. Accessed March 23, 2012.

Dehydration and Hypovolemia

- Excessive intracellular fluid loss usually due to hypovolemia
  - Usually due to excess fluid loss from GI tract, skin, and kidneys
- Highest morbidity and mortality in pediatric populations
- Types of hypovolemia:
  - Hypertonic/hypernatremic (GI losses, fever, diabetes, renal disease)
    - Net loss of extracellular water, or gain of sodium; Na > 145 mmol/L
  - Isotonic (hemorrhage, GI losses, trauma)
    - Loss of sodium is proportional to water; Na 135 to 145 mmol/L
  - Hypotonic/hyponatremic (GI losses, pancreatitis, heart failure, ascites, adrenal insufficiency, psychogenic polydipsia, salt wasting nephropathy)
    - Net loss of sodium relative to extracellular water; Na <135 mmol/L
- **Signs and Symptoms**
  - Dry mucosa
  - Thirst
  - Concentrated urine
  - Decreased sweating
  - Dizzy
  - Flushed
  - Resting tachycardia/weak pulse
  - Hypotension
  - Delayed capillary refill
  - Coma

- ■ **Risk factors**
  - Extremes of age, pregnancy (treat aggressively)
  - Acute illness, for example, debilitating pneumonia
  - Cognitive impairment: Delirium, sedation, psychosis
  - Limited fluid intake: Dysphagia, fear of incontinence, limited mobility
  - Increased fluid losses: Illness (especially GI), environment, diuretics, hemorrhage, trauma
  - Altered thirst: CNS lesions, medications, hyperglycemia
  - Iatrogenic: Peritoneal drainage
- ■ **Diagnosis**
  - History: Consider vomiting, diarrhea, fluid intake, urine output, postural dizziness, medications
    - ◦ Pediatrics (see Table 4-5): Number of wet diapers, crying tears, sunken eyes, recent weight when well

TABLE 4-5 Degree of Dehydration Assessment in Pediatrics

CLINICAL EXAMINATION	MILD (3%-5%)	MODERATE (6%-9%)	SEVERE (≥10%)
Heart rate	Normal, good volume	Rapid	Rapid, weak
Systolic pressure	Normal	Normal to low	Low
Respirations	Normal	Deep, rate may be increased	Deep, tachypnea
Mucosa	Tacky or slightly dry	Dry	Parched
Anterior fontanelle	Normal	Sunken	Markedly sunken
Eyes	Normal	Sunken	Markedly sunken
Skin turgor	Normal	Reduced	Tenting
Skin	Normal	Cool	Cool, mottled, acrocyanosis
Urine output	Normal or mildly reduced	Markedly reduced	Anuria
Systemic signs	Increased thirst	Listlessness, irritability	Grunting, lethargy, coma

- ■ **Physical examination**
  - Heart rate, blood pressure, capillary refill, skin turgor, sunken eyes, respiratory pattern, mucus membranes, overall appearance, and active/lethargic
- ■ **Investigations**
  - Serum
    - ◦ Electrolytes, urea, creatinine, glucose, calcium, osmolality
  - Urine
    - ◦ Increased urine specific gravity
    - ◦ Increased urine osmolality
- ■ **Causes**
  - GI losses—Nausea and vomiting
  - Dermal losses—Sweating, burns
  - Vascular losses—Trauma, hemorrhage
  - Diuretics
  - Pancreatitis
  - Heart failure
  - Cirrhosis with ascites
  - Renal disease
  - Diabetes/hyperglycemia
  - Psychogenic polydipsia
  - SIADH
  - Salt wasting nephropathy
  - Adrenal insufficiency

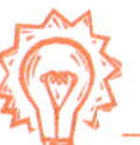

Hourly maintenance fluid: 4-2-1 Rule

4 mL/kg/h for 0 to 10 kg (first 10 kg of patient weight)

+

2 mL/kg/h for 10 to 20 kg (second 10 kg of patient weight)

+

1 mL/kg/h for each kg over 20 kg (eg, 60 kg person has a maintenance fluid rate of 100 mL/h)

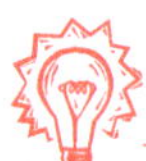

ONGOING LOSSES

One large vomit or one large diarrhea = 8 mL/kg body weight

Consider public health notification, for example, if restaurant related, large outbreak, nursing home

DIARRHEA RED FLAGS

- Fever
- Unintentional weight loss >10 lb
- Anemia
- Hematochezia or melena
- Positive fecal occult blood test
- Pus in stool
- Nocturnal defecation
- Symptoms refractory to treatment
- Family history of colon cancer or inflammatory bowel disease

Fever and diarrhea: Associated with invasive bacteria (eg, *Salmonella*, *Shigella*, *Campylobacter*), enteric viruses, and cytotoxic bacteria (eg, *Clostridium difficile*, *Entamoeba histolytica*)

Bloody diarrhea: associated with *Escherichia coli*, *Entamoeba histolytica*, Shigella, *Campylobacter*, Salmonella.

- **Treatment**
  - Fluid replacement
    - Oral fluids for mild-to-moderate dehydration and patient can tolerate po
    - IV fluids for severe dehydration, shock, and if oral not possible (eg, vomiting, altered level of consciousness)
  - Need to (1) replace deficit, (2) provide maintenance fluids, and (3) replace ongoing losses
    - Deficit replacement can be calculated with various formulas:
      - Deficit = (pre-illness weight) − (post-illness weight)
      - Deficit = (% deficit) × (10 ml/kg) × (pre-illness weight)
      - Deficit = (0.6 × weight) × (serum Na − 140)/140
  - Replace 1/2 the fluids (deficit + maintenance + ongoing losses) in the first 8 hours and the remaining over 16 hours

Diarrhea

ACUTE DIARRHEA

- Defined as diarrhea of <14 days duration
- **Risk factors**
  - Food, travel, medications, outbreaks, malignancy, IBD, IBS
- **Diagnosis**
  - Do not over investigate if no red flags
- **Investigations**
  - Assess for possible dehydration with physical examination
  - Stool:
    - Viral studies: If no blood or mucus or systemic signs
    - Gram stain, culture, and sensitivity: If immunocompromised, IBD, bloody diarrhea, or persistent
    - Ova, cysts, and parasites: If travel history or persistent diarrhea
    - *Clostridium difficile* toxin: if recent antibiotic use or persistent diarrhea
- **Treatment**
  - Rehydration and supportive care: avoid solid food or dairy
  - BRAT diet (banana, rice, apple sauce and toast)
  - Antibiotics should be considered if any of the following symptoms are present:
    - Severe traveller's diarrhea: >4 unformed stools/day, fever, and blood, pus or mucous in the stool
    - >8 stools per day
    - Symptoms for >1 week
    - Immunocompromised
    - Hospitalized patients
  - Probiotics
  - Loperamide (to reduce stool frequency)—Consider if no fever or bloody stool
- **Complications**
  - Hemolytic-uremic syndrome
  - *Clostridium difficile* infection
  - Toxic shock syndrome
  - Toxic megacolon

CHRONIC OR RECURRENT DIARRHEA

- Loose stools with or without increased stool frequency lasting 4 or more weeks
- Associated with multiple medical conditions
  - Consider: Malabsorption, inflammatory bowel disease, irritable bowel syndrome, infectious, maldigestion, laxative abuse, drugs/osmotic agents, disordered motility, neuroendocrine tumours, colon cancer, HIV, recent cholecystectomy, hyperthyroidism
- **Physical examination**
  - Signs of IBD (eg, mouth ulcers, skin rash, episcleritis)
  - DRE to assess for anal fissure or fistula (may indicate IBD), anal tone, and reflexes
  - Evidence of malabsorption (eg, wasting)
  - Abdominal masses
  - Lymphadenopathy
  - Thyroid
- **Investigations**
  - Blood work: CBC, TSH, electrolytes, albumin, creatinine, vitamin B_{12}, folate
  - Stool:
    - Leukocytes, occult blood, gram stain, culture and sensitivity, ova/cysts/parasites, *C. difficile*, pH, fat content
  - Also consider as prompted by history:
    - Serologic testing for Celiac disease, endoscopy, HIV serology, further stool testing
- **Diagnosis**
  - In elderly, diarrhea is more likely to be due to underlying pathology which may require investigation.
  - Initial test may include CBC, electrolytes, stool studies for occult blood, leukocytes, osmotic gap, pH, or fat.
  - Watery stool:
    - Osmotic (fecal osmotic gap >125 mOsm/kg): Fasting may resolve symptoms if dietary, breath hydrogen testing may detect lactose intolerance, celiac disease screening, check stool magnesium for laxative abuse
    - Secretory (fecal osmotic gap <50 mOsm/kg): stool culture, ova and parasites, look for metabolic causes
  - Fatty (fecal fat): May require imaging for structural disease or pancreatic insufficiency
  - Inflammatory (leukocytes and blood): Structural disease or infectious causes (*C. difficile*)
- **Treatment**
  - Will be indicated by history, examination, and investigation findings
  - Probiotics
  - Loperamide
  - Consider empiric metronidazole

MALDIGESTION/MALABSORPTION

- Malabsorption refers to impaired nutrient absorption.
- Maldigestion refers to impaired nutrient digestion.

- Normal nutrient absorption relies on:
  - (1) processing by brush border, (2) absorption into intestinal mucosa, and (3) transport into circulation
- Global malabsorption:
  - Mucosa is diffusely involved; or there is a decrease in absorptive surface, for example, celiac disease.
- Partial or isolated malabsorption:
  - Specific nutrient absorption is affected, for example, cobalamin malabsorption.
- **Presentation**
  - Usually vague symptoms, may have abdominal distention, flatulence, anorexia.
  - Global malabsorption: Pale, greasy, foul-smelling stools, weight loss.
  - Partial malabsorption: Related to specific nutrient; for example, cobalamin malabsorption will lead to pernicious anemia.
  - Assess for dehydration and effects of vitamin/mineral deficiencies
- **Diagnosis**
  - CBC, electrolytes, iron studies, vitamin B_{12}, folate, calcium, magnesium, phosphate, albumin, liver function tests
  - Tests for specific malabsorption
    - Fat malabsorption: Fecal fat
    - Carbohydrate malabsorption: D-xylose, lactose intolerance
    - Protein malabsorption: α1-antitrypsin clearance, stool chymotrypsin for pancreatic insufficiency
    - Vitamin B_{12}: Schilling test
  - Imaging: Abdominal US and endoscopy
- **Treatment**
  - Will be based on diagnosis

CELIAC DISEASE

- A malabsorption syndrome due to gluten intolerance
  - Gliadin is a fraction of gluten mainly responsible for triggering an immune reaction in genetically susceptible individuals
  - Small bowel effects include villous atrophy, mucosal inflammation, crypt hyperplasia; these changes resolve on removal of gluten from the diet.
- **Risk factors**
  - Family history, diabetes mellitus type II, persistent unexplained elevated AST and ALT on liver panel, HLA-DQ2, HLA-DQ8, possibly related to exposure to gluten in first 3 months of life.
  - Female > Male (2:1)
- **Complications**
  - Nutritional deficiencies (vitamin D, iron, calcium), intestinal ulcers or strictures, low bone mineral density, delayed puberty and menarche, decreased fertility until diagnosed and treated, low birth weight babies in untreated mothers
  - Increased risk of autoimmune disorders, malignancy, and specifically of T-cell lymphoma
- **Presentation**
  - Typically nonspecific with fatigue, chronic diarrhea, anorexia, bloating, weight loss, foul-smelling stool
  - Children often present with failure to thrive

■ **Extraintestinal manifestations**
- Skin: Dermatitis herpetiformis (pruritic papulovesicular rash on extensor surfaces)
- CNS: Cerebellar ataxia, peripheral neuropathy, irritability
- Heme: Iron or folate deficiency anemia (consider celiac in patients with refractory iron deficiency anemia), vitamin B_{12} deficiency

■ Associated conditions
- Autoimmune conditions: type 1 DM, autoimmune thyroiditis
- Genetic: HLA DQ2 and DQ8, trisomy 21, Turner syndrome, IgA deficiency

■ **Diagnosis**
- Clinical diagnosis is made based on history and positive serology; for confirmation, endoscopic biopsy is required.
- For testing a patient MUST be on a gluten-containing diet for at least 3 months.
- Response to a gluten-free diet is not diagnostic as this may be gluten sensitivity.
- Serology:
  ○ IgA tissue transglutaminase (tTG)—best single serological test
  ○ IgA antiendomysial antibody (EMA)
  ○ Both tTG and EMA have high sensitivity (89%-94%) and specificity (98%-99%)
- If serology is positive, refer to gastroenterology for biopsy.

■ **Treatment**
- Avoid gluten-containing foods lifelong: Barley, wheat, and rye; oats in diet appear safe but introduce with caution
- Treat nutritional deficiencies: Iron, folate, vitamin D, vitamin B_{12}.
- Dietician referral.
- Bone mineral density testing
  ○ Monitor symptoms resolution and repeat serology in 6 months.
  ○ Level 2 evidence for budesonide in addition to gluten-free diet resulting in decreased symptoms.

Bibliography

Bonis PAL, LaMont JT. Approach to the adult with chronic diarrhea in developed countries. In: Basow DS, ed. *UpToDate*. Waltham, MA; 2012. Retrieved from http://www.uptodate.com/. Accessed March 23, 2012.

DynaMed. *Acute Diarrhea in Adults*. Ipswich, MA: EBSCO Publishing; 2016. Retrieved from http://search.ebscohost.com.cyber.usask.ca/login.aspx?direct=true&site=DynaMed&id=113862. Accessed March 23, 2012.

DynaMed. *Celiac Disease*. Ipswich, MA: EBSCO Publishing; 2016. Retrieved from http://search.ebscohost.com.cyber.usask.ca/login.aspx?direct=true&site=DynaMed&id=113862. Accessed March 23, 2012.

DynaMed. *Chronic Diarrhea*. Ipswich, MA: EBSCO Publishing; 2016. Retrieved from http://search.ebscohost.com.cyber.usask.ca/login.aspx?direct=true&site=DynaMed&id=113862. Accessed March 23, 2012.

Kelly CP. Diagnosis of celiac disease. In: Basow DS, ed. *UpToDate*. Waltham, MA; 2012. Retrieved from http://www.uptodate.com/. Accessed March 23, 2012.

Schuppan D, Dieterich W. Pathogenesis, epidemiology, and clinical manifestations of celiac disease in adults. In: Basow DS, ed. *UpToDate*. Waltham, MA; 2012. Retrieved from http://www.uptodate.com/. Accessed March 23, 2012.

Wanke CA. Approach to the adult with acute diarrhea in developed countries. In: Basow DS, ed. *UpToDate*. Waltham, MA; 2012. Retrieved from http://www.uptodate.com/. Accessed March 23, 2012.

Dyspepsia

- Dyspepsia is a symptom and **not** a diagnosis.
- Differential diagnosis of patients presenting with dyspepsia includes:
  - Functional dyspepsia (ie, no organic pathology): Up to 60% of patients with typical symptoms
    - Rome III criteria for functional dyspepsia
      - >1 of the following for ≥3 months and onset ≥6 months prior to diagnosis
        - Bothersome postprandial fullness
        - Early satiety
        - Epigastric pain or burning
      - No evidence of structural disease to explain symptoms
  - Peptic ulcer disease: Up to 25% of dyspepsia
  - Gastritis
  - Gastroesophageal reflux disease (GERD)
  - Medications: Steroids, nonsteroidal anti-inflammatory drugs (NSAIDs) including COX-2 inhibitors and ASA, bisphosphonates, calcium channel blockers, digoxin
  - Irritable bowel syndrome
  - Pancreatitis
  - Biliary disease
  - Cancer
  - Consider cardiac chest pain!
- **Presentation**
  - Three common patterns (with a lot of overlap)
    - Ulcer-type/acid dyspepsia
      - Burning epigastric pain, relieved with antacids, food
      - Obtain history of NSAID use
    - Dysmotility type
      - Nausea, bloating, anorexia
    - Unspecified
- **Physical examination**
  - Should be normal, although may have epigastric tenderness
  - Look for abdominal masses, signs of anemia, signs of weight loss
  - Rectal examination or fecal occult blood if suggested by history
- **Investigations**
  - Will be based on age and presence of alarm symptoms
  - No investigations:
    - In patients with no alarm symptoms, no NSAID use, and a classic history of GERD-type symptoms.
    - In patients with NSAID use and no alarm symptoms.
  - *Helicobacter pylori* testing:
    - In patients with no alarm symptoms, and symptoms are not typical of GERD, and in patients with failed trial of acid suppression therapy
      - If testing is positive, treat with *H. pylori* eradication.
      - If testing is negative, trial PPI for 4 to 6 weeks.

DYSPEPSIA ALARM SYMPTOMS: VBAD

V—Vomit
B—Blood (hematemesis or melena)
A—Abdominal mass/anemia/age > 50
D—Dysphagia
Others: Weight loss, early satiety, refractory to treatment

- Endoscopy:
  - For any patient over 50, alarm symptoms, family history of cancer, or not responding to therapy

■ **Treatment**
- See discussion under GERD and PUD sections.
- Lifestyle modifications are number one!
  - Exercise, decrease alcohol, quit smoking, avoid spicy foods, decrease caffeine, avoid overeating especially in the evenings
  - Discontinue NSAIDs, or combine with acid suppression as discussed later if unable to discontinue.
- Acid suppression
  - Histamine-type 2 receptor blockers (H_2 blockers)
    - Standard dose PPI is more efficacious than H_2 blocker.
  - Proton pump inhibitors
    - Good evidence in heartburn and epigastric pain predominant dyspepsia.
    - Standard dose PPI is more efficacious than H_2 blocker.
    - Ineffective in patients with dysmotility (belching, bloating) type symptoms.
  - Bismuth salts
  - Antacids: Often used as self-medication; provide rapid, but less sustained symptom relief
- Prokinetics: Some evidence in functional and nonulcer dyspepsia
- Herbals: Peppermint, caraway, turmeric

PEPTIC ULCER DISEASE

■ Includes gastric and duodenal ulcers
- An increase in gastric acid secretion and a weakening of the mucosal barrier can result in ulcer formation.

■ **Risk factors**
- *Helicobacter pylori* infection and NSAID use are most common risk factors.
  - Note that most individuals infected with *H. pylori* do not develop ulcers.
- Other: Smoking, steroids, bisphosphonates, tumours, Crohn disease, gastritis (can be secondary to alcohol), radiation damage, CMV infection.

■ **Complications**
- Bleeding
- Penetration: Retroperitoneal
- Perforation: More common with duodenal ulcers
- Gastric outlet obstruction
- MALT lymphoma

■ **Presentation**
- Episodic epigastric pain.
- Symptom relief with eating, antacids, or acid suppression medications.
- Gastric ulcers more likely to have pain soon after eating.
- Duodenal ulcers—Pain relieved with food, pain during sleep, pain 3 hours after eating.
- Chronic ulcers—Asymptomatic, especially if NSAID-induced.

- **Investigations**
  - CBC, FOBT
  - *Helicobacter pylori* testing
    - Urea breath test—For active infection, useful for pre and posttreatment.
    - Serology (antibody testing)—Not useful if have been treated previously.
    - Fecal antigen testing—For active infection, less well-validated than breath test.
  - Endoscopy
    - Required if any family history of cancer, alarm symptoms, or if over 50 years old
    - For failed *H. pylori* eradication or not responding to treatment
  - Biopsy
    - Recommended for all gastric ulcers; duodenal ulcers are less likely to be malignant.
- **Treatment**
  - Lifestyle modifications
    - Exercise, decrease alcohol, quit smoking, eats small frequent meals, avoid spicy foods, decrease caffeine, avoid overeating especially in the evenings
    - Discontinue NSAIDs, or combine with acid suppression as discussed later if unable to discontinue
  - *Helicobacter pylori* eradication
    - First line: Triple therapy for 10 to 14 days
      - Proton pump inhibitor
      - Clarithromycin
      - Amoxicillin or metronidazole
    - Second line: Quadruple therapy for 10 to 14 days
      - Proton pump inhibitor or H_2 blocker
      - Bismuth subsalicylate
      - Metronidazole
      - Tetracycline
    - Patients with gastric ulcer may benefit from 3 weeks of PPI following eradication; however, evidence is lacking
  - For *H. pylori*-negative ulcers: Treat with PPI for 4 to 8 weeks.
  - Surgical treatment may be necessary in patients in whom medical therapy fails or perforated ulcer.

Helicobacter pylori serology can be positive for 1 to 2 years after treatment.

GASTROESOPHAGEAL REFLUX DISEASE

- Occurs when stomach contents reflux into the esophagus due to an inappropriate relaxation of the lower esophageal sphincter (LES), decreased LES tone, and delayed gastric emptying
  - Reflux contents may be gastric or bile (duodenogastroesophageal reflux)
- **Risk factors**
  - Increased intra-abdominal pressure, for example, pregnancy, obesity, chronic cough.
  - Smoking, alcohol ingestion, eating spicy, fatty, citrus foods.
  - Medications that decrease LES pressure:
    - Calcium channel blockers, anticholinergics, theophylline, nitrates, sildenafil, albuterol
  - *Helicobacter pylori* infection is not associated with GERD, in fact there is a lower prevalence of *H. pylori* in patients with GERD.

- ■ **Complications**
  - Barrett esophagus, esophageal adenocarcinoma, chronic laryngitis, asthma, dental erosions
- ■ **Presentation**
  - Heartburn sensation (aka acid brash or water brash)—Burning or discomfort behind sternum, rising into neck, worse after meals, worse when lying flat, relieved with antacids
  - Regurgitation—Flow of acid secretions into mouth
  - Atypical presentations include: Cough, laryngitis, hoarse voice, halitosis, chest pain
- ■ **Physical examination**
  - Typically normal
  - May see evidence of dental erosions, nasopharyngeal sinusitis, nasal or pharyngeal polyps
- ■ **Alarm symptoms**
  - Vomiting, blood loss, age > 50 years, abdominal mass, dysphagia, weight loss
- ■ **Diagnosis**
  - Presumptive diagnosis based on history, lack of alarm symptoms, and <50 years
    - Confirmed with symptomatic improvement with 4 to 6 week trial of acid suppression treatment
  - If no symptomatic relief, consider alternate diagnosis, may require endoscopy (see "Dyspepsia")
- ■ **Treatment**
  - Lifestyle modifications
    - Elevate head of bed, avoid acidic foods, avoid large meals
    - Exercise, decrease alcohol, quit smoking, avoid spicy foods, decrease caffeine, avoid overeating especially in the evenings
  - Proton pump inhibitor or H_2-receptor blocker
    - Standard dose PPI is more efficacious than H_2 blocker.
  - Reassess therapy at **4 to 8 weeks**
    - If no response, consider increased dose, or change to PPI if on H_2 blocker.
    - If no symptomatic relief still, consider alternate diagnosis, may require endoscopy (see "Dyspepsia").
  - Reassess need for long-term therapy periodically and wean to minimum effective dose (or discontinue if symptoms do not recur).
  - May consider on-demand PPI use in patients who have had good response to PPI therapy.
  - Consider endoscopy to assess for Barrett esophagus if patient has been on therapy for 10 years.
  - Long-term risks of PPI use: *C. difficile*, hip fracture, pneumonia, hypoparathyroid, vitamin B_{12} deficiency, iron deficiency anemia

Must use urea breath test if testing for cure. Do test 4 weeks after treatment is completed, if indicated.

Bibliography

Canadian Agency for Drugs and Technologies in Health. Screening and diagnostic tests before endoscopy: clinical evidence and guidelines. 2011. Retrieved from http://www.cadth.ca/media/pdf/htis/oct-2011/RB0434-000%20Endoscopy%20Guidelines.pdf. Accessed March 23, 2012.

DynaMed. *Functional Dyspepsia.* Ipswich, MA: EBSCO Publishing; 2016. Retrieved from http://search.ebscohost.com.cyber.usask.ca/login.aspx?direct=true&site=DynaMed&id=113862. Accessed March 23, 2012.

DynaMed. *Peptic Ulcer Disease.* Ipswich, MA: EBSCO Publishing; 2016. Retrieved from http://search.ebscohost.com.cyber.usask.ca/login.aspx?direct=true&site=DynaMed&id=113862. Accessed March 23, 2012.

Longstreth GF. Approach to the patient with dyspepsia. In: Basow DS, ed. *UpToDate*. Waltham, MA; 2012. Retrieved from http://www.uptodate.com/. Accessed March 23, 2012.

Schuster B. Gastrointestinal-acid suppression drugs: evidence, tips and pearls. *RxFiles Drug Comparison Charts*. 10th ed. Saskatoon, SK: Saskatoon Health Region; 2010:63-64.

Schuster B. *H. pylori. RxFiles Drug Comparison Charts*, 10th ed. Saskatoon, SK: Saskatoon Health Region; 2010: 65.

Gastrointestinal Bleeding

TABLE 4-6	Upper and Lower GI Bleed	
	UPPER GI BLEED	**LOWER GI BLEED**
Definition	• Bleeding from the gastrointestinal tract proximal to the ligament of Treitz	• Bleeding from the gastrointestinal tract distal to the ligament of Treitz

Etiology	• Peptic ulcer disease
	• Varices
	• Gastritis (eg, NSAID/ETOH induced)
	• Esophagitis
	• Mallory-Weiss tear
	• Vascular anomalies
	• Malignancy
		• Hemorrhoids
		• Anal fissure
		• Diverticular bleeding
		• Ischemic bowel disease
		• Inflammatory bowel disease
		• Colonic ulcer
		• Malignancy
		• Vascular lesions
		• Pediatric
		  • Intussusception
		  • Meckel diverticulum

Presentation	• Melena—Black tarry stool indicates digested upper GI blood • Hematochezia—Bright rectal bleed indicates profuse upper GI bleed • Hematemesis—Bright red indicates fresh bleed • Coffee ground emesis—Indicates digested blood	• Hematochezia • Melena
Investigations	• CBC • INR and PTT • Electrolytes, urea, creatinine, LFTs • ECG • Type and crossmatch • Esophagoduodenoscopy	• CBC • INR and PTT • Electrolytes, urea, creatinine, LFTs • ECG • Type and crossmatch • Sigmoidoscopy and/or colonoscopy(may start with sigmoid in unprepared bowel) • Angiography if bleeding >0.5 mL/min
Treatment	• Proton pump inhibitor • NPO +/− NG tube • Esophagoduodenoscopy (both diagnostic and therapeutic) • For suspected varices: Somatostatin analog (eg, octreotide), and continue for 3-5 days post confirmation • *Helicobacter pylori* testing and treatment if peptic ulcers diagnosed • Antibiotics in patients with cirrhosis	• NPO +/− NG tube (rule out upper GI cause) • Identify and treat source of bleeding • Consider risks/benefits of anticoagulants, NSAIDs, aspirin, steroids, SSRIs

■ **Risk factors**

- Alcohol, smoking, liver cirrhosis, *H. pylori* infection, chronic renal insufficiency, ICU admission, previous GI bleed
- Medications: Anticoagulant therapy, NSAIDs, steroids, calcium channel blockers, SSRIs
- Modify treatment to reduce risk (eg, cytoprotection)

■ Be sure to inquire about diet and medications which can cause red or black stool

- Beets, iron, Pepto-Bismol

- **Presentation**
  - Depends on degree of bleeding
    - Differentiate between upper and lower GI bleed if possible.
      - Upper GI bleed: Black stools/melena but still may have bright red blood if profuse.
      - Lower GI bleed: Bright red blood.
    - Recognize causes before shock and resuscitate as needed.

ESOPHAGEAL VARICEAL BLEEDING

- Consider in all patients with upper GI bleeding and a history of liver cirrhosis
- **Risk factors**
  - Cirrhosis with portal hypertension and development of gastric or esophageal varices, ascites, active alcohol use.
- Regular endoscopies to monitor varices and prevent bleeds.
- Consider antibiotic prophylaxis if upper GI bleed and cirrhosis to prevent spontaneous bacterial peritonitis.
- **Treatment**
  - Acute: Somatostatin analogue, for example, octreotide
  - Chronic: Nonselective β-blocker, for example, propranolol to decrease heart rate by 25% and prevent rebleeding

TABLE 4-7 Degree of Blood Loss in Adults

FIT MALE, 70 KG (5 L OF BLOOD WHEN WELL)	CLASS I	CLASS II	CLASS III	CLASS IV
Blood loss	750 mL	750-1000 mL	1500-2000 mL	>2000 mL
HR	Normal	100-120	>120	>140
BP	Normal	Normal, postural hypotension	Often Normal, may see narrow pulse pressure	↓↓
CNS	Normal	Anxious	Agitated	↓ consciousness
Respiratory rate	Normal	↑	↑↑	↑↑↑
Urine output	↓	↓↓	Minimal	None
Replacement fluid	Normal Saline	Normal Saline/ Ringer's lactate	Mix—crystalloid, colloid, plasma	Blood ± colloid

Bibliography

DynaMed. *Acute Lower Gastrointestinal Bleeding*. Ipswich, MA: EBSCO Publishing; 2016. Retrieved from http://search.ebscohost.com.cyber.usask.ca/login.aspx?direct=true&site=DynaMed&id=113862. Accessed March 23, 2012.

DynaMed. *Acute Upper Gastrointestinal Bleeding*. Ipswich, MA: EBSCO Publishing; 2016. Retrieved from http://search.ebscohost.com.cyber.usask.ca/login.aspx?direct=true&site=DynaMed&id=113862. Accessed March 23, 2012.

Leddin DJ, Enns R, Hilsden R, et al. Canadian Association of Gastroenterology position statement on screening individuals at risk for developing colorectal cancer: 2010. *Can J Gastroenterol.* 2010;24(12):705-714.

CHAPTER 5

Pediatrics

In Newborns

Priority Topic 67

IMPORTANT POINTS

- Always look for subtle physical anomalies that may hint toward an association with other anomalies or syndromes. For example, low-set ears, sacral dimples, jaundice, cyanosis, head circumference, fontanelle size, cleft lip/palate, murmurs, hips, palmar creases.
- When assessing newborns with nonspecific concerns from the caregiver, **always** think of sepsis as a differential and look for signs as it may not present as in adults. For example, feeding difficulties, respiratory changes, irritability, maternal GBS status, maternal fever, maternal history of recent STI, PROM, and other signs and symptoms of sepsis.
- Stay up to date with neonatal resuscitation guidelines if you have newborns in your practice.
- Encourage breastfeeding for newborn babies, but do not criticize a parent's decision to bottle feed.
- Continually monitor for abnormalities such as hip abnormalities, hearing difficulties, heart murmurs, as they may not be immediately obvious.
  - Well baby checks begin routinely at 1 to 2 weeks of age, following the Rourke baby record.
- Educate parents on signs and symptoms of impending illness when discharging newborns from hospital and ensure that they are aware of how to access care.
  - Fever in newborns <3 months warrants evaluation. If changes are noted in eating, sleeping, bowel or bladder habits of the babies, they should be assessed.

Bibliography

Working Group on the Certification Process. *Priority Topics and Key Features with Corresponding Skill Dimensions and Phases of the Encounter.* The College of Family Physicians of Canada.

Well Baby Care
Priority Topic 99

- Assess development, weight, height, and head circumference at every visit and chart on growth scale (WHO Canadian Growth Chart).
- Provide anticipatory information for developmental milestones.
- Always ask about family adjustment, include mood disorders.
- Always have child abuse as a differential, especially for unusual symptoms or injuries.
- Discuss the importance of vaccination, and address parental questions/hesitancy toward vaccines.
- Be aware of cultural factors and resources available (eg, circumcision).
- Screen for anemia at 6 to 12 months in at-risk populations (eg, lower socioeconomic status, Asians, First Nations, low birth weight babies, infants fed with whole cow's milk within the first year of life).
- Acetaminophen can be used as antipyretic—10 to 15 mg/kg/dose every 4 to 6 hours. Ibuprofen can also be used >6 months—4 to 10 mg/kg/dose every 6 to 8 hours.

Address all of following at each visit:

A. General questions
- Note risk factors, family history, pregnancy history, delivery history (including resuscitation).
- Address parental concerns at every visit.

B. Feeding
- Exclusive breastfeeding is recommended for the first 6 months by Health Canada, and should be encouraged and supported in those mothers who choose to do so.
- Breastfed babies should receive 400 IU daily vitamin D supplementation.
  - Of note, the CPS recommends 800 IU daily particularly for those in northern communities due to decreased sun exposure.
- No honey in the first year.
- No beets, carrots, spinach, or turnips before 6 months (contain nitrates).
- Encourage parents to start with iron-containing foods when introducing first solids, although no specific recommendations on order of foods being introduced exist.
- Avoid dry, solid, round, smooth, or sticky foods that can cause choking and sugary foods and drinks.
- Introduce new foods one at a time, with at least 3 days in between to monitor for reactions.
- According to the CPS, there is no evidence that delaying any foods beyond 6 to 12 months decreases the risk of forming allergies. This holds true for children deemed to be high risk as well (those with siblings or parents with allergies/asthma/atopic dermatitis/allergic rhinitis).

C. Developmental milestones
- Should be monitored closely.
- Delay in achieving age-appropriate milestones may unmask an underlying developmental/learning disorder.

Use ROURKE in clinical practice http://www.rourkebabyrecord.ca/.

Well baby checks are recommended at 1 week, 2 months, 4 months, 6 months, 12 months, 18 months, 2 to 3 years, and 4 to 5 years. Some family physicians also do visits at 2 weeks, 9 months and 15 months as well. Add additional visits if the child is unwell or needs closer monitoring.

TABLE 5-1	Baby's First Foods
0-6 months	Recommend exclusive breastfeeding for the first 6 months of life with 400 IU of vitamin D supplementation • Can express breast milk, can freeze for up to 6 months, and refrigerate for up to 3 days • Warm milk by placing in warm water (microwaving can destroy vitamins) If feeding with formula, use iron-fortified formulas, 5 oz/kg/day for first 2 weeks then increase
6-9 months	Start with iron-fortified infant cereals, grain products such as dry toast or crackers pureed cooked yellow, green, orange vegetables, pureed cooked fruits, ripe mashed fruits pureed cooked meat, fish, chicken, tofu, mashed beans, egg yolk
9-12 months	Plain cereals, whole grain bread, rice, pasta soft mashed, cooked vegetables, soft fresh fruits, peeled, seeded, diced, canned fruits (in water or juice) minced/diced meat, fish, chicken, tofu At 9 months, offer high fat yogurt, cottage cheese, grated hard cheese, **introduce whole milk from 9-12 months**, limit milk products to 720 mL/day (risk of iron deficiency anemia)

http://www.caringforkids.cps.ca/handouts/feeding_your_baby_in_the_first_year. See introducing solid foods.

TABLE 5-2	Developmental Milestones			
AGE	**GROSS MOTOR**	**FINE MOTOR**	**LANGUAGE**	**SOCIAL/COGNITION**
1 month	Focus gaze, startles with loud noises	Sucks well on nipple		Calms when comforted
2 months	Lifts head/chest when lying on stomach	Vision tracks past midline	Coos, reacts to sounds	Recognizes parent, smiles socially; comforted by touching and rocking
4-5 months	Rolls from front to back and vice versa, can hold head steady when chest supported while sitting	Can grip toys such as rattles, can follow movements with their eyes	Laughs, squeals, starts to make sounds of consonants, can orient to voices	Likes to look around, laughs
6 months	Sits with support, rolls from back to side	Transfers between hands, raking grasp	Babbles	Stranger anxiety, turns head toward sounds, voices pleasure/displeasure
9-10 months	Sits without support, stands with support	Three-finger pincer grasp	Mama/dada nonspecific, first word ~ 11 months	Can wave bye-bye, can play pat-a-cake, looks for an object that is seen hidden, responds differently with different people
12 months	Can throw things, crawls/bum shuffle, pulls to stand/walks	Two-finger pincer grasp	3+ words (do not have to be clear), can follow 1-step commands	Imitates, has separation anxiety, responds to own name
18 months	Walks alone, (walks sideways while holding onto furniture at 15 months)	Feeds self with spoon with little spilling	Learning body parts, responds when name is called, points to what is wanted, 20+ words, imitates sounds/speech	Behaviour is usually manageable, interested in other kids, soothes easily, seeks out comfort when distressed
2 years	Jumps, walks up/down stairs with help, walk backward 2 steps without help, tries to run	Can build tower of 6 cubes, puts objects into small container	Two-word phrases	Obeys 2-step commands, removes clothes alone
3 years	Can ride tricycle, climb stairs with support of railing	Uses cutlery and utensils, can copy a circle, can twist a lid off a jar, turns pages one at a time	Five-word sentences	Can brush teeth assisted, can wash and dry hands, understands 2+3 step commands, shares some of the time
4 years	Can hop on two feet, can climb stairs with alternating feet	Can copy a cross and a square (closer to 4.5 years), undoes buttons and zippers	Recognizes colours and some numbers	Can play cooperatively, and play board games, asks a lot of questions, tries to comfort someone that is upset
5 years	Can skip and walk backward, can hop on one foot	Can copy a triangle, can tie shoelaces, can recognize right vs left, can print letters, can throw/catch a ball	Speaks clearly most of the time in adult-like sentences	Can play dress-up and domestic role playing

Chart adapted from Le T, et al. High Yield Facts in Pediatrics: Development. *First Aid for the USMLE Step 2 CK*. 8th ed. McGraw-Hill, New York; NY: 2012. Updated to correlate with the Rourke Baby Record, 2014 National English Edition.

D. Education
- Car seat, helmets
- Bath safety
- Second-hand smoke
- Sleeping position, crib safety, safe toys
- Fever advice
- Child proofing, keep over the counter meds and poisons out of reach

E. Physical examination
- Measure height, weight, and head circumference at every visit (WHO Canadian Growth Chart)
- Correct percentiles if born at <37 weeks, until 24 to 36 months
- Check skin, fontanelles, red reflex, heart, lungs, abdomen, umbilicus, hips, tone, testicles, foreskin

Bibliography

The Canadian Pediatric Society. *Dietary exposures and allergy prevention in high-risk infants.* 2013 (reaffirmed 2016). http://www.cps.ca/documents/position/dietary-exposures-and-allergy-prevention-in-high-risk-infants.

The Canadian Pediatric Society. *Pregnancy and babies—feeding your baby in the first year.* 2006. http://www.caringforkids.cps.ca/handouts/feeding_your_baby_in_the_first_year.

The Canadian Pediatric Society. *Vitamin D supplementation: Recommendations for Canadian mothers and infants.* 2007 (reaffirmed 2015). http://www.cps.ca/documents/position/vitamin-d.

Health Canada—Food and Nutrition. *Nutrition for healthy term infants—statement of the Joint Working Group: Canadian Paediatric Society, Dieticians of Canada and Health Canada.* 2007. http://www.hc-sc.gc.ca/fn-an/pubs/infant-nourrisson/nut_infant_nourrisson_term-eng.php.

Le T, Bhushan V, Lee K, et al. Developmental milestones. *First Aid for the USMLE Step 2 CK.* 5th ed. New York, NY: McGraw-Hill; 2005:302.

Leslie R, Denis L, James R, *Rourke Baby Record—Evidence-based infant/child health maintenance guide.* 2014. http://www.rourkebabyrecord.ca/.

In Children
Priority Topic 50

IMPORTANT POINTS

- Always keep your differential broad to include common medical problems such as UTIs, pneumonia, depression, appendicitis, as they may present differently in children. For example, depression can present with more aggression, anger, acting out in children and adolescents.
- At every visit, try to ask about other aspects of their lives—school performance, relationships, friends, home life, bullying, modifiable risk factors such as exercise or diet, and practicing preventative measures such as wearing helmets and seatbelts.
- Ask directly about risky behaviours such as drug use, smoking, driving, and sex.
- Advise adolescents that their visits are confidential but try to encourage them to openly discuss issues with their parents/guardians such as sex, birth control, bullying, drugs, pregnancy, suicide, depression.
- Always have child abuse as a differential, especially for unusual symptoms or injuries.
- Always use age-appropriate language, and try to talk to children and adolescents directly, rather than just to their parents.

- When communicating with children, come to their eye level.
- Do not limit investigations if they are needed just because they may cause distress for the patient or parents.

Bibliography

Chen YA, Tran C. Chapters 23 (Pediatrics) and 26 (Psychiatry). *Toronto Notes—Comprehensive Medical Reference & Review for MCCQE I and USMLE II*. Toronto, Canada: Toronto Notes for Medical Students Inc; 2011.

Working Group on the Certification Process. Priority topics and key features with corresponding skill dimensions and phases of the encounter. The College of Family Physicians of Canada; 2010.

HEADSS mnemonic—cover these points when assessing children and adolescents
- Home life
- Education
- Activities/social
- Drugs
- Sex
- Smoking

Learning
Priority Topic 57

IMPORTANT POINTS

- Early detection improves outcome. Routinely ask about a child's performance at school.
- Always consider hearing and visual difficulties and psychiatric disease when children present with learning difficulties.
- Try to always ask about learning difficulties at routine visits.
- Five areas of potential difficulty: Intelligence, academic achievement, attention/concentration, perceptual (visual/motor) function, and behaviour.
- Can also have difficulty with listening, speaking, writing, reasoning, or computing.
- Always assess the impact of disability on family and child.
- Use history, examination, and investigations to identify/exclude medical causes (eg, otitis media, iron deficiency, hearing difficulty), detect trauma, perinatal events, pregnancy history, school performance, hobbies, family history of similar problems, behavioural problems, substance, verbal, physical abuse, developmental delay.
- Educate parents to their level of understanding about their child's condition.
- Try to organize community resources for family.
  - Multidisciplinary team members can include family doctors, pediatricians, parents, psychologist, teachers, nurses, educators, counsellors, administrators, social workers, occupational therapists, physiotherapy, speech and language specialist.

AUTISM SPECTRUM DISORDER

- DSM - V diagnostic criteria was introduced in 2013 for autism spectrum disorder, and integrated the other learning disorders (Asperger syndrome, pervasive developmental disorder, and childhood disintegrative disorder).
- Diagnosis is now based on *4 domains* of symptoms, and is further classified based on level of severity/level of support needed (1 mild, 2 moderate, 3 severe).
  1. *Impairment in social interaction and communication* (needs impairment in all 3: Social and emotional reciprocity, nonverbal communication, creating and maintaining relationships)
  2. *Abnormal and repetitive behaviour, interest, activities* (2/4 subtypes needed: Stereotyped speech and behaviour, resistance to change, fixated interests, hyper[or hypo] sensitivity to sensory input)
  3. *Presentation in early childhood development*
  4. *Limited and hindered everyday activities*

- A validated screening tool now exists, called M-CHAT, which consists of 23 yes/no questions and provides a low/moderate/high risk of ASD being present. There is additionally a follow-up questionnaire available for those in the moderate risk group.

- Hearing screening, along with screening labs (CBC, iron studies, TSH, etc.) should be completed when considering a diagnosis of ASD.

- When concerns are identified, consultation with pediatric developmental specialists, or child psychiatrists is recommended to assess and manage their developmental follow-up needs.

- These children will benefit from a multidisciplinary approach (PT, SLP, OT, psychologist, social worker).

- Advise the parents on peer-support groups available for autism (such as Autism Society).

Bibliography

Augustyn M, et al. Clinical features of autism spectrum disorders. 2011. http://www.uptodate.com/-contents/clinical-features-of-autism-spectrum-disorders?view=print.

Lee PF, Thomas R, Lee PA, et al. Canadian Family Physician. *Approach to autism spectrum disorder*. 2015. http://www.cfp.ca/content/61/5/421.full.pdf+html.

Chen YA, Tran C. Chapters 23 (Pediatrics) and 26 (Psychiatry). *Toronto Notes—Comprehensive Medical Reference & Review for MCCQE I and USMLE II*. Toronto, Canada: Toronto Notes for Medical Students Inc; 2011.

Phillips DM, Longlett SK, Mulrine C, et al. School problems and the family physician. *Am Fam Physician*. 1999;59(10):2816-2824. http://www.aafp.org/afp/1999/0515/p2816.html.

Robins Diana L. *M-CHAT*. 2016. http://mchatscreen.com/.

Von Hahn L, et al. Specific learning disabilities in children: Evaluation. 2010. http://www.uptodate.com/contents/specific-learning-disabilities-in-children-evaluation?

Von Hahn L, et al. Specific learning disabilities in children: Role of the primary care provider. 2011. http://www.uptodate.com/contents/specific-learning-disabilities-in-children-role-of-the-primary-care-provider?

Immunizations

Priority Topic 49

IMPORTANT POINTS

- Document **all** vaccinations.

- Inquire about immunization status if presenting with infectious disease as treatment options might be different if unvaccinated.

- Vaccination is not a guarantee of protection!

- Should **not** be delayed in mild acute illness, concurrent antibiotic use, or seizure.

- There are very few TRUE contraindications/precautions to vaccinations (per the National Advisory Committee on Immunizations [NACI]).

  - Anaphylaxis to vaccine or component previously.

  - SEVERE asthma (optimize before vaccinating, live attenuated influenza vaccine [LAIV] should not be given to those with severe asthma and those attended medically with wheeze).

  - Congenital malformation of GI tract, or history of intussusception (rotavirus vaccination is contraindicated in these children).

  - Guillain–Barre syndrome onset within 6 weeks of vaccination (reported with TD and influenza).

- Immunocompromised individuals (no live vaccinations, unless not severely immunocompromised then can consider) (review vaccination status prior to starting immunosuppressant therapy if able).
- Pregnancy (live vaccines contraindicated).
- TB, active and untreated (measles/mumps/rubella [MMR], MMRV, varicella, herpes zoster contraindicated as precautionary measure).

■ Vaccines and autism—Most recent research suggests **NO** link between development of autism and vaccines (2006 Immunization Guide—*Health Canada*).

TABLE 5-3 Specific Groups Benefitting from Vaccination

GROUP	RECOMMENDED VACCINATIONS
>65 years	Pneumococcal × 1 (or more often if at high risk), yearly influenza vaccine
Sickle cell/β-thalassemia	Pneumococcal (both polysaccharide and conjugated), *Haemophilus influenzae* B, meningococcal, influenza (yearly)
Chronic liver disease	Hepatitis A and B, +/− pneumococcal, influenza
Health-care workers	Hepatitis A and B, yearly influenza
HIV	No live vaccinations (MMR, varicella, yellow fever, oral typhoid, rotavirus, FluMist, BCG, zoster, smallpox) Pneumococcal, influenza (yearly), meningococcal
Chronic disease (COPD, DM, CKD)	Pneumococcal, yearly influenza
G or C—females 9-26 years, may be given to females >26 years G—males 9-26 years, males >9 years who have sex with men	HPV (Gardasil [G])—HPV types 6,11,16, 18, Cervarix (C)—HPV types 16 and 18 **Gardasil 9 has been approved by Health Canada and targets 9 strains of HPV
Travellers	Yellow fever, typhoid, Japanese encephalitis, Dukoral (*Vibrio cholerae* and ETEC), RotaTeq (rotavirus), hepatitis (Twinrix), measles, mumps, rubella, pertussis, typhoid, tetanus, diphtheria, meningococcal (Saudi Arabia), rabies, malaria oral prophylaxis depending on destination

Rules for Vaccinating Certain Populations

1. Allergy—Thimerosal, egg, latex, preservatives
   - Eggs—Do not give yellow fever vaccinations
   - Streptomycin/neomycin—Do not give inactivated poliomyelitis (IPV), measles/mumps/rubella (MMR)
2. Live vaccines—Give 1 month apart, or at separate sites
3. Pregnancy—No live vaccinations (MMR, varicella, LAIV)
4. Breastfeeding—Safe to vaccinate except smallpox and yellow fever
5. Preterm infants:
   - Vaccinate based on chronological age, not from birth date
   - Must be >2 kg for first hepatitis B vaccination
6. Anaphylaxis/encephalopathy/CNS complication with DTaP—Can give only DT (no pertussis)
7. Previous vaccination reaction—There are **no** contraindications for further vaccinations. Note vaccination reaction:
   - Temperature <40.5°C
   - Redness, swelling, sore at injection sit
8. Asplenia—Requires pneumococcal, HiB, meningococcal, influenza

Egg allergy is no longer a contraindication to influenza vaccine. Please see www.publichealth.gc.ca. for details.

9. Influenza—Those receiving their first ever vaccination, between 6 months and 9 years require two immunizations at a minimum of 4 weeks apart. Any time thereafter can be a solo injection. Also, live attenuated vaccination is contraindicated in those under 2 years of age, due to increased incidence of wheezing.

- Of note: Potential up-coming vaccine: Bexsero. It is a multicomponent vaccine for meningococcal serogroup B (4CMenB). Men B is now the most prevalent serogroup (which has no current vaccine coverage, beside Bexsero), due to declining incidence of Men C from vaccination efforts. This vaccination can be considered in certain situations, mainly those individuals at highest risk of contracting invasive meningococcal disease. However, Bexsero is not yet recommended for routine use by National Advisory Committee on Immunization.

- Also Gardasil 9 has been approved by Health Canada and may become more readily available in the near future as it covers 9 strains of HPV rather than the previous 4 strains.

The immunization schedule details vary in each province in Canada. Please see provincial guidelines.

TABLE 5-4	Routine Adult Vaccines
RECOMMENDED VACCINE	**DOSAGE**
Tetanus, diphtheria, pertussis	Td every 10 years, Tdap if not given before × 1
Measles, mumps, rubella	Once in adulthood if born after 1970
Varicella	Not if history of chickenpox, two doses in adulthood if not immune (especially immigrants, females of childbearing age, immunocompromised, cystic fibrosis)

TABLE 5-5	Vaccine Classifications
Live attenuated	MMR, oral polio, typhoid, yellow fever, anthrax, intranasal influenza, varicella
Killed	Salk polio (IPV)
Inactivated	Hepatitis B vaccine, DTaP (DT-inactivated toxin, P is inactivated cells)
Capsular polysaccharide	Pneumococcal, *H. influenzae*

TABLE 5-6	Pediatric Immunization Schedule Summarized[†]
AGE	**VACCINES NEEDED**
2 months[*] 4 months[*] 6 months[*] 18 months[*]	Tdap Pneumoccocal HiB IPV
12 months	MMR VZV Meningococcal
18 months	MMR VZV
4-6 years	Tdap IPV
>6 years	HPV (>9 yo, routine in females, recommended by NACI in males) Meningococcal

[*]Each age requires all vaccinations in right column.
[†]May differ based on individual provincial schedules.

Bibliography

Government of Canada. *Canadian Immunization Guide: Part 2 – Vaccine Safety*. 2016. http://healthycanadians.gc.ca/publications/healthy-living-vie-saine/2-canadian-immunization-guide-canadien-immunisation/index-eng.php?page=3.

Government of Canada. *Canadian Immunization Guide: Part 4 – Active Vaccines*. Updated September 2016. http://healthycanadians.gc.ca/publications/healthy-living-vie-saine/4-canadian-immunization-guide-canadien-immunisation/index-eng.php?page=9#p4c8a3.

Government of Canada. *Canadian Immunization Guide: Part 4 – Active Vaccines: Human Papillomavirus Vaccine*. Updated July 2016. Public Health Agency of Canada. Canada communicable disease report—Volume 38, ACS-1—update on human papillomavirus virus (HPV) Vaccines. Jan 2012. http://www.phac-aspc.gc.ca/publicat/ccdr-rmtc/12vol38/acs-dcc-1/index-eng.php#a3-3.

Public Health Agency of Canada. *Canadian Immunization Guide*. 7th ed. 2006. http://www.phac-aspc.gc.ca/publicat/cig-gci/.

Public Health Agency of Canada. The Recommended Use of the Multicomponent Meningococcal B (4CMenB) Vaccine in Canada. 2014. http://www.phac-aspc.gc.ca/naci-ccni/mening-4cmenb-exec-resum-eng.php#toc_5.

Public Health Agency of Canada. Travel vaccines. 2007. http://www.phac-aspc.gc.ca/im/travelvaccines-eng.php.

Rx Files Academic Detailing Program. *Rx Files—Drug Comparison Charts: Vaccinations*. 10th ed. 73; 2014.

CHAPTER 6

Psychiatry

Depression

Priority Topic 24

MAJOR DEPRESSIVE EPISODE (MDE)

For at least 2 weeks, the patient experiences at least five depressive symptoms (depressed mood or decreased interest, plus four others)

Risk Factors for MDE

- Neuroticism (negative affectivity)
- Recent stressful life event, injury, or illness
- Chronic pain, fatigue, or insomnia
- Chronic medical illnesses
- Other psychiatric disorders (eg, substance use, anxiety)
- Adverse childhood experiences
- First-degree family history of MDE (heritability is 40%)[1]

Treatment

- Assess suicide risk at every evaluation.
- Monitor treatment response using validated outcome measures, such as Patient Health Questionnaire 9 (PHQ-9).
- Aim for remission of symptoms to baseline psychological function [eg, PHQ-9 score of <5].
- Plan two phases of treatment:
  - Acute—To achieve remission (8-12 weeks duration, visits every 1-2 weeks).
  - Maintenance—To prevent relapse/recurrence (at least 6 months, but often longer)
- Follow-up weekly or biweekly, depending on severity, until clear improvement identified. After that, visits can be reduced to monthly and then less often.

Therapies

- Combination psychotherapy and pharmacotherapy is more effective than either treatment alone [1-4].
- Psychotherapy and pharmacotherapy monotherapies appear to be equivalent in efficacy [5].

DEPRESSIVE SYMPTOMS (MSIGECAPS)

- **M**—Depressed mood
- **S**—Sleep disturbance
- **I**—Interest reduced
- **G**—Guilt and self-blame
- **E**—Energy loss and fatigue
- **C**—Concentration problems
- **A**—Appetite change
- **P**—Psychomotor changes
- **S**—Suicidal thoughts

COMMON ANTIDEPRESSANT SIDE EFFECTS

(1) Nausea

(2) Insomnia/agitation

(3) Weight gain (eg, mirtazapine, trazodone)

(4) Somnolence (eg, trazodone)

(5) Orthostatic hypotension

(6) Headache

(7) Sexual dysfunction (eg, SSRIs)

- No one psychotherapy appears to be more efficacious than the others [6,7] (eg, CBT, interpersonal therapy). Choose based on availability.
- Second-generation selective serotonin reuptake inhibitors (SSRIs) do not clinically differ in efficacy, and should be selected based on adverse events and onset of action [8,9].
- Tricyclic antidepressants (TCAs) and monoamine oxidase inhibitors (MAOIs) are second-line treatments because of safety and tolerability issues.
- For antidepressant treatment, expect the usual trajectory of response:
  - Initial mild symptom improvement (eg, >20% improvement in PHQ-9) within 2 to 4 weeks
  - Good clinical response (eg, >50% improvement in PHQ-9) within 4 to 8 weeks
  - Remission of symptoms (eg, PHQ-9 <5) by 8 to 12 weeks

MAINTENANCE PHARMACOTHERAPY

- The antidepressant dosage in the maintenance phase should be the same as in the acute phase.
- All patients should be maintained on antidepressants for at least 6 months after clinical remission.
- Patients with the following risk factors should be maintained on antidepressants for at least 2 years: Older age, psychotic features, chronic episodes, recurrent episodes (three or more in lifetime), frequent episodes (two or more in 5 years), difficult-to-treat episodes, and severe episodes.
- Taper antidepressants slowly to avoid relapse. Provide regular follow-up every 2 to 3 months for the first 6 months. Psychotherapy is helpful to prevent relapse.

MANAGING NONRESPONSE TO ANTIDEPRESSANT THERAPY

- If improvement is not following usual trajectory of response (as above), the following are indicated in the order listed:
  - Optimize the antidepressant by increasing the dose as tolerated.
  - Switch to an antidepressant with a different neurochemical action.
  - Augment with lithium or triiodothyronine (T_3).
  - Switch to an antidepressant with a similar neurochemical action.
  - Augment with buspirone or an atypical antipsychotic such as olanzapine.
  - Combine with another antidepressant.
- Consider psychiatry referral for electroconvulsive therapy (ECT).

PERSISTENT DEPRESSIVE DISORDER (DYSTHYMIA)

For at least 2 years, the patient experiences depressive symptoms (decreased mood/interest, plus two others), but does not meet criteria for MDE. No manic/hypomanic episode present during this 2-year period.

Treatment same as for MDE.

References

1. Cuijpers P, Dekker J, Hollon SD, et al. Adding psychotherapy to pharmacotherapy in the treatment of depressive disorders in adults: A meta-analysis. *J Clin Psychiatry.* 2009;70(9):1219-1229.

2. Cuijpers P, van Straten A, Warmerdam L, et al. Psychotherapy versus the combination of psychotherapy and pharmacotherapy in the treatment of depression: A meta-analysis. *Depress Anxiety.* 2009;26(3):279-288.

3. Cuijpers P, Reynolds CF 3rd, Donker T, et al. Personalized treatment of adult depression: medication, psychotherapy, or both? A systematic review. *Depress Anxiety.* 2012;29(10):855-864.

4. Cuijpers PP, Sijbrandij M, Koole SL, et al. Adding psychotherapy to antidepressant medication in depression and anxiety disorders: a meta-analysis. *World Psychiatry.* 2014;13(1):56-67.

5. Cuijpers P, van Straten A, van Oppen P, et al. Are psychological and pharmacologic interventions equally effective in the treatment of adult depressive disorders? A meta-analysis of comparative studies. *J Clin Psychiatry*. 2008;69(11):1675-1685; quiz 1839-1841.

6. Shinohara K, Honyashiki M, Imai H, et al. Behavioural therapies versus other psychological therapies for depression. *Cochrane Database Syst Rev*. 2013;(10):. CD008696.

7. Cuijpers P, van Straten A, Andersson G, et al. Psychotherapy for depression in adults: a meta-analysis of comparative outcome studies. *J Consult Clin Psychol*. 2008;76(6):909-922.

8. Gartlehner G, Hansen RA, Morgan LC, et al. *Second-generation antidepressants in the pharmacologic treatment of adult depression: An update of the 2007 comparative effectiveness review*. Agency for Healthcare Research and Quality (US); Rockville, MD: 2011.

9. Gartlehner G, Hansen RA, Morgan LC, et al. Comparative benefits and harms of second-generation antidepressants for treating major depressive disorder: an updated meta-analysis. *Ann Intern Med*. 2011;155(11):772-785.

Bibliography

American Psychiatric Association. *Diagnostic and Statistical Manual of Mental Disorders*. 5th ed. Washington DC: American Psychiatric Publishing, Inc; 2013.

Chen YA, Tran C. *Toronto Notes–Comprehensive Medical Reference & Review for MCCQE I and USMLE II*. Toronto, Canada: Toronto Notes for Medical Students, Inc; 2011.

Kaplan HI, Sadock BJ, Sadock VA. *Kaplan and Sadock's Synopsis of Psychiatry: Behavioural Sciences/Clinical Psychiatry*. 10th ed. New York, NY: Lippincott Williams and Wilkins; 2007.

RxFiles. Antidepressant comparison chart. *Drug Comparsion Charts*. 8th ed. Saskatoon, SK. Saskatoon Health Region; 2010:105.

BIPOLAR DISORDER (SUPPLEMENTARY TOPIC)

Definitions

Bipolar type I

- At least one manic episode with or without an episode of major depression

Bipolar type II

- At least one hypomanic episode and one MDE

Manic Episode

- For at least 7 days, the patient experiences elevated mood plus at least three manic symptoms.

Hypomanic Episode

- For 4 to 6 days, the patient experiences elevated mood plus at least three manic symptoms

Treatment

- Assess suicide risk, homicide risk.
- Treat substance abuse.
- Severely ill patients require combination pharmacotherapy initially, such as lithium plus an antipsychotic [1-3]. Benzodiazepines are generally added for agitation, anxiety, and insomnia.
- Before starting on lithium, screen for pregnancy, order TSH, electrolytes, lipids, BUN, Cr, and complete an ECG.
- Hypomania or mild mania may be treated with monotherapy antipsychotics such as risperidone or olanzapine [4].
- Network meta-analysis (n >14,000) ranked the following antipsychotics as the most efficacious for managing mania, in order: risperidone, haloperidol, and olanzapine [5].

MANIC SYMPTOMS (DIGFAST)
- **D**—Distractibility
- **I**—Impulsivity
- **G**—Grandiosity
- **F**—Flight of ideas
- **A**—Activities increased
- **S**—Sleep, decreased need
- **T**—Talkative

Long-term lithium use can lead to diabetes insipidus (DI) and hypothyroidism.

CYCLOTHYMIC DISORDER

For at least 2 years, the patient experiences hypomanic and depressive symptoms, but does not meet criteria for mania or MDE.

References

1. Grunze H, Vieta E, Goodwin GM, et al. The World Federation of Societies of Biological Psychiatry (WFSBP) guidelines for the biological treatment of bipolar disorders: update 2009 on the treatment of acute mania. *World J Biol Psychiatry.* 2009;10(2):85-116.

2. American Psychiatric Association. Practice guideline for the treatment of patients with bipolar disorder (revision). *Am J Psychiatry.* 2002;159(4 Suppl):1-50.

3. Yatham LN, Kennedy SH, Schaffer A, et al. Canadian Network for Mood and Anxiety Treatments (CANMAT) and International Society for Bipolar Disorders (ISBD) collaborative update of CANMAT guidelines for the management of patients with bipolar disorder: update 2009. *Bipolar Disord.* 2009;11(3):225-255.

4. Kendall T, Morriss R, Mayo-Wilson E, et al. Assessment and management of bipolar disorder: summary of updated NICE guidance. *BMJ.* 2014;349:g5673.

5. Yildiz A, Nikodem M, Vieta E et al. A network meta-analysis on comparative efficacy and all-cause discontinuation of antimanic treatments in acute bipolar mania. *Psychol Med.* 2015;45(2):299-317.

Bibliography

American Psychiatric Association. *Diagnostic and Statistical Manual of Mental Disorders.* 5th ed. Washington, DC: American Psychiatric Publishing, Inc; 2013.

Chen YA, Tran C. *Toronto Notes–Comprehensive Medical Reference & Review for MCCQE I and USMLE II.* Toronto, Canada: Toronto Notes for Medical Students, Inc; 2011.

Kaplan HI, Sadock BJ, Sadock VA. *Kaplan and Sadock's Synopsis of Psychiatry: Behavioural Sciences/ Clinical Psychiatry* 10th ed. New York, NY: Lippincott Williams and Wilkins; 2007.

RxFiles. Antidepressant comparison chart. Drug Comparsion Charts. 8th ed. Saskatoon, SK. Saskatoon Health Region; 2010:105.

GENERALIZED ANXIETY DISORDER SYMPTOMS (BE SKIM)

- **B**—Blank mind, poor concentration
- **E**—Easily fatigued
- **S**—Sleep disturbance
- **K**—Keyed up, restlessness
- **I**—Irritability
- **M**—Muscle tension

Anxiety Disorders

Priority Topic 6

GENERALIZED ANXIETY DISORDER

Excessive worry that is difficult to control. The symptoms persist for at least 6 months and include at least three of the following symptoms:

- Rule out other physiologic/psychologic conditions with the help of history (eg, nicotine, caffeine, alcohol, recreational drugs) and laboratory investigations (eg, TSH, urine toxicology, electrolytes, blood glucose, U/A, CBC)

Risk Factors

- Female.
- Neuroticism (negative affectivity).
- Harm avoidance, parental overprotection in childhood.
- Stressful life event and/or traumatic event, including abuse.
- Family history of anxiety (1/3 of generalized anxiety disorder [GAD] risk is genetic).
- Comorbid psychiatric disorder (particularly depression).

Treatment

- Assess suicide risk at every encounter.
- Monitor treatment response using validated outcome measures, such as GAD-7 [1].
- Mild GAD with no functional impairment may be observed, with follow-up every 6 months.

Acute Therapy

Benzodiazepines may be used if symptoms are severe (eg, lorazepam). Usually for short-term use due to side effects (including sedation), potential cognitive impairment in the elderly, dependence, and withdrawal issues.

Chronic Therapy

- Meta-analyses have found pharmaco and psychotherapy to be equivalent in efficacy [2].
- Psychotherapy is primarily via cognitive behavioural therapy (CBT), which has strong evidence [2-4].
- First-line pharmacotherapy is via SSRIs and SNRIs (eg, escitalopram, paroxetine, sertraline, venlafaxine XR). Antidepressants treat ruminative worry (the core feature of GAD) much more effectively than do benzodiazepines.
- If an SSRI is ineffective after optimization, switch to an alternate SSRI or an agent with a different mechanism of action (an SNRI).
- Second-line pharmacotherapies include benzodiazepines, bupropion-extended release, buspirone, imipramine, and pregabalin due to their side-effect profile.

NOTE: SSRIs may increase anxiety in the first 2 weeks of treatment.

POST TRAUMATIC STRESS DISORDER

Avoidance, hyperarousal, and reexperiencing of a traumatic, life-threatening event. Patient often relives the experience through hallucinations or flashbacks and they often avoid stimuli that they associate with the trauma. These symptoms persist for at least 1 month.

Treatment is with psychotherapy (trauma-focused CBT), pharmacotherapy (SSRIs, SNRIs), or a combination. No one option has been shown to be more empirically effective than the others [5].

OBSESSIVE COMPULSIVE DISORDER

A compilation of obsessions (intrusive, recurrent, undesired thoughts), and/or compulsions (repetitive behaviours or rituals). These symptoms cause significant distress in a patient's life and at some point the patient recognizes that their obsessions/compulsions are excessive.

Treatment is with psychotherapy (exposure–response prevention CBT), pharmacotherapy (SSRIs), or a combination. Meta-analysis shows SSRIs to be more effective than placebo [6], and exposure-response prevention CBT to be more effective than SSRIs or placebo [7].

SPECIFIC PHOBIAS

Marked fear of a specific thing or situation. This involves high levels of anxiety and avoidance of the feared object, to the point that it affects the patient's life.

Common phobias:
- Animals (snake, spider)
- Natural environments (heights, water)
- Medicine (injections, blood)

Treatment is with psychotherapy (exposure-based CBT). Short-term, unavoidable phobias (eg, flying) may be treated with benzodiazepines.

PANIC DISORDER

Involves recurrent and unexpected panic attacks. There is a significant fear that these panic attacks will recur and this fear has persisted for at least 1 month.

Treatment is with psychotherapy (CBT), pharmacotherapy (SSRIs, SNRIs, benzodiazepines), or both.

PANIC ATTACK SYMPTOMS (STUDENTS)
S—Sweating
T—Trembling
U—Unsteadiness
D—Derealization
E—Excessive heart rate
N—Nausea
T—Tingling
S—Shortness of breath
Symptoms usually peak within 10 minutes.

A fear of being somewhere when escape might be difficult. The patient will often avoid the situations that bring on this fear. As per the DSM-V, patient must demonstrate fear in at least two of the following five situations:

1. Using public transportation
2. Being in open spaces
3. Being in enclosed spaces
4. Being in a crowd
5. Being outside the home alone

Treatment is the same as for panic disorder.

References

1. Spitzer RL, Kroenke K, Williams JB, et al. A brief measure for assessing generalized anxiety disorder: the GAD-7. *Arch Intern Med*. 2006;166(10):1092-1097.
2. Mitte K. Meta-analysis of cognitive-behavioral treatments for generalized anxiety disorder: a comparison with pharmacotherapy. *Psychol Bull*. 2005;131(5):785-795.
3. Norton PJ, Price EC. A meta-analytic review of adult cognitive-behavioral treatment outcome across the anxiety disorders. *J Nerv Ment Dis*. 2007;195(6):521-531.
4. Hofmann SG, Smits JA. Cognitive-behavioral therapy for adult anxiety disorders: a meta-analysis of randomized placebo-controlled trials. *J Clin Psychiatry*. 2008;69(4):621-632.
5. Hetrick SE, Purcell R, Garner B, et al. Combined pharmacotherapy and psychological therapies for post traumatic stress disorder (PTSD). *Cochrane Database Syst Rev*. 2010;(7):CD007316.
6. Soomro GM, Altman D, Rajagopal S, et al. Selective serotonin re-uptake inhibitors (SSRIs) versus placebo for obsessive compulsive disorder (OCD). *Cochrane Database Syst Rev*. 2008(1):CD001765.
7. Foa EB, Liebowitz MR, Kozak MJ, et al. Randomized, placebo-controlled trial of exposure and ritual prevention, clomipramine, and their combination in the treatment of obsessive-compulsive disorder. *Am J Psychiatry*. 2005;162(1):151-161.

Bibliography

American Psychiatric Association. *Diagnostic and Statistical Manual of Mental Disorders*. 5th ed. Washington, DC: American Psychiatric Publishing, Inc; 2013.

Chen AY, Tran C. *Toronto Notes*. Toronto, ON: Type & Graphics, Inc; 2011.

Kaplan HI, Sadock BJ, Sadock VA. *Kaplan and Sadock's Synopsis of Psychiatry: Behavioural Sciences/ Clinical Psychiatry*. 10th ed. New York, NY: Lippincott Williams and Wilkins; 2007.

Rx Files. Anxiety disorder medication chart. *Drug Comparison Charts*. 8th ed. Saskatoon, SK: Saskatoon Health Region; 2010:100.

Suicide

Priority Topic 90

SUICIDE RISK FACTORS (SAD PERSONS)

S—Sex—male

A—Age >60 or <18

D—Depression

P—Previous attempts

E—Ethanol abuse

R—Rational thinking loss

S—Suicide in family

O—Organized plan

N—No spouse/lack of support system

S—Serious illness/intractable pain

- Assess suicidal ideation in all patients presenting with **any** mental illness.
- Know your community resources (eg, suicide hotline, local mental health clinic).
- If the patient is suicidal, assess the need for admission (voluntary or involuntary).
- If the patient is suicidal, but has a low risk of completing the act, they may be treated as an outpatient. However, create a **safety plan** [1] with the patient and provide very close follow-up. Risk stratifies based on risk factors:

Reference

1. Stanley B, Brown GK. Safety planning intervention: a brief intervention to mitigate suicide risk. *Cogn Behav Pract*. 2012;19(2):256-264.

Bibliography

Chen YA. *Toronto Notes 2011: Comprehensive Medical Reference Review for MCCQE I USMLE II*. 27th ed. Toronto, ON: Toronto Review Notes; 2011.

Filate W, Ng D, Leung R, Sinyor M. *Essentials of Clinical Examination Handbook*. 5th ed. University of Toronto: The Medical Society Faculty of Medicine; 2005.

Counselling

Priority Topic 18

- Allow adequate time when counselling patients.
- Identify the patient's understanding of his/her problem before beginning counselling.
- Clinician must recognize his/her own beliefs and emotions may interfere with counselling.
- Clinicians must recognize when they are exceeding boundaries (eg, transference, counter-transference) or limits (problem is more complex than initially thought) and refer appropriately.

Transference—Unconscious redirection of feelings from one person to another.
Counter-transference—Redirection of a therapist's feelings toward a client.

Bibliography

Working Group on the Certification Process. Priority topics and key features with corresponding skill dimensions and phases of the encounter. The College of Family Physicians of Canada; 2010. http://www.cfpc.ca/uploadedFiles/Education/Certification_in_Family_Medicine_Examination/Definition%20of%20Competence%20Complete%20Document%20with%20skills%20and%20phases.pdf.

Eating Disorders

Priority Topic 34

TABLE 6-1	Anorexia vs Bulimia: Characteristics, Diagnosis, and Treatment	
	ANOREXIA NERVOSA	**BULIMIA NERVOSA**
Definition	**An obsession with controlling food intake.**	**Characterized by repeated cycles of binge eating followed by purging.**
Symptoms	Fear of gaining weight and/or obsession with becoming thinner. Signs of starvation = hypotension, bradycardia, amenorrhea, constipation, dry skin, brittle nails, lanugo hair, osteoporosis, prerenal failure	Repeated cycles of binging followed by purging. A feeling of loss of control over eating behaviour. Russell sign = calloused knuckles from repeated self-induced vomiting. Dental issues, renal failure, Mallory–Weiss tear, Abnormal lab values (metabolic alkalosis, hypokalemia, hyponatremia, hypochloremia).
Risk factors	Female, between the ages of 15 and 19, obesity, concurrent mental illness, competitive athlete, history of sexual abuse, and family history of mood or eating disorder	Female (90% of cases occur in women). Mood disorders, history of sexual or physical abuse, drug use, and childhood obesity. Typically within normal BMI
Diagnosis	The following criteria must be met: • Restriction of energy intake leading to weight that is less than minimally normal (ie, BMI < 18.5) • Intense fear of gaining weight • Unrealistic evaluation of body image	The following criteria must be met: • Eat large quantities of food in discrete intervals of time with lack of control over eating (binge eating) • Repetitive behaviour to prevent weight gain (laxatives, vomiting, exercise) • Binge/purge at least two times/week for 3 months • Self-worth unduly influenced by body shape and weight • Symptoms do not occur during episodes of anorexia
Subtypes	Restrictive—Dieting, fasting, excessive exercise only Binge-purge—Purge following meals, sometimes without prior binge	Purging—Purge following meals Nonpurging—Utilize other methods of expending calories (eg, excessive exercise following a large meal)
Treatment	• Monitor closely for relapse, as it is very common. • Establish a therapeutic relationship. • Use multidisciplinary approach (psychologist, dietician, psychiatrist). • Monitor lab values for complications for electrolyte abnormalities, low bone density of eating disorder. • Provide close follow-up. • Consider admission to hospital if low body weight, abnormal lab values, abnormal vitals, or actively suicidal. • Early intervention is proven more effective for both anorexia and bulimia. • Cognitive behavioural therapy. • Combination CBT + antidepressants are more effective than antidepressants alone.	

Need to rule out anorexia and bulimia when considering diagnosis of body dysmorphic disorder.

BODY DYSMORPHIC DISORDER

Definition

- Preoccupation with perceived defect in physical appearance

Diagnosis

- Repetitive behaviours (eg, mirror checking, excessive grooming, skin picking, reassurance seeking) or mental acts (eg, comparing his or her appearance with that of others) in response to the appearance concerns.
- Causes clinically significant distress or impairment.
- Other eating disorders have been ruled out.

Management

- Pharmacotherapy (SSRIs such as fluoxetine [1-3]) or psychotherapy (CBT [4]), or both.

KEY POINTS

- Disorders of self-image.
- Therapeutic relationship with patient is essential.
- Multidisciplinary approach is required for treatment.
- Anorexia has a better prognosis than bulimia.

References

1. Phillips KA, Albertini RS, Rasmussen SA. A randomized placebo-controlled trial of fluoxetine in body dysmorphic disorder. *Arch Gen Psychiatry*. 2002;59(4):381-388.
2. Phillips KA, Hollander E. Treating body dysmorphic disorder with medication: evidence, misconceptions, and a suggested approach. *Body Image*. 2008;5(1):13-27.
3. Phillips KA. Pharmacotherapy for body dysmorphic disorder. *Psychiatr Ann*. 2010;40(7):325-332.
4. Veale D, Anson M, Miles S, et al. Efficacy of cognitive behaviour therapy versus anxiety management for body dysmorphic disorder: a randomised controlled trial. *Psychother Psychosom*. 2014;83(6):341-353.

Bibliography

American Psychiatric Association. *Diagnostic and Statistical Manual of Mental Disorders*, 5th ed. Washington, DC: American Psychiatric Publishing, Inc; 2013.

BMJ Clinical Evidence. http://clinicalevidence.bmj.com.cyber.usask.ca/x/systematic-review/1009/overview.html. Accessed March 30, 2012.

Bacaltchuk J, Hay P, Trefiglio R. Antidepressants versus psychological treatments and their combination for bulimia nervosa. *Cochrane Database Syst Rev*. 2001;(4)CD003385.

DynaMed [database online]. Anorexia Nervosa. EBSCO Publishing. http://web.ebscohost.com/dynamed/detail?sid=4a423eb2-9470-4d0e-886f-fc25c5e74c61%40sessionmgr114&vid=4&hid=108&bdata=JnNpd GU9ZHluYW1lZC1saXZl#db=dme&AN=114614. Accessed March 30, 2012.

DynaMed [database online]. Bulimia Nervosa. EBSCO Publishing. http://web.ebscohost.com/dynamed/detail?vid=3&hid=108&sid=4a423eb2-9470-4d0e-886f-fc25c5e74c61%40sessionmgr114&bdata=JnNpd GU9ZHluYW1lZC1saXZl#db=dme&AN=114924. Accessed March 30, 2012.

Kaplan HI, Sadock BJ, Sadock VA. *Kaplan and Sadock's Synopsis of Psychiatry: Behavioural Sciences/Clinical Psychiatry*. 10th ed. New York, NY: Lippincott Williams and Wilkins; 2007.

National Eating Disorder Information Centre. nedic.ca. Accessed March 29, 2012.

National Guideline Clearinghouse. Practice guideline for the treatment of patients with eating disorders. http://www.guideline.gov/content.aspx?id=9318. Accessed March 30, 2012.

Personality Disorders

Priority Topic 72

- Pervasive and inflexible pattern of behaviour that is inconsistent with the norms of the individual's culture.
- Leads to distress or impairment.
- Begins by early adulthood.
- Patients have intact reality testing and abstract abilities without any thought disorder.
- Divided into three clusters:

CLUSTER A — "WEIRD"

- Odd, eccentric (see Table 6-2)

TABLE 6-2	**Cluster A Personality Disorders**		
	PARANOID	**SCHIZOID**	**SCHIZOTYPAL**
Characteristics for diagnosis (DSM-V)	Four or more of: (SUSPECT) **S**—Spousal infidelity suspected **U**—Unforgiving (bears grudges) **S**—Suspicious **P**—Perceives attacks (and reacts quickly) **E**—Enemy or friend? (doubts loyalty of friends) **C**—Confiding in others is feared **T**—Threats perceived in benign events	Four or more of: (DISTANT) **D**—Detached or flattened affect **I**—Indifferent to criticism or praise **S**—Sexual experiences of little interest **T**—Tasks done solitarily **A**—Absence of close friends **N**—No desire for or joy in close relationships **T**—Takes pleasure in few activities	Five or more of: (ME PECULIAR) **M**—Magical thinking **E**—Experiences unusual perceptions **P**—Paranoid ideation **E**—Eccentric behaviour or appearance **C**—Constricted or inappropriate affect **U**—Unusual thinking or speech **L**—Lacks close friends **I**—Ideas of reference **A**—Anxiety in social situations **R**—Rule out developmental disorder
Description	Distrustful and suspicious nature Socially isolated Brief episodes of psychosis with persecutory delusion	Socially detached and emotionally restricted "Happy loners" Disinterested in others, praise, or criticism Dysphoria	Eccentric Discomfort with social relationships Odd behaviour, appearance, speech, and perceptions Odd and magical thinking
Risk factors	Family h/o schizophrenia Family h/o delusional d/o, paranoid type.	Male Family h/o schizophrenia	Family h/o schizophrenia
Management	Cognitive behavioural therapy (CBT) and insight-oriented counselling	Tx of choice = insight psychotherapy Supportive therapy, eg, ID emotions	Tx like residual schizophrenia Insight-oriented, supportive therapy, milieu therapy

CLUSTER B — "WILD"

- Dramatic, emotional, erratic, and attention seeking (see Table 6-3)
- Associated with substance abuse/dependence

TABLE 6-3	**Cluster B Personality Disorders**			
	BORDERLINE	**HISTRIONIC**	**NARCISSISTIC**	**ANTISOCIAL**
Characteristics for diagnosis (DSM-V)	Five or more of: (DESPAIRER) **D**—Disturbance of identity **E**—Emotionally labile **S**—Suicidal behaviour **P**—Paranoia or dissociation **A**—Abandonment (frantic efforts to avoid) **I**—Impulsive **R**—Relationships (unstable, polarizing) **E**—Emptiness (feelings of) **R**—Rage (inappropriate)	Five or more of: (ACTRESSS) **A**—Appearance focused **C**—Centre of attention **T**—Theatrical (exaggerated behaviour) **R**—Relationships (believed to be more intimate than they really are) **E**—Easily influenced **S**—Seductive behaviour **S**—Shallow emotions **S**—Speech (impressionistic and vague)	Five or more of: (GRANDIOSE) **G**—Grandiose **R**—Requires admiration **A**—Arrogant **N**—Need to be special **D**—Dreams of success and power **I**—Interpersonally exploitative **O**—Others (lacks empathy) **S**—Sense of entitlement **E**—Envious	Three or more of: (CORRUPT) **C**—Cannot conform to law **O**—Obligations ignored **R**—Reckless disregard for safety **R**—Remorseless **U**—Underhanded (deceitful) **P**—Planning insufficient (impulsive) **T**—Temper (irritable and aggressive)
Description	Instability eg, relationships, self-image, affect Marked impulsivity **Red flags:** Doctor shopping/legal suits against doctor; suicide attempts	Excessive emotionality and attention-seeking behaviour Unlike other PD, these patients will often seek treatment, but are emotionally needy and hesitant to stop therapy	Grandiosity, need for admiration, and lack of empathy	Disregard for, and violation of, the rights of others Onset <15 years old = conduct d/o, but labelled antisocial PD when ≥18 years old.
Risk factors	Childhood abuse and neglect; abandonment. 5× more likely if d/o present in first-degree relative		Childhood abuse and neglect	Family history of antisocial PD Lower SES; abandonment or abuse; repeated harsh punishments 100% conduct d/o as child
Management	CBT Psychiatric consult Assess suicide risk often	Insight-oriented psychotherapy Assess suicide risk	CBT	CBT Assess for associated conditions: spousal/child abuse, drunk driving

CLUSTER C — "WORRIED AND WIMPY"

- Anxious, fearful (see Table 6-4)

TABLE 6-4	Cluster C Personality Disorders		
	OBSESSIVE-COMPULSIVE	**AVOIDANT**	**DEPENDENT**
Characteristics for diagnosis (DSM-V)	Presence of obsessions, Compulsions, or both: Obsession—Recurrent, unwanted thoughts that cause distress Compulsion—Repetitive behaviours or mental acts that the individual feels driven to perform	Four or more of: (CRINGES) **C**—Criticism/rejection preoccupies thoughts in social situations **R**—Restraint in relationships due to fear of shame **I**—Inhibited socially by sense of inadequacy **N**—Needs to be sure of being liked before engaging socially **G**—Gets away from occupational activities which require interpersonal contact **E**—Embarrassment (risk of) prevents from taking risks **S**—Self viewed as unappealing or inferior	Five or more of: (RELIANCE) **R**—Reassurance required for daily decisions **E**—Expressing disagreement difficult **L**—Life responsibilities assumed by others **I**—Initiating projects difficult **A**—Alone (feels helpless and uncomfortable when alone) **N**—Nurturance (goes to excessive lengths to obtain) **C**—Companionship sought urgently when a relationship ends **E**xaggerated fears of being left to care for self
Description	Preoccupation with orderliness, perfectionism and control Perform compulsions to relieve distress of obsessions	Social inhibition, feelings of inadequacy and hypersensitivity to criticism and rejection Similar to schizoid PD but *wants* relationships	Submissive and clingy behaviour related to an excessive need to be taken care of At risk for spousal abuse
Risk factors	Genetic: Monozygotic >dizygotic twins, first-degree relative with OCD or Tourette syndrome	Childhood abuse or neglect	Chronic physical illness in childhood or separation anxiety Early childhood parental loss
Management	CBT—Improves up to 70% of patients. R/o coexisting Tourette syndrome	Tx of choice is individual psychotherapy (improve self-esteem) Behaviour therapy—Systematic desensitization, social skills, assertiveness training	Tx of choice is insight-oriented CBT Anxiety management, assertive training Set limits Relatively favourable prognosis

KEY POINTS

- Chronic disorders with no cure, and their ego-syntonic nature makes them difficult to treat.
- Psychotherapy (CBT) is first-line therapy, as it is the most effective [1-3].
- Currently no medications approved by US FDA for treatment of personality disorders.
- Treat comorbid conditions appropriately, with pharmacotherapy as indicated (eg, depression)
- Also see Table 6-5.

TABLE 6-5	Personality Disorders—Cluster-Specific Key Points		
	CLUSTER A (WEIRD)	**CLUSTER B (WILD)**	**CLUSTER C (WORRIED AND WIMPY)**
Disorders	Paranoid, schizoid, schizotypal	Antisocial, borderline, histrionic, narcissistic	Avoidant, dependent, obsessive-compulsive
Key points	Odd, eccentric	Dramatic, emotional, erratic, attention seeking Associated with substance abuse/dependence	Anxious, fearful
Treatment	Psychotherapy	Psychotherapy	Psychotherapy

References

1. Leichsenring F, Leibing E. The effectiveness of psychodynamic therapy and cognitive behavior therapy in the treatment of personality disorders: a meta-analysis. *Am J Psychiatry*. 2003;160(7):1223-1232.

2. Leichsenring F, Rabung S. Effectiveness of long-term psychodynamic psychotherapy: a meta-analysis. *JAMA*. 2008;**300**(13):1551-1565.

3. Matusiewicz AK, et al. The effectiveness of cognitive behavioral therapy for personality disorders. *Psychiatr Clin North Am*. 2010;33(3):657-685.

Bibliography

American Psychiatric Association. *Diagnostic and Statistical Manual of Mental Disorders*. 5th ed. Washington, DC: American Psychiatric Publishing Inc; 2013.

Angstman KB, Rasmussen NH. Personality disorder: Review and clinical application in daily practice. Am Fam Physician. 2011;84(11):1253-1260.

Caplan JP, Stern TA. Mnemonics in a mnutshell: 32 aids to psychiatric diagnosis. *Current Psychiatry*. 2008;7(10):27-33.

Devens M. Personality disorders. *Prim Care Clin Office Prac*. 2007;34:623-640.

DynaMed [database online]. Antisocial personality disorder. EBSCO Publishing. http://web.ebscohost .com.cyber.usask.ca/dynamed/detail?vid=16&hid=9&sid=5fdbf4ec-bc94-440b-af64-b72b84140 e48%40sessionmgr4&bdata=JnNpdGU9ZHluYW1lZC1saXZlJnNjb3BlPXNpdGU%3d#db=dme &AN=114962. Accessed March 24, 2012.

DynaMed [database online]. Avoidant personality disorder. EBSCO Publishing. http://web.ebscohost .com.cyber.usask.ca/dynamed/detail?vid=20&hid=9&sid=5fdbf4ec-bc94-440b-af64-b72b84140 e48%40sessionmgr4&bdata=JnNpdGU9ZHluYW1lZC1saXZlJnNjb3BlPXNpdGU%3d#db=dme &AN=114108. Accessed March 24, 2012.

DynaMed [database online]. Borderline personality disorder. EBSCO Publishing. http://web.ebscohost .com.cyber.usask.ca/dynamed/detail?vid=9&hid=9&sid=5fdbf4ec-bc94-440b-af64-b72b84140e 48%40sessionmgr4&bdata=JnNpdGU9ZHluYW1lZC1saXZlJnNjb3BlPXNpdGU%3d#db=dme &AN=116319. Accessed December 5, 2012.

DynaMed [database online]. Dependent personality disorder. EBSCO Publishing. http://web.ebscohost .com.cyber.usask.ca/dynamed/detail?vid=22&hid=9&sid=5fdbf4ec-bc94-440b-af64-b72b84140 e48%40sessionmgr4&bdata=JnNpdGU9ZHluYW1lZC1saXZlJnNjb3BlPXNpdGU%3d#db=dme &AN=114240. Accessed March 24, 2012.

DynaMed [database online]. Histrionic personality disorder. EBSCO Publishing. http://web.ebscohost .com.cyber.usask.ca/dynamed/detail?vid=18&hid=9&sid=5fdbf4ec-bc94-440b-af64-b72b84140 e48%40sessionmgr4&bdata=JnNpdGU9ZHluYW1lZC1saXZlJnNjb3BlPXNpdGU%3d#db=dme &AN=114862. Accessed March 13, 2012.

DynaMed [database online]. Narcissistic personality disorder. EBSCO Publishing. http://web.ebscohost .com.cyber.usask.ca/dynamed/detail?vid=14&hid=9&sid=5fdbf4ec-bc94-440b-af64-b72b84140 e48%40sessionmgr4&bdata=JnNpdGU9ZHluYW1lZC1saXZlJnNjb3BlPXNpdGU%3d#db=dme &AN=116855. Accessed March 13, 2012.

DynaMed [database online]. Paranoid personality disorder. EBSCO Publishing. http://web.ebscohost .com.cyber.usask.ca/dynamed/detail?vid=3&hid=9&sid=5fdbf4ec-bc94-440b-af64-b72b84140e 48%40sessionmgr4&bdata=JnNpdGU9ZHluYW1lZC1saXZlJnNjb3BlPXNpdGU%3d#db=dme &AN=114532. Accessed March 15, 2012.

DynaMed [database online]. Schizoid personality disorder. EBSCO Publishing. http://web.ebscohost .com.cyber.usask.ca/dynamed/detail?vid=7&hid=9&sid=5fdbf4ec-bc94-440b-af64-b72b84140e 48%40sessionmgr4&bdata=JnNpdGU9ZHluYW1lZC1saXZlJnNjb3BlPXNpdGU%3d#db=dme &AN=114747. Accessed March 15, 2012.

DynaMed [database online]. Schizotypal personality disorder. EBSCO Publishing. http://web.ebscohost .com.cyber.usask.ca/dynamed/detail?vid=5&hid=9&sid=5fdbf4ec-bc94-440b-af64-b72b84140e 48%40sessionmgr4&bdata=JnNpdGU9ZHluYW1lZC1saXZlJnNjb3BlPXNpdGU%3d#db=dme &AN=116517. Accessed March 15, 2012.

Ferri F. *Ferri's Clinical Advisor*. 2011

Paris J. Pharmacological treatments for personality disorders. *Int Rev Psychiatr*. 2011;23:303-309.

Stein DJ, Denys D, Gloster AT, et al. Obsessive-compulsive disorder: diagnostic and treatment issues. *Psychiatr Clin N Am*. 2009;2:665-685.

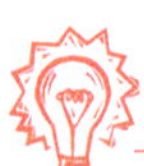

SUBSTANCE DISORDER SYMPTOMS (STOP AND CIWA)

S—Significant amount of time spent using, recovering from, or obtaining substance

T—Tolerance increased

O—Obligations unfulfilled due to substance use

P—Physically hazardous environments substance is used in

A—Activities/hobbies given up because of substance use

N—No control (uses larger amounts than initially intended)

D—Desire to cut down, unsuccessfully

C—Cravings

I—Interpersonal problems as result, but continues to use substance

W—Withdrawal symptoms upon cessation

A—Aware substance damages them, but continues to use it

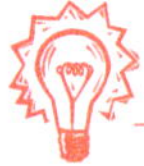

STAGES OF CHANGE

Stage 1: Precontemplation

Stage 2: Contemplation

Stage 3: Preparation

Stage 4: Action

Stage 5: Maintenance

Substance Abuse

Priority Topic 89

SUBSTANCE USE DISORDER

Definition

- Replaces DSM-IV substance abuse, substance dependence.
- Cluster of cognitive, behavioural, and physiological symptoms indicating the individual continues using the substance despite significant substance-related problems.
- Substance-related disorders encompass 10 classes of drugs: Alcohol; caffeine; cannabis; hallucinogens; inhalants; opioids; sedatives, hypnotics, and anxiolytics; stimulants (amphetamine-type substances, cocaine, and other stimulants); tobacco; and other (or unknown) substances.
- For a substance listed above (except caffeine, which the DSM-V does not identify as a substance use disorder), substance use disorder is diagnosed by two or more substance disorder symptoms within the past 12 months.

Risk Factors

- Mental illness, chronic disability, lower socioeconomic class
- Comorbid conditions = sexually transmitted infections, cirrhosis, HIV, hepatitis C

Management of Substance Use Disorder

- Psychotherapy.
- Assessing stage of change may be useful.
- Offer services such as alcoholics anonymous, detoxification centre, and halfway house.
- Schedule regular follow-up appointments.
- Pharmacotherapy may include SSRI, naltrexone, disulfiram, depending on specific substance use disorder (eg, opioid, cocaine, EtOH). The individual pharmacotherapies are beyond the scope of this text.

Alcohol Use Disorder

- As per criteria above
- One of the most common substance use disorders, with important sequelae

Alcohol Withdrawal

Stage 1: Tremor, sweating, anorexia, diarrhea, agitation

Stage 2: Hallucinations

Stage 3: Seizures

Stage 4: Delirium tremens, autonomic hyperactivity

- Most likely to occur in those who routinely consume more than four to five drinks per day.
- Treat alcohol withdrawal with supportive care, benzodiazepines, and thiamine following a validated protocol, such as the Clinical Institute Withdrawal Assessment for Alcohol (CIWA-Ar) [1].

Key Points

- Substance use disorder can occur with a variety of substances.
- Screen for and treat comorbid conditions.
- Psychotherapy is the mainstay of treatment for all substance use disorders.
- Pharmacotherapy is substance-specific.

Reference

1. Mayo-Smith MF. Pharmacological management of alcohol withdrawal. A meta-analysis and evidence-based practice guideline. American Society of Addiction Medicine Working Group on Pharmacological Management of Alcohol Withdrawal. *JAMA*. 1997;278(2):144-151.

Bibliography

American Psychiatric Association. *Diagnostic and Statistical Manual of Mental Disorders*. 5th ed. Washington DC: American Psychiatric Publishing Inc; 2013.

Centre for Addiction and Mental Health. Canada's Low-Risk Alcohol Drinking Guidelines. http://www.camh.net/About_Addiction_Mental_Health/Drug_and_Addiction_Information/low_risk_drinking_guidelines.html. Accessed April 4, 2012.

Chen AY, Tran C. *Toronto Notes*. Toronto, ON: Type & Graphics, Inc; 2011.

Dhalla S, Kopec JA. The CAGE questionnaire for alcohol misuse: a review of reliability and validity studies. *Clin Invest Med*. 2007;30(1):33-41.

DynaMed [database online]. Alcohol Withdrawal. EBSCO Publishing. http://web.ebscohost.com/dynamed/detail?vid=3&hid=118&sid=6d7eb159-b513-4455-a850-7f34b384dc23%40sessionmgr104&bdata=JnNpdGU9ZHluYW1lZC1saXZlJnNjb3BlPXNpdGU%3d#db=dme&AN=114807. Accessed April 4, 2012.

Kaplan HI, Sadock BJ, Sadock VA. *Kaplan and Sadock's Synopsis of Psychiatry: Behavioural Sciences/Clinical Psychiatry*. 10th ed. New York, NY: Lippincott Williams and Wilkins; 2007.

Somatoform Disorders

Priority Topic 86

- Somatoform disorders are conditions involving multiple somatic complaints in multiple organ systems that cannot be explained by a general medical condition.
- Symptoms are produced unconsciously and they cause significant distress or impairment in functioning.

SOMATIC SYMPTOM DISORDER

Symptoms

- Common symptoms include (but not limited to) headache, abdominal pain, back pain, pelvic pain, dizziness, numbness, weakness, fatigue, shortness of breath, vomiting, dysphagia, and sexual symptoms.

Diagnosis

- One or more somatic symptoms that result in significant disruption of daily life for ≥6 months
- At least one of the following:
  - Disproportionate thoughts about seriousness of the symptoms
  - Persistently high anxiety about symptoms
  - Excessive time and energy devoted to these symptoms

Management

- See later

Key Points

- Tends to be chronic in nature.
- Somatization can be present in a patient who has a diagnosed medical condition.

FUNCTIONAL NEUROLOGIC SYMPTOM DISORDER (CONVERSION DISORDER)

Definition

- Symptoms affecting voluntary motor (weakness) or sensory systems (loss of sensation).
- Symptoms often suggest neurologic disease, but does not fit any neurologic disorder.
- Stress is trigger for symptoms.

Diagnosis

- Diagnosis depends on four features:
  1. ≥1 symptoms involving motor or sensory systems.
  2. No clinical findings to support the diagnosis of a neurologic condition.
  3. Symptoms are not better explained by another disorder.
  4. Symptoms cause clinically significant distress.

Management

- See later

Key Points

- Spontaneous remission in most cases

ILLNESS ANXIETY DISORDER

Definition

- Preoccupation with fear of having or acquiring a serious illness

Diagnosis

- Somatic symptoms are not present, or only mild
- High level of anxiety about health
- Excessive health-related behaviours (eg, repeated self-examinations, medical appointments)
- Duration ≥6 months
- Not better explained by another illness

Management

- See later

Key Points

- Belief is not delusional. The patient realizes they have an unrealistic thought.

MANAGEMENT PRINCIPLES FOR SOMATOFORM DISORDERS

- Create strong doctor–patient relationship.
- Avoid multiple physicians being involved.
- Set limits on number of visits, encourage regular scheduled visits.
- Focus on psychosocial, not physical symptoms.
- Avoid unnecessary testing.
- Use multidisciplinary approach (biofeedback, acupuncture, psychotherapy, group therapy).
- Treat comorbid psychiatric illnesses if present.
- Avoid anxiolytics (if needed use only in short-term).
- Help patients develop their problem-solving skills.

KEY POINTS

- Empathy is important when working with patients with somatoform disorders.
- Somatoform disorders can lead to many unnecessary tests, surgeries, and drug dependence.
- Need to rule out depression and substance abuse.

Bibliography

American Psychiatric Association. *Diagnostic and Statistical Manual of Mental Disorders*. 5th ed. Washington, DC: American Psychiatric Publishing, Inc; 2013.

Buhlmann U, Winter A. Perceived ugliness: an update of treatment-relevant aspects of body dysmorphic disorder. *Curr Psychiatry Rep*. 2011;13:283-288.

Chen AY, Tran C. *Toronto Notes*. Toronto, ON: Type & Graphics, Inc; 2011.

Conversion disorder: advanced in our understanding. *CMAJ*. 2011;183(8).

DynaMed [database online]. Body Dysmorphic Disorder. EBSCO Publishing. http://web.ebscohost.com/dynamed/detail?vid=8&hid=108&sid=4a423eb2-9470-4d0e-886f-fc25c5e74c61%40sessionmgr114&bdata=JnNpdGU9ZHluYW1lZC1saXZlJnNjb3BlPXNpdGU%3d#db=dme&AN=116253. Accessed April 2, 2012.

DynaMed [database online]. Somatization Disorder. EBSCO Publishing. http://web.ebscohost.com/dynamed/detail?vid=6&hid=108&sid=4a423eb2-9470-4d0e-886f-fc25c5e74c61%40sessionmgr114&bdata=JnNpdGU9ZHluYW1lZC1saXZlJnNjb3BlPXNpdGU%3d#db=dme&AN=116198. Accessed April 2, 2012.

Kaplan HI, Sadock BJ, Sadock VA. *Kaplan and Sadock's Synopsis of Psychiatry: Behavioural Sciences/Clinical Psychiatry*. 10th ed. New York, NY: Lippincott Williams and Wilkins; 2007.

MD Consult. Search for Somatization Disorder. http://home.mdconsult.com/das/book/63108090-5/view/1353. Accessed April 2, 2012.

Nicholson TR, Stone J, Kanaan RA. Conversion disorder: a problematic diagnosis. *J Neurol Neurosurg Psychiatry*. 2011;82:1267-1273.

Schizophrenia

Priority Topic 80

Definition

Two or more of the following for ≥1 month, with continuous disturbance in functioning for ≥36 months:

- Delusions—Fixed, false beliefs (eg, persecutory, grandiose, referential, erotomanic)
- Hallucinations (ie, perceptions that occur without an external stimulus; often auditory)
- Disorganized thinking/speech (eg, loose associations, tangentiality, word salad)
- Disorganized/catatonic behaviour (ie, marked decrease in reactivity to environment)
- Negative symptoms (eg, diminished emotional expression, avolition, alogia, anhedonia)

Symptoms produce disordered social functioning.

Must exclude mood disorders, substance abuse, and general medical conditions as cause of psychosis.

Risk Factors

- Strong genetic component
- First-degree relative affected by bipolar disorder, depression, autism spectrum disorder
- Increasing paternal age
- Cannabis use
- Birth in winter or early spring

Schizophreniform disorder—same criteria as schizophrenia, but duration is 1 to 6 months.

Treatment: Nonpharmacological

- Encourage abstinence from drugs and alcohol.
- Psychosocial supports—Housing, family support, disability issues, and vocational retraining.
- For stable patients with schizophrenia (not floridly psychotic) assess at every visit:
  - Positive and negative symptoms
  - Suicidal, homicidal ideation
  - Performance of activities of daily living
  - Level of social functioning
  - Medication compliance and side effects
- For decompensating patients determine if related to:
  - Substance use/abuse
  - Medication compliance and side effects
  - Change in psychosocial supports

Typical Antipsychotics (eg, Haloperidol, Chlorpromazine):

Goal of antipsychotic treatment is to increase functioning, minimize side effects, maximize compliance, and prevent relapse.

Typical Antipsychotics (eg, haloperidol, chlorpromazine)

- Mechanism of action: Dopaminergic blockade.
- Side effects are due to low dopamine; **extrapyramidal side effects** are more common.

Atypical antipsychotics (eg, risperidone, olanzapine, quetiapine, clozapine)

- Mechanism of action: More complex, act on dopamine and serotonin receptors
- Treats negative symptoms more effectively
- Side effects: Cardiometabolic more common

Side Effects

1. Extrapyramidal side effects: More common with typical antipsychotics or high dose atypical (risperidone >8 mg/day)
   - Dystonia: Sustained muscle spasm, often involves neck, eyes-oculogyric crisis
   - Akathisia: Feeling of internal restlessness; increased risk of suicide
   - Pseudoparkinsonism: Tremor, rigidity, akinesia, postural instability (TRAP)
   - **Tardive dyskinesia:**
     - Caused by long-term usage (≥6 months); often irreversible
     - Hyperkinetic disorder, involuntary irregular choreoathetoid movement
     - Most commonly face and mouth including chewing, sticking out tongue, and grimacing
     - Lifetime risk: 25% with typical; 10% with atypical antipsychotics
2. Hyperprolactinemia (more common with typical)
   - Men: Gynecomastia, decreased libido
   - Women: Lactation, amenorrhea, infertility
3. Increased cardio-metabolic risk (more common with atypical medications)
   - Weight gain, insulin resistance and diabetes, dyslipidemia
4. Anticholinergic side effects
5. Antihistamine side effects:
   - Sedation
6. Antiadrenergic side effects (alpha 1):
   - Orthostatic hypotension

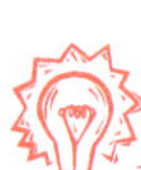

COMMON ANTIPSYCHOTIC DRUG SIDE EFFECTS

Typical—Extrapyramidal side effects

Atypical—Increased cardio-metabolic risk

ANTICHOLINERGIC TOXIDROME/ SIDE EFFECTS

- Hot as a hare—fever/sweating.
- Blind as a bat—visual disturbance.
- Mad as a hatter—confusion.
- Dry as a bone.
- Bowel and bladder lose their tone.

7. **Neuroleptic malignant syndrome:**
   - It is a *life-threatening* complication that can occur *at any time* during treatment.
   - Cause: Massive dopamine blockade, develops over 24 to 72 hours
   - Lab result:
     - ↑ WBC, ↑ CK, ↑ liver enzymes, ↑ plasma myoglobin, myoglobinuria
   - Risk factors:
     - Sudden increase in dosage or starting a new drug
     - Patient: Young, male, medical illness, dehydration, and poor nutrition
     - External heat load (hot summer days)
   - Treatment:
     - Admit to ICU.
     - **Stop** antipsychotic immediately (and any other DA blockers, ie, antiemetics).
     - Treat fever, hydrate, and use cooling blankets.
     - Dantrolene: A muscle relaxant, or benzodiazepines.
     - Bromocriptine: A dopamine agonist.

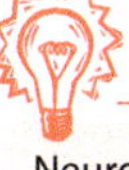

Neuroleptic Malignant Syndrome (FARM)
F—Fever
A—Autonomic (↑HR, ↑BP, sweating)
R—Rigidity
M—Mental status changes

Key Points

- Schizophrenia is a **chronic disease** that involves one or more psychotic episodes.
- There is often a **prodromal period** of decline lasting months to years: increasing impairment in work, school, or home life followed by social withdrawal and finally overt psychosis.
- Generally patients with schizophrenia have **poor insight**. This can lead to the patients stopping their medicines. It is important to discuss the disease and the rationale behind the treatment plan with the patient.
- Consider schizophrenia in adolescents presenting with behavioural problems.
- Get collateral history from family, social workers.
- Screen for alcohol and drug use.
- Mental illnesses are highly prevalent in this population and increase morbidity and early mortality

Bibliography

Ables AZ, Nagubilli R. Prevention, recognition, and management of serotonin syndrome. *Am Fam Physician*. 2010;81(9):1139-1142.

American Psychiatric Association. *Diagnostic and Statistical Manual of Mental Disorders*. 5th ed. Washington, DC: American Psychiatric Publishing, Inc; 2013.

Chen AY, Tran C. *Toronto Notes*. Toronto, ON: Type & Graphics Inc; 2011.

DynaMed [database online]. Schizophrenia. EBSCO Publishing. http://web.ebscohost.com/dynamed/det ail?vid=3&hid=111&sid=23399d76-7182-4457-97ed-f542627c53a8%40sessionmgr110&bdata=JnNpd GU9ZHluYW1lZC1saXZlJnNjb3BlPXNpdGU%3d#db=dme&AN=115234. Accessed April 5, 2012.

McPhee SJ, Papadakis MA, eds. *Current Medical Diagnosis and Treatment*. 49th ed. New York, NY: McGraw Hill Medical; 2010.

Viron M, Baggett T, Hill M, Freudenreich O. Schizophrenia for primary care providers: how to contribute to the care of a vulnerable patient population. *Am J Med*. 2012;125:223-230.

Grief

Priority Topic 43

Key Points

- Grieving is a normal human reaction to loss. Prepare patients for emotional and physical responses they will be having when experiencing loss (eg, of a loved one, a job, a pet).
- Assess what stage of grief the patient is in.

FIVE STAGES OF GRIEF
(1) Denial
(2) Anger
(3) Bargaining
(4) Depression
(5) Acceptance

- Inquire about depression and suicidal ideation in grieving patients, especially in those with prolonged grief reactions.
- Very young or elderly may have atypical grief reactions.
- Diagnosis of MDE is usually withheld until at least 2 months after a loss as normal bereavement can last this long. However, there is no concrete definition as to how long a "normal" grief reaction can last.

Bibliography

Kaplan HI, Sadock BJ, Sadock VA. *Kaplan and Sadock's Synopsis of Psychiatry: Behavioural Sciences/ Clinical Psychiatry*. 10th ed. New York, NY: Lippincott Williams and Wilkins; 2007.

Kübler-Ross E. *On Death and Dying*. Routledge: Simon and Schuster;1969.

Working Group on the Certification Process. Priority topics and key features with corresponding skill dimensions and phases of the encounter. The College of Family Physicians of Canada; 2010. http://www .cfpc.ca/uploadedFiles/Education/Certification_in_Family_Medicine_Examination/Definition%20 of%20Competence%20Complete%20Document%20with%20skills%20and%20phases.pdf.

Can have teachers and parents fill out Swanson, Nolan, and Pelham IV Form (SNAP-IV Form) to assist in diagnosis.

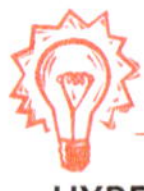

INATTENTIVE SYMPTOMS (FDDLE FAST)

F—Focus—cannot remain focused

D—Distractible

D—Does not listen when spoken to directly

L—Loses things easily

E—Errors with details

F—Forgetful

A—Avoids tasks which require sustained focus

S—Sidetracked easily

T—Time management is poor

HYPERACTIVE-IMPULSIVE SYMPTOMS (IF TWO RIPS)

I—Interrupts conversations

F—Fidgety

T—Talks excessively

W—Waiting in lines is difficult

O—On the go, uncomfortable being still

R—Runs or climbs when inappropriate

I—Intrudes into others games, activities

P—Playing silently not an option

S—Seat—Can't stay seated when expected to do so

Conduct disorder—If diagnosed before age 18

Antisocial personality disorder—If diagnosed after age 18

Behavioural Problems

Priority Topic 10

ATTENTION DEFICIT/HYPERACTIVITY DISORDER

- Affects 5% to 12% of school-aged kids. Male to female ratio is 4:1
- Associated higher risk of conduct disorder, oppositional defiant disorder, and substance abuse
- 70% to 80% continue into adolescence, and 65% into adulthood

Diagnosis

- Requires ≥6 symptoms of inattention, or ≥6 of hyperactivity-impulsivity
- Symptoms must:
  - Have onset prior to 12 years of age
  - Be present for ≥6 months
  - Be present in ≥2 environments (eg, school and home)

Treatment

- Preschool-aged children (4-5 years)—Behavioural therapy [1,2]
- School-aged children (6+ years)—Combination behavioural and pharmacotherapy [1,2]
- Behavioural therapy may include [1]:
  - Maintaining a daily schedule, minimize distractions, limit choices, use charts, and checklists
- Response rate to stimulant pharmacotherapy is ~70% [3]
- Methylphenidate, dexmethylphenidate, and amphetamines have similar efficacy and side-effect profiles [4,5]

CONDUCT DISORDER

Definition

Persistent pattern of behaviour that violates the rights of others as well as age-appropriate social norms. Behaviours include aggression to people and animals, destruction of property, deceitfulness or theft, and violation of rules. Patient must demonstrate ≥3 behaviours in past 12 months, and ≥1 in past 6 months. The behaviours must cause a significant impairment in the patient's life.

Treatment

- Early intervention with aid of CBT, parenting skills, anger management, family therapy, employment programs, and social skills training

OPPOSITIONAL DEFIANT DISORDER

Definition

Pattern of negative/hostile and defiant behaviour for ≥6 months with significant impairment in the patient's life

Treatment

- Parenting skills, psychoeducation, individual/family therapy, establish generational boundaries

KEY POINTS

- Keep broad differential diagnosis, as behavioural issues are often multifactorial, including medical conditions (eg, hearing problems, depression, abuse, drug use).
- Use multiple sources when gathering data on behaviour concerns.
- Use multidisciplinary approach.

References

1. Wolraich M, et al. ADHD: clinical practice guideline for the diagnosis, evaluation, and treatment of attention-deficit/hyperactivity disorder in children and adolescents. *Pediatrics.* 2011;128(5):1007-1022.

2. Dulcan M. Practice parameters for the assessment and treatment of children, adolescents, and adults with attention-deficit/hyperactivity disorder. American Academy of Child and Adolescent Psychiatry. *J Am Acad Child Adolesc Psychiatry.* 1997;36(10 Suppl):85S-121S.

3. Schachter HM, Pham B, King J, et al. How efficacious and safe is short-acting methylphenidate for the treatment of attention-deficit disorder in children and adolescents? *A meta-analysis. CMAJ.* 2001;165(11):1475-1488.

4. Jadad AR, et al. Treatment of attention-deficit/hyperactivity disorder. *Evid Rep Technol Assess (Summ).* 1999;(11):i-viii, 1-341.

5. Faraone SV, Biederman J, Roe C. Comparative efficacy of Adderall and methylphenidate in attention-deficit/hyperactivity disorder: a meta-analysis. *J Clin Psychopharmacol.* 2002;22(5):468-473.

Bibliography

American Psychiatric Association. *Diagnostic and Statistical Manual of Mental Disorders.* 5th ed. Washington, DC: American Psychiatric Publishing, Inc; 2013.

Kaplan HI, Sadock BJ, Sadock VA. *Kaplan and Sadock's Synopsis of Psychiatry: Behavioural Sciences/Clinical Psychiatry.* 10th ed. New York, NY: Lippincott Williams and Wilkins; 2007.

Tao L, Dehlendorf C, Mendoza M, Ohata C. *First Aid for the Family Medicine Boards.* New York, NY: McGraw Hill; 2008.

Working Group on the Certification Process. Priority topics and key features with corresponding skill dimensions and phases of the encounter. The College of Family Physicians of Canada; 2010. http://www.cfpc.ca/uploadedFiles/Education/Certification_in_Family_Medicine_Examination/Definition%20of%20Competence%20Complete%20Document%20with%20skills%20and%20phases.pdf.

Yingming A. Chen. *Toronto Notes 2011: Comprehensive Medical Reference Review for MCCQE I USMLE II,* 27th ed. Toronto, ON: Toronto Review; 2008.

CHAPTER 7

Chronic Disease

Chronic Disease

Priority Topic 14

- Chronic diseases are illnesses that are prolonged in duration and are rarely cured completely.
- Chronic diseases such as heart disease, stroke, cancer, chronic respiratory diseases, and diabetes, are the leading causes of death and disability. According to the CDC, chronic diseases (as a group) are responsible for 7 of 10 deaths each year (Chronic Disease Prevention and Health Promotion, 2016). Chronic diseases are common, and costly, and yet in many respects—largely preventable.
- Inquire about: (a) psychological impact of their diagnosis and treatment, (b) functional impairment, (c) depression or risk of suicide, and (d) underlying substance abuse, as these patients are at greater risk.
- Patients may seek medical attention for acute symptoms of their chronic disease such as:
  (a) Acute complications of chronic disease (eg, diabetic ketoacidosis [DKA] in DM or compression fracture in osteoporosis)
  (b) Acute exacerbations of the disease (eg, asthma exacerbation, acute arthritis, AECOPD)
  (c) A new, unrelated condition (eg, MI in a patient with underlying panic attacks with chest pain as a symptom)
- Pain is often a predominant symptom in chronic disease. Actively inquire about pain and treat it appropriately by titrating medication to the patient's pain. Consider nonpharmacologic treatment and adjuvant therapies (eg, cognitive behavioural therapy, physiotherapy, acetaminophen combined with opioids for synergistic effects).
- Regularly reassess adherence to the treatment plan (including medication) and in a nonadherent patient, explore the reasons why, with the goal to improve future adherence. Some example questions to ask are: "Do you sometimes forget to take your medication?" "Have you been regularly attending your physiotherapy/counselling appointments?"

STRATEGIES TO IMPROVE ADHERENCE INCLUDE

- Regularly scheduled visits (eg, DMII visits every 3 months)
- Bubble packing medications
- Two-in-one drug combinations
- Long-acting drug formulations

Bibliography

Centers for Disease Control: Chronic Disease Overview [Internet]. http://www.cdc.gov/chronicdisease/overview/index.htm.

The College of Family Physicians Canada: Priority Topics and Key Features with Corresponding Skill Dimensions and Phases of the Encounter [Internet]. http://www.cfpc.ca/uploadedFiles/Education/Priority%20Topics%20and%20Key%20Features.pdf.

World Health Organization: Noncommunicable Diseases [Internet]. http://www.who.int/mediacentre/factsheets/fs355/en/.

Asthma

Priority Topic 7

Definition

Chronic inflammatory disease of the airways characterized by reversible airflow limitation and a variable degree of hyperresponsiveness of airways to stimuli.

Symptoms

- Wheeze, cough, or sputum production, difficulty breathing, chest tightness.
- Symptoms are frequent, recurrent, and often worse at night and in the early morning.
- Typically exacerbated by exercise, allergen exposure (eg, house dust mites, pets, pollens, moulds, spores), viral infections, cigarette smoke, cold or damp air, or emotions.
- History of improvement in symptoms or lung function in response to trial of beta-agonists or inhaled corticosteroids (ICSs).

Risk Factors

- Personal history of atopic disorder
- Family history of atopic disorder and/or asthma

Diagnosis/Investigation

- Rule out other disorders: For example, tumours in adults or foreign body in children
- Diagnosis:
  - In adults and children ≥6 years of age: Spirometry
    - Spirometry measures presence and severity of airflow obstruction, as well as reversibility of obstruction.
    - As demonstrated in the Canadian Thoracic Society Guidelines (2):

TABLE 7-1	**Spirometry Diagnostic Criteria for Asthma***	
	CHILDREN ≥6 YEARS	ADULTS
Reduced pre bronchodilator FEV$_1$/FVC	Less than the lower limit of normal (approx. <0.8-0.9)	Less than the lower limit of normal (approx. <0.75-0.8)
Post bronchodilator improvement (FEV$_1$)	≥12%	≥12% (and a minimum of 200 mL)

*If spirometry results are nondiagnostic, but there is still suspicion of asthma, consider peak expiratory flow variability, methacholine challenge test, exercise challenge test, ± inhaled corticosteroid trial for 4 to 6 weeks.

- In children, <6 years of age (Canadian Thoracic Society [CTS] and Canadian Paediatric Society [CPS]):
  - Clinical diagnosis based on asthma-like episodes.
    - Episodes should demonstrate airflow obstruction (wheeze) and reversibility (improvement with short-acting bronchodilator +/− corticosteroid), when no alternative diagnosis is suspected.
  - When it is not possible to have a healthcare practitioner demonstrate asthma-like episode, convincing parental report will suffice (1).
- Chest x-ray is NOT required for diagnosis of asthma; consider if need to rule out other causes of wheezing, or further complications such as pneumonia on a background of asthma (1).

General Management

- Most people with asthma should have minimal to no impact on their quality of life.
- As demonstrated in the 2012 CTS guidelines, well-controlled asthma is defined as (2):
  - Daytime symptoms <4 days/week
  - Night-time symptoms <1 night/week
  - Use of reliever/rescue treatment <4 doses/week
  - No limitation of activities or absence from work/school due to asthma
  - Good lung function (PEF or FEV_1 ≥90% personal best), with minimal PEF diurnal variation (<10%-15%)
  - Mild, infrequent exacerbations at most
- Asthma control should be assessed q3 to 4 months (1):
  - Exacerbations or poor baseline control → consider more intensive management
  - Minimal symptoms → consider step-down/reduced therapy
- Allergens and irritants (1):
  - Evaluate and assess impact and exposure.
  - Consider allergy testing in children with persistent symptoms.
- Recommend complete cessation of smoking and avoidance of environmental tobacco smoke.
- Recommend annual influenza vaccination for patients and their families.

Pharmacological Management

- Devices:
  - Children: Metered dose inhaler (MDI) → First line (with an age-appropriate spacer)
  - Adults: Dry powdered device (DPI) → Efficacious and often more convenient
    - Can also be used in children >6 years (typically second line).
- General measures:
  - Review medication adherence and inhaler technique frequently.
  - Reconsider diagnosis if poor response to therapy.
  - Develop asthma action plan with the patient (http://www.Asthma-ActionPlan.com): See CTS 2012 guidelines for further information (2).
- Stepwise approach:
  - A stepwise approach should be taken to pharmacotherapy.
  - Start treatment at the step that is most appropriate to the initial severity of asthma.
- Pharmacology as per CTS 2012 guidelines (2):
  - For mild, infrequent symptoms: Use inhaled SABA PRN.
  - Any indicator of poorly controlled asthma warrants daily ICS at the lowest effective dose.

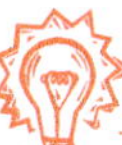

Recall that many children will outgrow symptoms by age 6, but if untreated while symptomatic, may have *permanently reduced lung function*—thus, should be treated early and until they outgrow it (if they outgrow it).

Below is the list of definitions that are used commonly throughout the asthma and chronic obstructive pulmonary disease (COPD) chapter. Some trade names are listed to further facilitate recognition. This list is not meant to be all-inclusive:
- SABA: Short-acting beta-agonist, such as salbutamol (Ventolin, Airomir) or terbutaline (Bricanyl)
- LABA: Long-acting beta-agonist, such as formoterol (Oxeze, Foradil) or salmeterol (Serevent)
- SAMA: Short-acting muscarinic antagonist, such as ipratropium (Atrovent)
- LAMA: Long-acting muscarinic antagonist, such as tiotropium (Spiriva)
- LTRA: Leukotriene receptor antagonist, such as montelukast (Singulair)
- ICS, such as fluticasone (Flovent), budesonide (Pulmicort), beclomethasone (Qvar), mometasone (Asmanex), ciclesonide (Alvesco)
- Some ICS/LABA combinations include Advair, Symbicort, Breo, Zenhale

Children 6 to 11 Years

If low dose ICS is inadequate → Increase to medium dose ICS before considering adjunctive therapy with LABA or LTRA.

Adults and Children ≥12 Years

If low dose ICS is inadequate → LABA added as first-adjunctive therapy (preferably in a combination inhaler with the ICS).*

- A figure demonstrating the above asthma management continuum, as well as additional details, may be found in the CTS 2012 guidelines (2).

Acute ER Treatment

- Oxygen: Supplemental oxygen to keep O_2 saturations ≥94% to 95%
- Bronchodilators:
  - MDI preferred if able to tolerate.
  - Severe exacerbations may require nebulizers (intermittent or continuous).
  - Inhaled salbutamol q20 mins × one to three doses, depending on severity, +/− add inhaled ipratropium to first three doses of salbutamol (depending on severity).
- Steroids:
  - Inhaled versus oral versus IV depending on severity (inhaled reserved only for very mild exacerbations)
  - If corticosteroid required in the ED, discharge home with:
    Adults: 30 to 50 mg prednisone po × 5 to 10 days
    Children: 1 to 2 mg/kg/day (max 50-60 mg) × 3 to 5 days
- Severe exacerbations +/− impending respiratory failure consider (3):
  - IV magnesium or
  - IV salbutamol, or
  - Medications such as aminophylline

References

1. Ducharme FM, Dell SD, Radhakrishnan D, et al. Diagnosis and management of asthma in preschoolers: A Canadian Thoracic Society and Canadian Paediatric Society position paper. *Can Resp J.* 2015;22(3):135-143.

2. Lougheed MD, Lemiere C, Ducharme FM, et al. Canadian Thoracic Society Asthma Clinical Assembly. Canadian Thoracic Society 2012 guideline update: Diagnosis and management of asthma in preschoolers, children and adults. *Can Resp J.* 2012;19(2):127-164.

3. Ortiz-Alvarez O, Mikrogianakis A. Canadian Paediatric Society. Acute Care Committee Position Statement: Managing the paediatric patient with an acute asthma exacerbation. *Paediatr Child Health.* 2012;17(5):251-255.

Bibliography

Evans M, Meuser J. *Mosby's Family Practice Sourcebook.* 4th ed. Ontario, Canada: University of Toronto; 2005.

Lougheed MD, Lemière C, Dell SD, et al. Canadian Thoracic Society Asthma Management Continuum—2010 Consensus Summary for children six years of age and over, and adults. *Can Resp J.* 2010;17(1):15-24.

---

* In patients ≥12 years the addition of a LABA to low dose ICS is more effective than simply increasing ICS dose from low to medium. There are concerns, however, regarding the safety of LABA (re: exacerbations, death); risks and benefits should be considered in the selection of either treatment option. This is an area that requires further research.

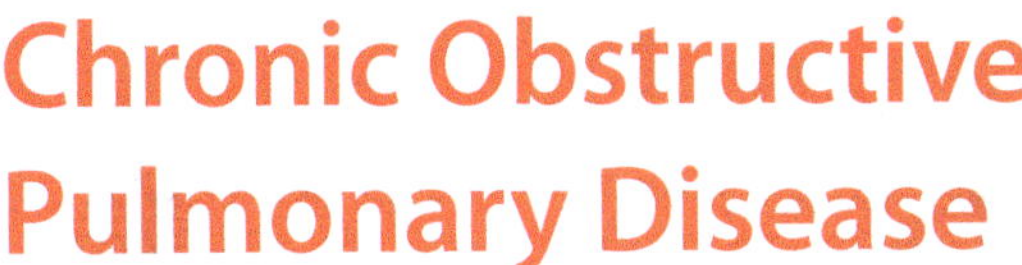

Chronic Obstructive Pulmonary Disease

Priority Topic 15

Definition

COPD encompasses both chronic bronchitis and emphysema. It is a chronic, slowly progressive disease characterized by airway obstruction that is largely fixed but may be partially reversible with bronchodilators.

Symptoms

Major symptoms include dyspnea (initially exertional), chronic/recurrent cough and/or sputum production, but may also include frequent infections, chest tightness or wheeze.

Risk Factors

- Smoking (80%-90% of cases)—Most important cause and contributing factor for COPD progression.
- Nonsmoking risk factors (10%-20%)— Mostly occupational or environmental exposures but also less common causes or risk factors such as α-1 antitrypsin deficiency (1%).

Diagnosis

- Definitive diagnosis requires spirometry: Post bronchodilator FEV_1/FVC <0.7 (indicates obstruction)
- Postbronchodilator FEV_1 % predicted used to stratify stage/severity of disease (1):
  - FEV_1 ≥80% predicted = mild
  - FEV_1 ≥50% but <80% predicted = moderate
  - FEV_1 ≥30% but <50% predicted = severe
  - FEV_1 <30% predicted = very severe
- Indications for spirometry include:
  - Smokers/ex-smokers ≥40 years of age PLUS one of the following:
    - Frequent respiratory infections
    - Dyspnea including SOBOE (eg, simple chores)
    - Chronic cough or sputum production
    - Wheeze (esp. at night or on exertion)
  - Select patients depending on exposures
- Mass screening of asymptomatic people with spirometry not recommended.
- Other investigations as required by history and physical examination (eg, CXR, further PFTs, stress test, ABG, sputum, echocardiogram, α-1 antitrypsin level if <45 years or nonsmoker, etc.)

As of 2016, the Canadian Task Force on Preventative Healthcare has recommended: Patients age 55 to 74, with ≥30 pack year smoking history, who are either current smokers or have quit in the past 15 years, may benefit from lung cancer screening with low dose CT scan annually, for up to 3 consecutive years. Note should be made that this is considered a "weak" recommendation, where both the benefits and harms of screening must be considered. Of additional interest: Chest radiography with or without sputum cytology, is not recommended for lung cancer screening. *Note that these recommendations apply to screening and thus, are not applicable if patients have signs or symptoms suggestive of lung cancer.*

Clinical Approach

- Quantify tobacco consumption and occupational or environmental exposures, and encourage minimizing exposures.
- Assess SOB and other symptoms:
  - Medical Research Council Dyspnoea Scale (mMRC)
  - COPD assessment tool (CAT)
- Assess frequency and severity of exacerbations.
- Assess for complications of COPD (eg, cor pulmonale).
- Assess for comorbidities (eg, Lung CA, CVD).
- Assess current therapy and need for further intervention.

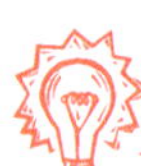

Goals of COPD management: Prevent progression, alleviate symptoms, improve exercise tolerance, reduce exacerbations, treat complications, improve health status, and reduce mortality.

Management

- COPD management should be based on symptoms + lung function/classification of airflow limitation + frequency/severity of exacerbations (consider the GOLD system to guide therapy).

  An ABCD grading system has been developed to guide therapy. Details can be found in the Global Initiative for COPD Reports (1).

- Drug and nondrug strategies can improve symptoms, activity levels, and quality of life.

(a) Smoking cessation

- Most effective intervention for preventing COPD progression, even in long-term smokers.
- Offer help to all smokers/families.
- Reinforce cessation at every contact.

(b) Education and self-management

- Focus on improving coping skills and quality of life.
- Encourage exercise—If activities are limited by symptoms, refer to an exercise training program.
- Refer to a pulmonary rehabilitation program/community respiratory services. Early participation has been shown to improve QOL.

(c) Drug management

Treatment regimen should be individualized considering severity of symptoms, degree of airflow limitation, and frequency of exacerbations.

- Bronchodilators:

  Short-acting bronchodilators
  - Regular and PRN use of short-acting bronchodilators improves symptoms.
  - SABA + SAMA combinations are superior to either medication alone.

  Long-acting bronchodilators
  - Regular use of long-acting bronchodilators improves symptoms and reduce rates of exacerbations (LAMA > LABA).
  - Combination therapy with both agents is superior to either medication alone.
- ICSs:
  - Main purpose → Reduce rates of exacerbation
  - Consider use if ≥1 to 2 COPD exacerbations per year

(d) Ongoing care

- Vaccinations:
  - Influenza—Annually
  - Pneumococcal—At least once per lifetime (consider repeat in 5-10 years)
- Long-term O_2 (typically for severe hypoxemia PaO_2 ≤55 mm Hg, or PaO_2 ≤60 mm Hg + bilateral ankle edema or cor pulmonale or hematocrit of >55%).
- In severe disease, discuss end-of-life issues, and patient's wishes on aggressive treatments.

Acute Exacerbations of COPD (AECOPD)

- Acute worsening of symptoms beyond day-to-day variation results in additional treatment; typically characterized by worsening dyspnea, sputum production or purulence and often in association with increased cough and/or wheeze.
- Triggers:
  - Viral or bacterial upper respiratory infection—Most common cause
  - Others: Irritants, PE, MI, anemia, CHF, systemic infection

- Short-acting beta-agonists (SABA) = salbutamol
- Short-acting anticholinergics/muscarinic Antagonists (SAMA) = ipratropium
- Long-acting beta-agonists (LABA) = salmeterol, formoterol
- Long-acting anticholinergics/muscarinic Antagonists (LAMA) = tiotropium

- Severe AECOPD can be a medical emergency;
  - Develop an exacerbation action plan (eg, CTS COPD action plan)
- Therapies include:

Bronchodilators

- Escalate use of short-acting bronchodilators to control symptoms (wheeze, dyspnea)
- May be adequate intervention for mild exacerbations

Systemic corticosteroids

- For moderate-to-severe exacerbations (good evidence)
- Typical regime = oral prednisone 25 to 50 mg/day (or equivalent) for 5 to 14 days (some sources suggest limiting use to 7 days maximum)

Antibiotics

- For moderate-to-severe exacerbations **or** if two of the following three symptoms:
  1. Increased dyspnea
  2. Increased sputum production
  3. Increased sputum purulence
- Antibiotic choice should be based on patient risk factors and local resistance patterns:
  - Multiple risk stratification tools exist for antibiotic selection in AECOPD.
  - For a simple exacerbation in a patient with COPD but without risk factors, first choices include doxycycline, TMP-SMX, amoxicillin, cephalosporins, and extended spectrum macrolides, depending on local resistance patterns.
  - In a patient with COPD and *risk factors**, the exacerbation is said to be complicated, and first choice may include a fluoroquinolone such as levofloxacin or moxifloxacin, or β-lactam/β-lactamase inhibitor such as amoxicillin-clavulin.
  - Alternatively, use appropriate antibiotics, such as ciprofloxacin, for suspected pseudomonas.

**Risk factors for complicated AECOPD as per CTS guidelines (2)*
- FEV1 <50% predicted
- Four or more exacerbations per year
- Use of home oxygen
- Use of chronic oral steroids
- Antibiotic use in the past 3 months
- Ischemic heart disease

**Risk factors for pseudomonas as per CTS guidelines (2):*
- Patients at risk of acquiring pseudomonas typically have very poor lung function (FEV$_1$ <35% predicted) or multiple risk factors from the above list. They have constantly purulent sputum; some have bronchiectasis.

References

1. Global Initiative for Chronic Obstructive Lung Disease: *Global Strategy for the Diagnosis, Management and Prevention of COPD*, 2017 Report. Available from: http://goldcopd.org/.

2. O'Donnell DE, Aaron S, Bourbeau j, et al. Canadian Thoracic Society Recommendations for management of chronic obstructive pulmonary disease—2003 update. *Can Resp J.* 2003;10(Supplement A):11A-33A.

Bibliography

Evans M, Meuser J. *Mosby's Family Practice Sourcebook.* 4th ed. University of Toronto: Ontario, Canada; 2005.

Kennedy S, Baerlocher MO. Screening for lung cancer. *CMAJ.* 2014;186(8):E296-E296.

O'Donnell DE, Aaron S, Bourbeau J, et al. Canadian Thoracic Society Recommendations for management of chronic obstructive pulmonary disease – 2007 update. *Can Resp J.* 2007;14(Supplement B): 5B-32B.

O'Donnell DE, Hernandez P, Kaplan A, et al. Canadian Thoracic Recommendations for management of chronic obstructive pulmonary disease – 2008 update. *Can Resp J.* 2008;15(Supplement A):1A-8A.

Singh S, Loke Y, Furberg C. Inhaled anticholinergics and risk of major adverse cardiovascular events in patients with chronic obstructive pulmonary disease: a systematic review and meta-analysis. *JAMA.* 2008;300(12):1439-1450.

Tsiligianni I, Goodridge D, Marciniuk D, Hull S, Bourbeau J. Four patients with a history of acute exacerbations of COPD: Implementing the CHEST/Canadian Thoracic Society guidelines for preventing exacerbations. *NPJ Prim Care Respir Med.* 2015;25:15023.

Hypertension

Priority Topic 47

Definitions

Note: All blood pressures noted are in mm Hg.

- **Hypertensive urgency:** Blood pressure ≥180/110 *without* signs of target end-organ damage.

- **Hypertensive emergency:** Blood pressure ≥180/110 with signs of target end-organ damage.

- **Hypertension:** Blood pressure ≥140/90 (classically), or a corresponding value depending on method of measurement (see thresholds in the diagnostic algorithm, Figure 7-1).

- **Hypertension (DM):** Blood pressure ≥130/80.

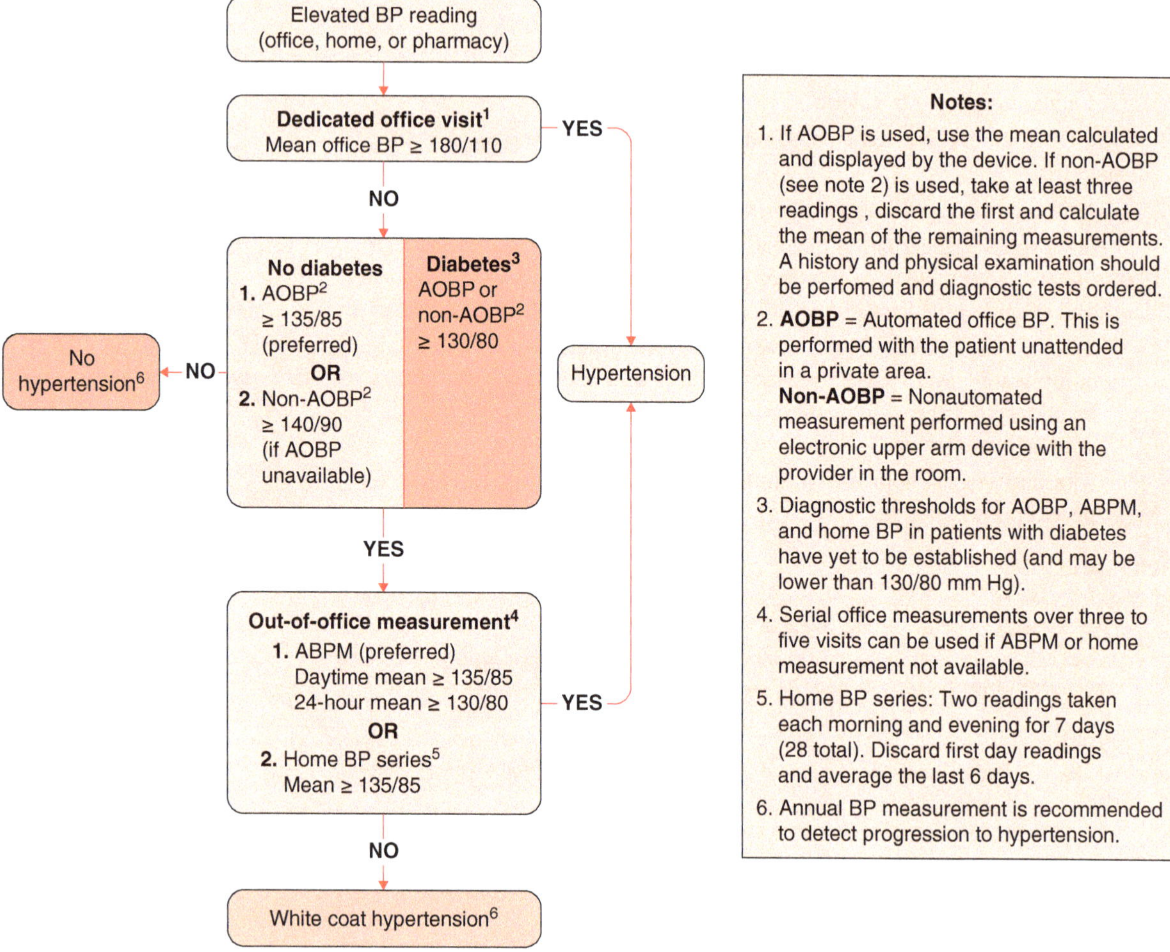

FIGURE 7-1:   From Leung AA, et al. *Can J Cardiol.* 2016;32(5):569-588, with permission from Elsevier.

Screen

- Screen routinely at least every 2 years, or annually if pre-hypertension (120-139/80-89) is identified.

- Screening may begin at 3 years of age.

BP Measurement Method (1)

- Diagnosis of hypertension depends on whether it is an ambulatory, home, or office value (attended or nonattended).

Out-of-office BP measurements

- Preferred to clinic measurements (ambulatory BP monitoring > home BP monitoring)
- Reasons for preference: White coat HTN, masked HTN, and better predictive value of hypertensive risks/complications

In-office BP measurements

- ≥2 readings should be taken during the same initial visit.
- Automated BP is preferred to auscultatory measurement (due to errors in auscultatory measurement).
- Unattended automatic BP measurement (without health provider interaction, using a fully automatic device in a quiet room or private area) is preferred to attended automatic BP measurement.
  - Attended readings—First value is discarded and latter readings averaged
    - HTN if ≥140/90
  - Unattended readings—The average BP should be calculated
    - HTN if ≥135/85

Diagnosis (1)

Due to the variability of values and white coat syndrome, it may take several visits before diagnosis.

Diagnostic algorithm may be obtained from the 2016 CHEP guidelines (1).

In-office measurements

A. Blood pressure ≥180/110 (hypertensive urgency or emergency) diagnose as hypertensive and manage immediately!

B. Blood pressure ≤180/110
  - Diagnosis of HTN is made from serial office visits.
  - Use the *average BP across all visits.*
  - Preferably, out-of-office BP measurements should be performed before visit 2 (ambulatory > home BP) using corresponding hypertensive thresholds.
  - Diagnose HTN in the following **in-office** scenarios:
    - Visit 2— Mean office BP ≥140/90 (systolic and/or diastolic) in patients with DM, chronic kidney disease (CKD) (GFR <60), or macrovascular target organ damage
    - Visit 3—Mean office BP ≥160/100 (systolic and/or diastolic)
    - Visit 5—Mean office BP ≥140/90 (systolic and/or diastolic)

Out-of-office BP measurements

  - Home BP and ambulatory BP (daytime readings)—HTN if average BP ≥135/85
  - 24-hour ambulatory readings—HTN if average BP ≥130/80

Evaluation (History, Physical, and Investigations)

Following diagnosis of hypertension: A history and physical examination +/− investigations should be performed immediately (within the same office visit), with a follow-up visit scheduled within 1 month.

■ **History (1)**

- Typically asymptomatic until complications arise.
- Inquire about cardiovascular risk factors (modifiable and nonmodifiable) for atherosclerosis—*refer to Ischemic Heart Disease section.*
- Inquire about signs and symptoms of target organ damage.
  - Cerebrovascular disease: TIA, prior stroke, and vascular dementia
  - Cardiovascular disease (angina, MI, LVH, or CHF)
  - Peripheral artery disease (intermittent claudication)

- ◦ Nephropathy (hx of CKD or albuminuria)
- ◦ Retinopathy (hx of hypertensive retinopathy)
- Rule out exogenous factors:
  - ◦ Prescription drugs (NSAIDs, steroids, venlafaxine, OCPs, decongestants, cold remedies which contain pseudoephedrine)
  - ◦ ETOH, stimulants (incl. cocaine), anabolic steroids, sodium intake

- **Physical examination**
  - Central and peripheral cardiovascular examination, abdominal examination, fundoscopy—looking for signs of target organ damage as outlined above.
  - **Features suggesting secondary hypertension (1):**
    - ◦ Sudden onset or worsening of hypertension and age >55 or <30 years
    - ◦ Hypertension resistant to three or more drugs
    - ◦ Renovascular symptoms:
      - ▫ Abdominal bruit
      - ▫ Rise in creatinine >30% with use of ACE-I or ARB
      - ▫ Pulmonary edema with hypertensive surges
      - ▫ Other atherosclerotic vascular disease
    - ◦ Renal insufficiency (including polycystic kidney)
    - ◦ Hyperaldosteronism features:
      - ▫ Unexplained spontaneous hypokalemia
      - ▫ Presence of an incidental adrenal adenoma
    - ◦ Pheochromocytoma features:
      - ▫ Headaches, palpitations
      - ▫ Sweating
      - ▫ Paroxysmal hypertension
      - ▫ Presence of an incidental adrenal adenoma
    - ◦ Thyroid disease
    - ◦ Cushing syndrome: Central obesity, moon face, striae, hirsutism, and acne
    - ◦ Obstructive sleep apnea: Daytime fatigue, snoring, and thick neck

- **Investigations**
  - Initial routine investigations (1):
    - ◦ Urinalysis (with urine albumin:creatinine ratio **if** DM or CKD)
    - ◦ Renal panel with creatinine and electrolytes (sodium, potassium)
    - ◦ Fasting glucose and/or HbA1c to test for concomitant DM
    - ◦ Lipid panel and triglycerides (fasting or non)—*refer to Hyperlipidemia Section*
    - ◦ 12-lead ECG
  - Appropriate investigations for secondary hypertension if indicated.
  - Appropriate investigations for complications if indicated (eg, echo if suspected LVH).
  - Follow-up lab monitoring dependent on clinical situation and choice of treatment.

Management

Assess overall cardiovascular risk (ie, vascular age, heart age)

Initiate lifestyle modification and/or pharmacotherapy as outlined below.

- **Lifestyle modifications** (1):
  - Weight loss targets:
    - ◦ BMI = 18.5 to 24.9 kg/m^2,
    - ◦ Waist circumference <102 cm for men, <88 cm for women

- DASH diet (dietary strategies against hypertension)
  - Emphasizes fruits and vegetables, fibre and whole grains, protein from plant sources, low fat dairy products, and overall reduction in saturated fat and cholesterol
- Low sodium intake (~2000 mg/d)
- Physical activity (30-60 min of moderate intensity dynamic exercise such as walking, cycling, swimming for 4-7 days/week + activities of daily living)
- Alcohol in moderation:
  - ≤ 2 drinks/day
  - Maximum: Men = 14 drinks/week, women = 9 drinks/week
- Stress management
- Smoking cessation
- Potassium
  - If NOT at risk of hyperkalemia → Increase dietary potassium to further reduce BP.
  - High risk of hyperkalemia includes patients with any of the following*:
    a. Baseline serum potassium >4.5 mmol/L
    b. CKD (GFR <60)
    c. Receiving renin-angiotensin-aldosterone inhibitors or other drugs known to cause hyperkalemia (eg, TMP-SMX, amiloride, triamterene…)

■ **Pharmacotherapy** (1):

1. Thresholds for *initiation* of drug therapy
   a. *Without* macrovascular target organ damage or other CVD risk factors

   BP ≥160/100 (systolic *or* diastolic)

   b. *With* macrovascular target organ damage or other independent CVD risk factors (including diabetes)

   BP ≥140/90 (systolic *or* diastolic)

   c. Frail elderly patients and anyone ≥80 years

   BP ≥160 SBP (assuming no DM or target organ damage)

2. HTN treatment targets (*once on pharmacotherapy*)**:
■ Most patients: ≤140/90
■ Age ≥80 years: SBP <150 mm Hg
■ DM: ≤130/80

3. Key points for HTN medication use
■ Start with monotherapy using a first-line medication. If adverse effects occur, another drug may be substituted.
■ Add a second medication if target BP levels are not achieved with standard dose monotherapy
■ *Consider* initiating treatment with two medications if systolic ≥20 mm Hg above target or diastolic ≥10 mm Hg above target.
■ First-line medications include—*Refer to first-line therapy for specific indications section (below)*:
  - ACE-I or ARB.
  - Thiazide.

ACRONYMS:
- ACE-I: Angiotensin Converting Enzyme Inhibition
- ARB: Angiotensin II Receptor Blockers
- BB: Beta Blocker
- CCB: Calcium Channel Blocker
- DHP CCB: Dihydropyridine Calcium Channel Blocker
- Non-DHP CCB: Non-Dihydropyridine Calcium Channel Blocker

---

* Assess and monitor closely before advising to increase potassium intake.

** Assessment of risks/benefits of lowering BP with medications must be considered prior to treatment or adjustment of medications.

- Long-acting CCB
- Beta-blocker (in patients <60 years) Often used for specific indications such as stable angina.

■ Multiple drug therapy is required in many patients.

■ Consider referral to a specialist if BP is not controlled with three antihypertensives.

4. First-therapy for specific indications (1)*:

Cardiovascular disease:

■ CAD: ACE-I or ARB; BB or CCB in patients with stable angina

■ Recent MI: BB + ACE-I (or ARBs if intolerant)

■ Heart failure: ACE-I/ARB + BB

■ Left ventricular hypertrophy: ACE-I (or ARB if intolerant), or long-acting CCB, or thiazide/thiazide-like diuretics

■ Previous stroke or TIA: ACE-I + thiazide/thiazide-like diuretic (note: combination drugs are available)

Diabetes (DM):

■ DM with microalbuminuria, renal disease, cardiovascular disease or associated risk factors: ACE-I or ARB

■ DM without above features: ACE-I (or ARB), or DHP-CCB or thiazide/thiazide-like diuretics

Non-diabetic CKD:

■ ACE-I (or ARB) if proteinuria

■ Diuretics as additive therapy

Follow-Up

■ If lifestyle modification only: Every 3 to 6 months (unless BP not well controlled, then q1-2 monthly depending on BP)

■ If anti-HTN drug treatment:

Every 1 to 2 months until two consecutive readings below target;

Every 3 to 6 months after BP target met (assuming BP remains in control)

Exception: Severe or symptomatic HTN should be seen more frequently.

■ As indicated in the investigations section, follow-up lab monitoring is dependent on clinical situation and choice of treatment

Management of Hypertensive Urgency/Emergency

■ Hypertensive urgency—Options for management include any of the following:
- Nicardipine, captopril, clonidine, and labetalol

■ Hypertensive emergency—Admit to hospital for IV medications to lower blood pressure

Hypertension in Pregnancy—Medications

■ Typical medications: Labetalol, methyldopa, or a long-acting DHP-CCB (nifedipine XL) (note: CCB are not to be used if giving magnesium)

Reference

1. Leung AA, Nerenberg K, Daskalopoulou SS, et al. Hypertension Canada's 2016 Canadian Hypertension Education Program Guidelines for Blood Pressure Measurement, Diagnosis, Assessment of Risk, Prevention, and Treatment of Hypertension. *Can J Cardiol*. 2016;32(5):569-588.

---

*See the latest CHEP 2016 guidelines (1) for additional detail on medical management, and for second-line therapies.

Bibliography

2015 Top Ten Canadian Clinical Guidelines: Hypertension [Internet]. http://www.top10guidelines.elsevier.ca/#/1-122.

DynaMed. Hypertensive Emergency. Ipswich, MA: EBSCO Publishing; 2011. http://search.-ebscohost.com.cyber.usask.ca/login.aspx?direct=true&site=DynaMed&id=113862. Accessed March, 2012.

Jensen B, Regier L, eds. RxFiles drug comparison charts. Oral Antihypertensives Summary/Guidelines Comparison Chart. 8th ed. Saskatoon, SK: Saskatoon Health Region: 6.

National Heart, Lung, and Blood Institute. Seventh report of the Joint National Committee on prevention, detection, evaluation and treatment of high blood pressure (JNC 7) express. *JAMA.* 2003;289:2560-2571.

Rabi DM, Daskalopoulou SS, Padwal RS, et al. The 2011 Canadian Hypertension Education Program recommendations for the management of hypertension: blood pressure measurement, diagnosis, assessment of risk, and therapy. *Can J Cardiol.* 2011;27(4):415-433.

United States Preventive Services Task Force. Screening for high blood pressure: U.S. preventive services task force reaffirmation recommendation statement. *Ann In Medicine.* 2007;147(11):783.

Hyperlipidemia

Priority Topic 46

Note should be made that certain aspects of hyperlipidemia diagnosis and management are somewhat controversial. This review presents a combination of information from the 2015 Canadian Family Physician (CFP) guidelines (1) and the 2016 Canadian Cardiovascular Society (CCS) guidelines (2).

Definition

Elevated total cholesterol, low-density lipoprotein cholesterol, or non-high-density lipoprotein cholesterol levels

Screening/Risk Factors

- In the *absence* of risk factors or conditions that ↑ risk of CVD, initiate screening in:

  CFP guideline: Men ≥40 years and women ≥50 years (1)

  CCS guideline: Both men and women ≥40 years (2)
  - Consider earlier screening in ethnic groups at ↑ risk (South Asian or First Nations)
  - Screen earlier if women are postmenopausal prior to age cut-offs.
  - Screen earlier in all patients with compelling risk factors for CVD.
- Compelling risk factors for CVD*:
  - Clinical evidence of atherosclerosis
  - Clinical signs of hyperlipidemia (arcus cornealis, xanthomas, xanthelasmas)
  - AAA
  - Erectile dysfunction
  - Hypertension
  - Diabetes mellitus
  - Obesity (BMI ≥30 kg/m^2)
  - CKD
  - Current cigarette smoking
  - HIV infection
  - Inflammatory disease (eg, IBD, SLE, rheumatoid arthritis…)—more evidence is needed to determine which inflammatory conditions are truly independently associated with elevated CVD risk
  - Family history of premature CAD
  - Family history of dyslipidemia

---

*Metabolic syndrome is an additional consideration for CVD risk—see Metabolic Syndrome at the end of the Hyperlipidemia section.

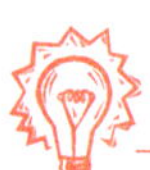

The Framingham risk score doubles if there is a history of premature CVD in a first-degree relative (<55 years for males, <65 years for females).

- Frequency of lipid screening:

Patient *NOT* on lipid lowering medication -

- Lipid panel—Typically adequate to test every 5 years* (CFP).
- CVD risk assessment (eg, modified Framingham risk score [3]) with blood testing and whenever a patient's expected risk status changes.

Lipid Testing

- Lipid values should be interpreted in the context of the patient's risk category. An LDL of ≥5.0 mmol/L alone is an indication for medical management. For LDL <5.0 mmol/L, the patient's overall risk must be considered. See *Pharmacotherapy* for detail.
- Lipid profile:
  - *Nonfasting lipid testing is acceptable*—does not significantly affect the overall risk assessment tools and ability to predict CVD events.
  - If patient has a history of triglyceride levels >4.5 mmol/L then fasting lipid testing recommended—studies in this group of patients are lacking.
- Rule out secondary causes of hyperlipidemia before making diagnosis.

Management/Treatment

- Lifestyle modifications
  - Smoking cessation
  - Diet (eg, mediterranean diet)
  - Exercise (≥150 minutes per week of moderate intensity, aerobic activity)
  - Other (moderate ETOH consumption, sufficient sleep, stress management, etc)
- Pharmacotherapy (when to start a statin):

Three major categories in which statins are considered (2):

1. **Statin-indicated conditions**—For these conditions prescribe statins, regardless of risk assessment (already considered high risk)
   a. Clinical atherosclerosis
      - Prior MI
      - Coronary revascularization (percutaneous coronary intervention, CABG, or other revascularization procedure)
      - Angina pectoris
      - Cerebrovascular disease (eg, TIA, CVA)
      - Peripheral vascular disease/peripheral artery obstructive disease (claudication and/or ABI <0.9)
   b. AAA (>3.0 cm diameter)
   c. DM plus one of the following:
      - Age ≥40 for T2DM or ≥30 for T1DM
      - >15 years duration
      - Microvascular disease
   d. CKD and age ≥50 (not recommended to initiate if already dialysis dependent, but not recommended to discontinue once becoming dialysis dependent)
   e. LDL ≥5.0 mmol/L
2. **Primary prevention**—Based on risk assessment (eg, Framingham) in the absence of a statin-indicated condition:
   a. Low risk (<10%)—No statin indicated

---

*Lipid levels change minimally over the short-term (1).

b. Intermediate risk (10%-19%)—Statin indicated if any one of the following:
   ◦ LDL ≥3.5 mmol/L
   ◦ Non-HDL ≥4.3
   ◦ Additional risk factors
c. High risk (≥20%): Statin indicated

3. Secondary prevention -
   - Start statin based on occurrence of previous event (such as MI or stroke)
   - Further risk assessment not necessary (already considered high risk)

- Pharmacotherapy/medication choices.
- Statin intensity refers to the potency of a particular statin type, and the dose of the statin.
- Statin intensity refers to the poten statin intensity based on what is necessary to reach treatment targets, based on lipid levels. Other guidelines argue that adjusting statin intensity to achieve treatment targets is unnecessary and that statin type and dose should depend on patient characteristics/risk categories.
   - Treatment based on risk category: Evidence favours the use of moderate- or high-intensity statin therapy in all patients, where high-risk patients benefit most from high-intensity therapy, and moderate-risk patients are good candidates for moderate-intensity therapy (1).
   - Treatment to target: ***Recommended target is LDL <2.0 mmol/L or >50% reduction of LDL*** (2)
- Reduction lipids.
- Refer to screening for patients not taking lipid therapy.
- Referr to screen lipid therapy:
   - The 2015 CFP guidelines recommend using lipid levels *prior* to statin therapy, and adjusting risk estimation by 25% to 35% reduction based on statin intensity (low intensity = 25% relative risk reduction, high intensity = 35% relative risk reduction) (1).
   - The 2016 CCS guidelines recommend monitoring lipid therapy lipids to ensure achieving treatment targets. It would be reasonable to check lipids 3 to 6 months after initiation of a medication or dose change. For every 1 mmol/L reduction of LDL, there is approximately a 20% to 22% risk reduction (2).

Important Points on Statin Use

- Statin use can be associated with muscle and liver injury, elevated glucose levels.
- Myalgia is a common adverse effect, but rhabdomyolsis is rare.
- Elevation in liver enzymes are common, but liver failure is rare.
- Testing CK and LFTs at baseline or for monitoring is not required but should be performed as clinically indicated.
   - One may choose to test CK and LFTs at baseline when starting a statin.
   - Some sources recommend testing CK and LFTs at 0, 3, 6 and 12 months, though this is likely unnecessary in many patients and has the potential to do harm (due to unnecessary cessation of statin therapy in asymptomatic patients); increases in CK and liver enzymes often occur in asymptomatic patients, and will often return to baseline with continued use.
   - One should consider patient characteristics and risk factors that may increase the chance of muscle and liver damage, when considering monitoring.
   - Annual CK and LFTs may be considered for patients on high-dose statins, or with risk factors for statin-induced adverse effects (ex. elderly, hypothyroid, high dose, alcoholism, drug interactions).
   - If muscle pain and weakness → check CK level. Concerning if CK >3 to 5 times normal levels.

Metabolic Syndrome

A group of risk factors that raise your risk of heart disease, stroke, and more.

Diagnosis

Harmonized definition (4)—Any three of the following:

1. Abdominal obesity (population and country-specific cut-offs)
2. TG ≥1.7 mmol/L or drug therapy for prior high triglycerides
3. HDL <1.0 (males), <1.3 (females) or drug therapy for prior low HDL
4. BP ≥130 systolic and/or ≥85 diastolic or drug therapy for prior elevated BP
5. Fasting glucose ≥5.6 mol/L or drug therapy for elevated fasting plasma glucose (FPG)

Treatment

Lifestyle modification, prevention of DM2 and CVD.

References

1. Allan GM, Lindblad AJ, Comeau A, et al. Simplified lipid guidelines: Prevention and management of cardiovascular disease in primary care. *Can Fam Physician*. 2015;61(10):857-867.
2. Anderson TJ, Grégoire J, Pearson GJ, et al. Canadian Cardiovascular Society Guidelines for the Management of Dyslipidemia for the Prevention of Cardiovascular Disease in the Adult. *Can J Cardiol*. 2016;32(11):1263-1282.
3. D'Agostino RB, Vasan RS, Pencina MJ, et al. General cardiovascular risk profile for use in primary care. The Framingham Heart Study. *Circulation*. 2008;117:743-753.
4. Alberti KG M, Eckel R, Grunsy S, et al. Harmonizing the metabolic syndrome. *Circulation*. 2009;120:1640-1645.

Bibliography

DynaMed. Hypercholesterolemia. Ipswich, MA: EBSCO Publishing; 2012, Feb 6. http://search.ebscohost.com.cyber.usask.ca/login.aspx?direct=true&site=DynaMed&id=113862. Accessed March, 2012.

Genest J, McPherson R, Frohlich J, et al. Canadian Cardiovascular Society/Canadian guidelines for the diagnosis and treatment of dyslipidemia and prevention of cardiovascular disease in the adult—2009 recommendations. *Can J Cardiol*. 2009;25(10):567-579.

Jensen B, Regier L, ed. RxFiles drug comparison charts. Lipid Lowering Therapy: Dyslipidemia *Comparison Chart*. 8th ed. Saskatoon, SK: Saskatoon Health Region; 2010:15.

Leung AA, Nerenberg K, Daskalopoulou SS, et al. Hypertension Canada's 2016 Canadian Hypertension Education Program Guidelines for Blood Pressure Measurement, Diagnosis, Assessment of Risk, Prevention, and Treatment of Hypertension. *Can J Cardiol*. 2016;32(5):569-588.

Diabetes

Priority Topic 25

Prevention: Reduction of Risk Factors

- Healthy diet and lifestyle with optimal BMI (target 18.5-24.9)
- Waist circumference (M <94 cm; F <80 cm)
- Encourage aerobic activity (30 minutes) most days of the week and resistance training three times per week
- Encourage smoking cessation

Use acarbose, metformin, or thiazolidinediones to reduce risk of developing T2DM in people with prediabetes.

TABLE 7-2	Symptoms/Characteristics
DM TYPE 1	**DM TYPE 2**
• Polyuria • Polydipsia • Polyphagia • Weight loss • Blurry vision • Dehydration • Neuropathy (late sign)	• Commonly asymptomatic • Acanthosis nigricans (sign of insulin resistance)

TABLE 7-3   Risk Factors for DM Type 2

• Dyslipidemia • Overweight • Abdominal obesity • Age 40-70 • HTN • First-degree relative with DM • Hx of IGT or IFG	• Schizophrenia • Steroid use • Second-generation antipsychotic use: (olanzapine, risperidone, clozapine, quetiapine) • High-risk population (Aboriginal, Hispanic, South Asian, African)	• Hx GDM • Delivery of a macrosomic infant • Acanthosis nigricans • Vascular Dz • DM-associated complications • PCOS

TABLE 7-4   Screening

DM TYPE 2	GDM
Fasting plasma glucose (FPG) • Q 3 years if >40 years, or sooner if risk factors • More frequent screening in those at very high risk, using a scoring system such as CANRISK	50 g OGTT (screen at 24-28 weeks) • <7.8 mmol/L = normal • 7.8-10.2 = do 75 g OGTT • >10.3 = GDM

TABLE 7-5   Diagnosis of Diabetes and Glucose Impairment

	GLUCOSE TEST		
DIAGNOSIS	FPG (MMOL/L)	75G OGTT	HbA1c (%)
Normal	<6.1	<7.8	< 6
DM	>7.0 on two occasions or Random glucose >11.1 with DM symptoms	>11.1	≥ 6.5
IFG (impaired fasting glucose)	6.1-6.9		
IGT (impaired glucose tolerance)		7.8-11.0	

TABLE 7-6   Type 2 Diabetes Medications

CLASS	ADVANTAGES	DISADVANTAGES
Biguanide • Metformin	• Weight neutral • ↓ Hypoglycemia	• GI side effects • CI: CrCL/eGFR <30 mL/min • Caution if liver failure or CrCL/eGFR <60 mL/min • Risk of lactic acidosis in HF, renal or liver disease, or hypoxemia
Insulin secretagogues: Sulfonylureas • Gliclazide • Glyburide	• Newer agents (Gliclazide) associated with ↓ hypoglycemia	• Weight gain (Glyburide) • CI: Sulfa allergy—rash, photosensitivity
Insulin secretagogues: Meglitinides • Repaglinide	• ↓ Hypoglycemia with missed meals • Better postprandial control	• TID to QID dosing
Insulin sensitizers: TZDs • Rosiglitazone	• ↓ Hypoglycemia • Good monotherapy	• 6-8 weeks to maximal effect • Weight gain (fluid retention), edema, rare CHF • Increased fracture risk • Avoid in HF, liver dysfunction • May increase the risk of ischemic events

TABLE 7-6	Type 2 Diabetes Medications (*Continued*)	
CLASS	ADVANTAGES	DISADVANTAGES
DPP-4 inhibitor • Sitagliptin (Januvia)	• Weight neutral • ↓ Hypoglycemia • Good postprandial control	• No long-term studies • Not for use in kidney or liver failure
Glucagon-like peptide-1 (GLP-1) receptor agonists Exenatide Liraglutide	• Weight loss • ↓ Hypoglycemia • Good postprandial control	• Subcutaneous injection • GI side effects • Contraindicated in those with hx/FHx of medullary thyroid carcinoma or MEN-2
Sodium-glucose co-transporter-2 (SGLT-2) inhibitors • Canagliflozin • Dapagliflozin	• Weight neutral • ↓ Hypoglycemia • Good postprandial control	• UTI and genital fungal infections side effects • Hypotension possible secondary to diuresis • Long-term safety unknown
Incretin mimetic • Liraglutide (Victoza)	• Glucose-dependent insulin secretion • ↓ Hypoglycemia • Improved postprandial control • Weight loss	• Injection • Nausea and diarrhea common, decreases with use • Minor hypoglycemia if used with sulfonylureas • Pancreatitis risk • CI: Fhx of MEN-2, medullary thyroid cancer
Alpha-glucosidase inhibitor • Acarbose	↓ Risk of hypoglycemia Weight neutral Good postprandial control	• GI side effects • Use in combination with another oral agent • Modestly effective in elderly • Hypoglycemia should be treated with glucose!
Insulin	Greatest A1C reduction No maximum dose	• Weight gain • Risk of hypoglycemia

FREQUENCY OF GLUCOSE SELF-MONITORING

DM Type 1
  Minimum 3×/day
DM Type 2

Insulin+/− oral:	>1×/day
Oral only:	1 to 2×/week*
Diet only:	Occasional testing

* Individualize recommendations based on risk of hypoglycemia and level of glycemic control. If poor control and/or risk of hypoglycemia, test more frequently (1).

DM TREATMENT GOALS (MMOL/L)

	NO CVD AND		
	DM	Frail*	young/safe
A1C (q3-6mo):	<7%	<8.5%	<6%
Q 3 to 6 months			
FPG:	4 to 7		4 to 6
2hr PPG	5 to 10		5 to 8
hours post			

Screening

- Not advised for type 1 diabetes
- FPG or HbA1c q3 years in individuals ≥ 40 years, or those at high risk (using a risk calculator, such as CANRISK) (2)
- 75 g oral glucose tolerance test (OGTT) in patients with impaired glucose tolerance:
  - FPG 6.1 to 6.9 mmol/L
  - HbA1c 6.0 to 6.4%

Diagnosis

- FPG ≥7.0 mmol/L
- HbA1c ≥6.5%
- Random plasma glucose (RPG) ≥11.1 mmol/L
- 2-hour-post 75 g OGTT ≥11.1 mmol/L

Pharmacologic Management

- See Figure 7-2.

Complications/Chronic Disease Monitoring

*Frail is defined as:

- Limited life expectancy
- High level of functional dependency
- Extensive CAD, at risk of ischemic event

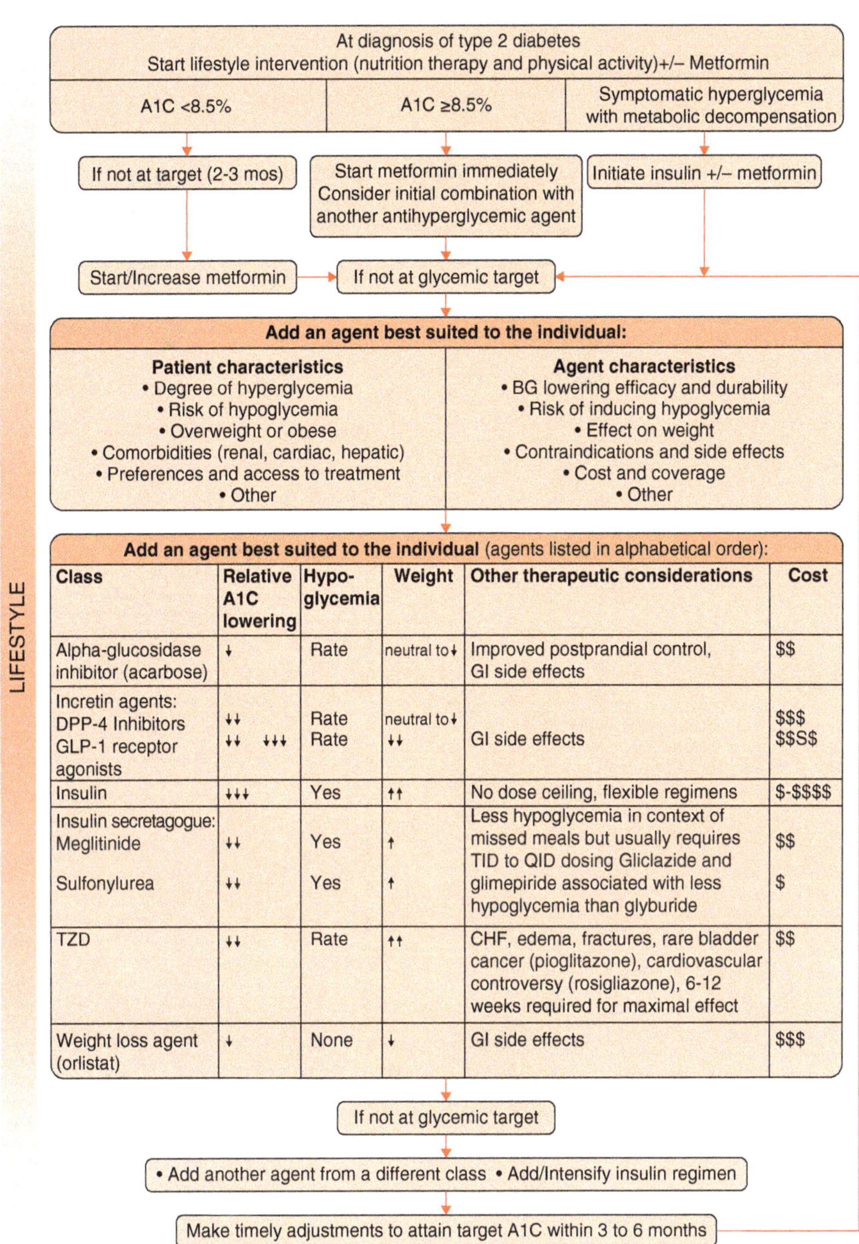

Add an agent best suited to the individual (agents listed in alphabetical order):

Class	Relative A1C lowering	Hypo-glycemia	Weight	Other therapeutic considerations	Cost
Alpha-glucosidase inhibitor (acarbose)	↓	Rare	neutral to↓	Improved postprandial control, GI side effects	$$
Incretin agents: DPP-4 Inhibitors	↓↓	Rare	neutral to↓	GI side effects	$$$
GLP-1 receptor agonists	↓↓ ↓↓↓	Rare	↓↓	GI side effects	$$$S$
Insulin	↓↓↓	Yes	↑↑	No dose ceiling, flexible regimens	$-$$$$
Insulin secretagogue: Meglitinide	↓↓	Yes	↑	Less hypoglycemia in context of missed meals but usually requires TID to QID dosing Gliclazide and glimepiride associated with less hypoglycemia than glyburide	$$
Sulfonylurea	↓↓	Yes	↑		$
TZD	↓↓	Rare	↑↑	CHF, edema, fractures, rare bladder cancer (pioglitazone), cardiovascular controversy (rosigliazone), 6-12 weeks required for maximal effect	$$
Weight loss agent (orlistat)	↓	None	↓	GI side effects	$$$

FIGURE 7-2:   Canadian Diabetes Association Clinical Practice Guidelines Expert Committee. Canadian Diabetes Association 2013 Clinical Practice Guidelines for the Prevention and Management of Diabetes in Canada. *Can J Diabetes*. 2013;37(suppl 1): S1-S212.

- Multiple comorbidities
- History of recurrent, severe hypoglycemia
- Hypoglycemia unawareness
- Long-standing diabetes with poor control, despite optimized treatment (1)

1. A1C (glycated hemoglobin):
   (a)   Test q 3 months
   (b)   Target: <7.0%
   (c)   Consider testing q 6 months if stable

IF DIABETIC PATIENT IS HIGH RISK OR HAS CVD:

Also start:

1. ACE-I/ARB (start also in your average-risk patient who is ≥55 years)
2. Statin (start also in your average-risk patient who is ≥40 years)
3. ASA/Plavix (not be used in average-risk patient for primary prevention)

TABLE 7-7	Emergency/Acute Complications of DM		
	SIGNS/SYMPTOMS	**LABS**	**TREATMENT**
Hypoglycemia <3.5 mmol/L	Tachycardia Sweating Tremulous Nausea/vomit Hunger Confusion Stupor	↓ glucose	Awake—Dextrose or 15 g glucose containing food q 15 minutes, until glucose > 5.0 mmol/L Unconscious—Glucagon IM or 50% glucose IV
Hyperglycemia	Abdominal pain Vomiting Lethargy Increased thirst Increased urination	↑ glucose	Insulin
DKA[a]	Tachycardia Vomiting Kussmaul breathing (rapid and deep) Fruity breath Lethargy Coma	↑ glucose ↑ osmolality ↑ anion-gap metabolic acidosis + Ketones ↑ K+ (falsely elevated)	Fluids K+ Insulin infusion
Hyperosmolar hyperglycemic syndrome[a]	Polyuria Polydipsia Polyphagia Weakness Lethargy Confusion Coma	↑↑ glucose ↑↑ osmolality ↑ anion-gap metabolic acidosis ↑ K+ (falsely elevated)	Fluids K+ Insulin infusion

[a]Often precipitated by infection, surgery, infarction, medical noncompliance.

2. **CKD**—Screen annually for:

		Normal	Micro	Macro
(a)	Proteinuria	<30 mg/day	30 to 300 mg/day	>300 mg/day
(b)	Urine ACR (albumin creatinine ratio):	M: <2; F: <2.8	<10× normal	>10 × normal

    (c) eGFR—CKD if <60 mL/min

3. Retinopathy (retinal examination):
   (a) DM type 2: At diagnosis then q1 to 2 years
   (b) DM type 1: 5 years postdiagnosis then q1 year

4. CAD:
   (a) ECG: q1 to 2 years (age >40 years or DM >15 years)
   (b) Lipids (TC, HDL-C, LDL-C, triglycerides):
   - Check lipid levels q1 to 3 years, if at target and no therapy.
   - If therapy indicated:
     ∘ CFP guidelines suggest NO repeat testing if patient is on the highest tolerated dose of statin therapy. (Low level evidence)
     ∘ Canadian Cardiovascular Society guidelines recommend a treat-to-target approach. Lipid targets as outlined below (strong recommendation, moderate quality evidence):

   High-risk lipid targets: LDL <2.0 mmol/L and TG/HDL <4.0 mmol/L

5. **Peripheral neuropathy:** Foot examination q1 year

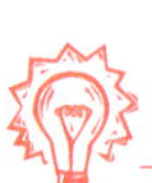

ACUTE ILLNESS IN DM—ADVISE FOR PATIENTS

- Can lead to DKA
- If preprandial glucose >14.0 mmol/L and symptoms—test urine/serum ketones
- Increase frequency of self-blood glucose testing
- Increased insulin requirements during illness/stress

Hypoglycemia (BG <4 mmol/L)

- Identified by the following symptoms: Palpitations, sweating, trembling, dilated pupils, blurred vision, nausea and/or vomiting, confusion, seizures, or coma.
- **Management**
  - Mild-to-moderate
    - 15 g carbohydrate PO (sucrose/glucose tablets/solution)
    - If still <4 mmol/L after 15 minutes, repeat
  - Severe, conscious
    - 20 g carb PO
    - If still <4 mmol/L after 15 minutes, repeat
  - Severe, unconscious
    - With IV access: 10 to 25 g glucose IV over 1 to 3 minutes (1 amp D50W = 25 g glucose)
    - No IV access: 1 mg glucagon subQ or IM (1)

Diabetic Ketoacidosis and Hyperosmolar Hyperglycemic State

- DKA and HHS are diabetic emergencies with overlapping features.
  - Insulin deficiency results in hyperglycemia. Hyperglycemia results in urinary losses of sodium, potassium, chloride, and water, leading to the resultant extra-cellular fluid volume depletion, metabolic acidosis, and a shift of potassium out of cells.
- **Hallmark of DKA= Ketoacidosis**
  - Ketoacidosis in type 1 diabetes occurs as a result of elevated glucagon levels and absolute insulin deficiency.
  - Ketoacidosis may occur in type 2 diabetes due to catecholamine release suppressing insulin secretion.
- **Hallmark of HHS = Fluid depletion and hyperosmolarity**
- **Management**
  - Larger focus on insulin administration in DKA versus HHS.
  - Crucial in management of both DKA and HHS are:
    - Fluid administration.
    - Monitoring of serum osmolarity to avoid rapid reductions.
    - Avoidance of hypokalemia.

Reference

1. Canadian Diabetes Association Clinical Practice Guidelines Expert Committee. Canadian Diabetes Association 2013 clinical practice guidelines for the prevention and management of diabetes in Canada. *Can J Diabetes*. 2013;37(suppl 1):S1-S212.

Bibliography

Allan GM, Lindblad AJ, Comeau A, et al. Simplified lipid guidelines: Prevention and management of cardiovascular disease in primary care. *Can Fam Physician*. 2015;61(10):857-867.

British Columbia Medical Association. Guidelines and protocols advisory committee. *Diabetes Care*. 2010. http://www.bcguidelines.ca/guideline_diabetes.html. Accessed November 18, 2011.

Canadian Cardiovascular Society. Canadian Cardiovascular Society guidelines for the management of dyslipidemia for the prevention of cardiovascular disease in the adult. *Can J Cardiol*. 2016;32:1263-1282.

Canadian Diabetes Association, Clinical Practice Guidelines Expert Committee. Prevention of diabetes. *Can J Diabetes*. 2008;32(suppl 1). http://www.diabetes.ca/files/cpg2008/cpg-2008.pdf. Accessed November 20, 2011.

McCulloch DK. Overview of medical care in adults with diabetes mellitus. In: Nathan DM, Mulder JE, eds. *Uptodate*; 2012. http://www.uptodate.com/contents/overview-of-medical-care-in-adults-with-diabetes-mellitus?source=search_result&search=diabetes&selectedTitle=1~150. Accessed December 5, 2011.

O'Connor NR. Diabetes type 2. In: Slawson D, French L, Lin K, eds. *Essential Evidence Plus*; 2011. https://www.essentialevidenceplus.com/content/eee/127. Accessed December 1, 2012.

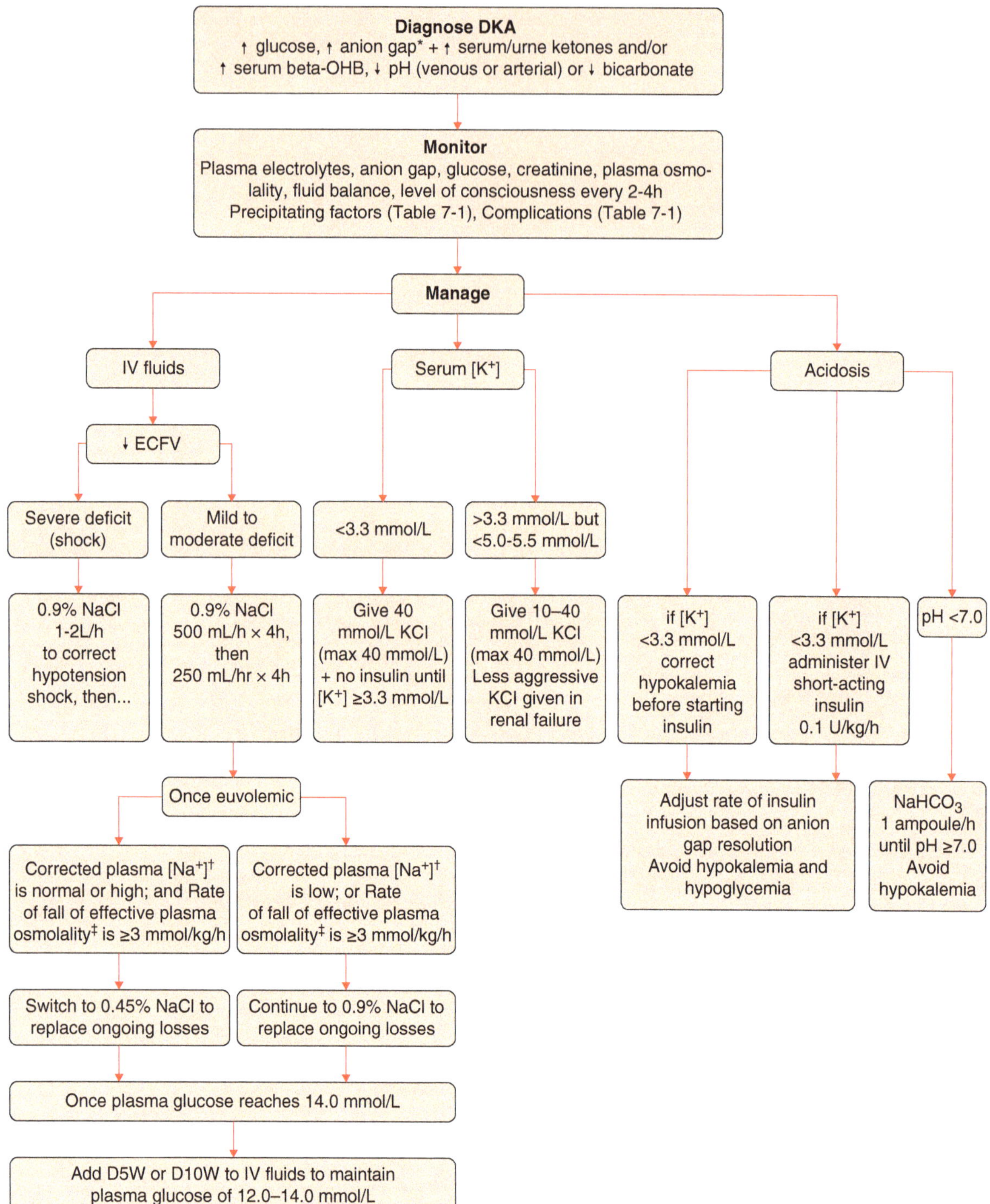

FIGURE 7-3: Canadian Diabetes Association Clinical Practice Guidelines Expert Committee. Canadian Diabetes Association 2013 Clinical Practice Guidelines for the Prevention and Management of Diabetes in Canada. *Can J Diabetes.* 2013;37(suppl 1):S1-S212.

Ischemic Heart Disease

Priority Topic 54

Definition

Atherosclerosis leading to narrowing of coronary arteries. Decreased blood flow leads to ischemia of heart muscle.

Symptoms

- Typical angina
  - Provoked by exertion or emotional stress
  - Chest heaviness or tightness
  - Relieved by rest or nitroglycerin
    - If all three characteristics met → Typical angina
    - May radiate to neck, jaw, arms, epigastric area, and back
- Atypical (more common in women, DM, young and low risk patients)
  - If two of the three characteristics → Atypical angina
  - If only one characteristic present → Not likely cardiac chest pain

Cardiovascular Risk Factors for Atherosclerosis

- Modifiable
  - Diabetes
  - Dyslipidemia
  - High stress
  - Poor diet
  - Abdominal obesity
  - Sedentary lifestyle
  - Tobacco use
  - Metabolic syndrome
  - Hypertension
  - Depression
  - CKD (microalbuminuria, proteinuria, or eGFR<60 mL/min/1.73 m^2)
  - Excess alcohol use
- Nonmodifiable
  - Age >55
  - Male
  - Family history of premature cardiovascular disease (males <55 years, females <65 years)
- Prior history of atherosclerotic disease
  - PVD
  - Previous stroke or TIA

Diagnosis

- Ischemic heart disease established if:
  - History of MI or acute coronary syndrome
  - Presence of obstructive lesions on angiographic imaging
- Ischemic heart disease presumed if:
  - Typical angina in a high-risk patient
    - Typical angina:
      - the presence of substernal chest pain or
      - discomfort provoked by exertion or emotional stress and
      - relieved by rest and/or nitroglycerin
  - Atypical angina or typical angina in an intermediate-risk patient, with positive functional testing (exercise stress test, perfusion imaging, or stress echocardiography)
  - Further testing should be sought in patients ≥30 years with typical angina features (above), as well as men ≥40 and women ≥60 with ≥1 typical angina symptom (1).

- **Management**
  - ◦ **Stable angina**
  - Management of modifiable risk factors
- Pharmacotherapy:
  Antianginal medications:
  - Beta-blocker (first-line therapy and mortality benefit)
  - Calcium channel blocker
  - Nitroglycerin (for symptom control)
  Risk-modifying medications:
  - ASA
  - ACE-I
  - Statin
  - Clopidogrel if recent acute coronary syndrome (NSTEMI—combination with ASA for 12 month; STEMI—ASA+ clopidogrel for 4 weeks if started in the first 24 hours of MI)
- Patient education and self-management
  - If angina, use sublingual nitro × 1. If no relief after 5 minutes, call emergency services immediately
  - If increased frequency of angina, call physician
  - If there is a change in symptoms, call physician
- Follow-up care
  - Symptom control
  - Medication adherence
  - Lifestyle modification
  - Impact on daily activity

Acute Coronary Syndrome

- ASA chewed (160-325 mg)
- Nitroglycerin (0.4 mg sublingually every 5 minutes for up to three doses)
  - Avoid if possibility of inferior MI, caution in low blood pressure.
- Oxygen if arterial saturation is <90%
- Beta-blocker and ACE-I to be considered after cardiology intervention/discussion
- Morphine
  - Caution in patients with low blood pressure, or the possibility of inferior MI

Post-MI Management: Secondary Prevention

- ACE-I (or ARB) indefinitely
  - Start low dose and titrate up to target dose
  - Mortality benefit
  - Prevents ventricular remodelling and decreases proteinuria
- Beta-blocker indefinitely
  - Start low dose and titrate up to target dose
  - Mortality benefit
  - Decreases reinfarction, arrhythmia, and sudden death
- Statin in all patients (even when baseline LDL <2.5 mmol/L)
  - Start at target dose, unless high risk of side effects
- ASA (75-162 mg) indefinitely
- Manage modifiable cardiovascular risk factors
  - Blood pressure: <140/90 (<130/80 with diabetes)
  - Lipids: LDL <2, total cholesterol/HDL <4

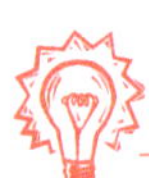

DRUGS WITH MORTALITY BENEFITS

MI: Beta-blocker, ASA, ACE-I, statin

CHF: Beta-blocker, ACE-I, spironolactone

COPD: Home O_2, smoking cessation

MODIFIABLE CARDIOVASCULAR RISKS

Risk factor	Target
Blood pressure	<140/90
	<130/80 (DM)
Lipids	LDL <2
	Tot Chol/HDL <4
Glucose	A1C <7%;
	FBG 4 to 7 mmol/L
2hr PPG	5 to 10 mmol/L
Smoking cessation	—

- Glucose: A1C <7%, FBG (fasting blood glucose) 4 to 7 mmol/L, postprandial blood glucose (2 hours) 5 to 10 mmol/L
- Smoking cessation counselling
■ Patient education to avoid NSAID/COX-2 inhibitors in post MI
■ Referral to cardiac rehabilitation program

Reference

1. Mancini GB, Gosselin G, Chow B, et al. Canadian Cardiovascular Society guidelines for the diagnosis and management of stable ischemic heart disease. *Can J Cardiol.* 2014;30(8):837-849.

Bibliography

DynaMed. Chest Pain. Ipswich, MA: EBSCO Publishing; 2012, March 15. http://search.ebscohost.com.cyber.usask.ca/login.aspx?direct=truse&site=DynaMed&id=113862. Accessed March, 2012.

DynaMed. Coronary Artery Disease (CAD). Ipswich, MA: EBSCO Publishing; 2012, March 2. http://search.ebscohost.com.cyber.usask.ca/login.aspx?direct=truse&site=DynaMed&id=113862. Accessed March, 2012.

Finnish Medical Society Duodecim. Coronary heart disease. 2010. http://www.guideline.gov/content.aspx?id=24713 Accessed March, 2012.

Jensen B, Regier L, eds. RxFiles drug comparison charts. *Post-MI—Drug & Dosage Considerations.* 8th ed. Saskatoon, SK: Saskatoon Health Region; 2010:12.

National Institute for Health and Clinical Excellence. Secondary prevention in primary and secondary care for patients following myocardial infarction. NICE Clinical Guideline 48. 2007. Accessed March 2012.

Safer Health Care Now. Improved care for acute myocardial infarction: Getting started kit. 2007. http://www.saferhealthcarenow.ca. Accessed March, 2012.

Congestive Heart Failure

Supplementary Priority Topic

Definition and Types

A clinical syndrome defined by symptoms suggestive of impaired cardiac output and/or volume overload with concurrent cardiac dysfunction.

■ **Systolic heart failure (SHF)**
  - Left ventricular ejection fraction <40%
  - Worse prognosis
■ **Heart failure with preserved systolic function (HFPSF; previously called diastolic heart failure)**
  - Left ventricular ejection fraction ≥40% (abnormal filling)
  - Half of all cases of HF

The most common cause of right ventricular failure is left ventricular failure.

TABLE 7-8	Heart Failure Causes	
CARDIAC		**NONCARDIAC**
SHF	**HFPSF**	
• Coronary artery disease • Hypertension • Valvular lesions (AS, AR, and MR) • Atrial fibrillation • Dilated cardiomyopathy	• Pericarditis • Hypertrophy • Fibrosis • Tamponade • Scarring	• Infiltrative disorders • HIV • Muscular dystrophy • Anemia • Thyrotoxicosis • Nonadherence with medications • Excess dietary sodium • Drugs (eg, alcohol, NSAIDs, cocaine, estrogens, corticosteroids)

Etiology

■ Ischemic heart disease (most common)
■ Hypertension
■ Valve disease

- Cardiomyopathy
- Arrhythmias
- Congenital heart defects
- Myocarditis
- Other (idiopathic, connective tissue disease, HIV, amyloidosis, hemochromatosis)

Evaluation

Assess volume status, risk factors, comorbid conditions, assign NYHA class.

Signs/Symptoms

- Fatigue (decreased exercise tolerance)
- Dyspnea, orthopnea, paroxysmal nocturnal dyspnea
- Fluid retention/weight gain/peripheral edema
- Cough
- Nocturia
- Rales
- Hepatomegaly
- Increased JVD
- S_3 gallop (systolic failure)
- S_4 (diastolic failure)

Investigations

- ECG
- Chest x-ray
- Transthoracic echocardiogram—Diagnostic in combination with clinical picture
- Labs: CBC, renal function, lytes, lipids, TSH, microalbuninuria (a marker of underlying endothelial dysfunction)
- BNP (if diagnosis is unclear)

Screening

- Not routine if asymptomatic
- Consider echocardiogram if multiple risk factors

Management

Chronic Heart Failure

- All patients:
  - Education.
  - Daily weights (report a weight gain of 2.5 kg/week).
  - Limit sodium intake (2-3 g/day; 6 g salt = 1 tsp salt = 2.4 g sodium).
  - Fluid restriction (1.5-2 L/day) for patients with fluid retention, significant renal impairment, or hyponatremia.
  - Decrease alcohol consumption (1 drink/day maximum).
  - Physical activity if stable HF.
  - Immunizations (one time pneumococcal and annual influenza).
  - **Treat all cardiac risk factors and underlying causes.**
- Pharmacotherapy:
  - NYHA I   – ACE-I (or ARB if intolerant)
  - NYHA II   – ACE-I, beta-blocker
  - NYHA III-IV   – ACE-I, beta-blocker, spironolactone, digoxin +/− nitrates
  - Loop diuretics if evidence of fluid retention/symptomatic.
  - Add low dose ASA if atherosclerosis.

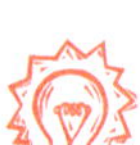

HF SYMPTOM TRIAD

Fatigue, dyspnea, fluid retention

EXTRA HEART SOUNDS

S_3—Dilated LV with rapid filling

S_4—Atrial contraction against a stiff ventricle

NEW YORK HEART ASSOCIATIONCLASSIFICATION

Class 1—Asymptomatic

Class 2—Symptomatic with ordinary activity

Class 3—Symptomatic with less than ordinary activity

Class 4—Symptomatic at rest

CHF RISK FACTORS

- Hypertension
- Ischemic heart disease
- Diabetes mellitus
- Dyslipidemia
- Smoking

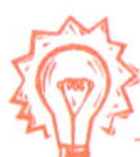

CHF DRUGS WITH MORTALITY BENEFITS

ACE-I/ARB

Beta-blocker

Spironolactone

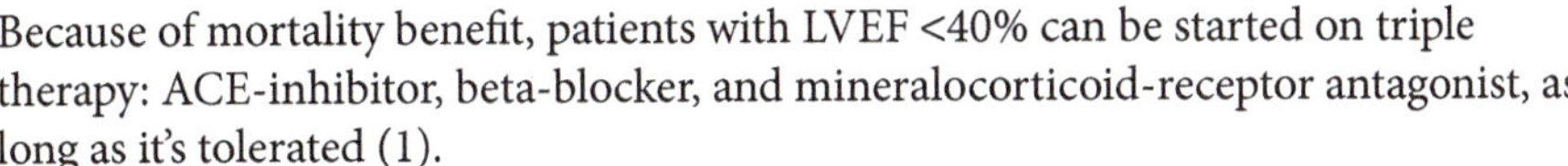

Because of mortality benefit, patients with LVEF <40% can be started on triple therapy: ACE-inhibitor, beta-blocker, and mineralocorticoid-receptor antagonist, as long as it's tolerated (1).

Acute Heart Failure

- Treat the precipitating causes
- Supplemental oxygen
- Assess perfusion and volume status
  - **Warm and wet** (well perfused and volume overloaded):
    - IV diuretic (2× usual PO dose and reassess after 60-90 min and titrate dose prn)
    - Vasodilator (nitroglycerin or nitroprusside)
    - Morphine
  - **Cold and wet** (cardiogenic shock):
    - Inotropes to stabilize (dopamine or dobutamine)
    - When stable, add diuretics and vasodilators (ACE-I, hydralazine, nitrates)

Prognosis

Poor prognostic factors include:

- Age >75
- Female
- Ventricular arrhythmias
- Atrial fibrillation
- NYHA Classes III and IV
- Left ventricular ejection fraction <35%
- Recurrent hospitalizations for acute HF
- High BNP
- Sodium <132 mmol/L
- Hypocholesterolemia
- Marked left ventricular dilation

Reference

1. Howlett JG, Chan M, Ezekowitz JA, et al. The Canadian Cardiovascular Society heart failure companion: bridging guidelines to your practice. Can J Cardiol. 2015;32(3):296-310.

Bibliography

DynaMed. Heart Failure. Ipswich, MA: EBSCO Publishing; 2012. http://search.ebscohost.com.cyber .usask.ca/login.aspx?direct=true&site=DynaMed&id=113862. Accessed March, 2012.

Guidelines and Protocols Advisory Committee (BC). Heart Failure Care. 2008. http://www.bcguidelines .ca/guideline_heart_failure_care.html#recommendation1.

Jensen B, Regier L (eds). (2010). RxFiles drug comparison charts. *Heart Failure—Treatment Overview,* 8th ed. Saskatoon, SK: Saskatoon Health Region; 12.

Fatigue

Priority Topic 38

Definition

Reduced ability to start and maintain activity, as well as difficulty with short-term memory and concentration

- 50% psychogenic
- 30% medical causes
- 20% idiopathic

ACE-I/ARB—Monitor creatinine and potassium upon initiation and within 7 to 10 days of starting or adjusting dose. If potassium at upper or lower limit of normal, monitor within 3 to 5 days of a dose adjustment (1).

Medical causes of fatigue: Patients often associate fatigue with activities they are no longer able to finish (decreased exertional capacity).

Psychogenic fatigue: Patients report being tired all of the time. Fatigue is not necessarily related to exertion, and does not improve after rest.

Ask open ended questions: "What do you mean by fatigue?"

Differential Diagnosis

TABLE 7-9	Causes of Fatigue—PS VINDICATE	
P	Psychogenic	Depression, dysthymia, anxiety, sleep disorder, CFS, life stress, fibromyalgia
S	Sedentary	Unhealthy/sedentary lifestyle
V	Vascular	Stroke
I	Infectious	Mononucleosis, TB, hepatitis, HIV
N	Neurogenic	Myasthenia gravis
	Neoplastic	Malignancy
	Nutrition	Anemia (iron deficiency, B_{12} deficiency)
D	Drugs	β-blockers, benzodiazepines, antihistamines, anticholinergics, etc.
I	Idiopathic	
C	Chronic illness	CHF, COPD, renal failure, chronic liver disease
A	Autoimmune	SLE, RA, polymyalgia rheumatica, mixed connective tissue disease
T	Toxin	Substance abuse (ie, ETOH, illicit drugs), heavy metal
E	Endocrine	Hypothyroidism, DM, pregnancy, adrenal insufficiency, Cushing syndrome

Adapted with permission from *Toronto Notes*.

FATIGUE: RED FLAGS!

- Weight loss
- Fever
- Night sweats
- Neurological defects
- Ill appearing

Approach to Patient with fatigue

First Visit

- Assess fatigue: Onset, duration, severity, exacerbation, and palliative factors, impact on function, PHQ-9, drug/ETOH screen, celiac screen, malignancy screen: **RED FLAGS!**
- Review current medications.
- Complete a physical examination.
- Initial testing can include CBC, TSH, ESR, glucose, renal panel, liver panel, U/A.
- Clinically indicated testing: CXR, BHCG, HIV, hepatitis, Lyme disease, tuberculin skin test, mononucleosis, ANA, RF, CK, cortisol, IgA tissue transglutaminase.

Second Visit

- Review labs: Any abnormal?
- Schedule frequent, brief follow-ups
- Patient education, support, and reassurance

Prognosis

Factors at presentation that predict persistent symptoms:

- Age >38 years
- More than 1.5 years of chronic fatigue
- History of dysthymia
- Less than 16 years of formal education
- Less than 8 years of medically unexplained physical symptoms

Management

- Schedule frequent, brief follow-ups.
- Patient education, support, and reassurance.
- Treat medical causes: Anemia, hypothyroid, depression.

Fatigue is more common in women than in men.

Patients who are experiencing domestic violence may initially present with fatigue.

- Consider trial of antidepressants for 6 to 8 weeks.
- Recommend: CBT, daily exercise, sleep hygiene, counselling, group therapy, nutritious diet.

FIBROMYALGIA

Definition/Diagnosis

Chronic widespread pain with:

- Characteristic tender points
- Pain for >3 months in four quadrants of the body
- Diagnosis of exclusion: Absence of identifiable disease

Labs:

  - Normal CBC, ESR, TSH, CK, renal, and liver function tests
- Multifactorial signs/symptoms:
  - Fatigue, impaired social and occupational function, sleep disturbance, depression/anxiety, hyperalgia, paresthesia, IBS, migraine

Treatment Combination Therapy to Reduce Key Symptoms

- Pharmacological (intended for relief of certain symptoms):
  - **Amitriptyline (TCA)**
  - Cyclobenzaprine (muscle relaxant)
  - SSRI for treatment of depression, anxiety
  - Zopiclone (nonbenzodiazepine sedative hypnotic) for sleep disturbance **short-term**
  - NSAIDs (anti-inflammatory)
  - Tramadol (opioid analgesic)
  - Acetaminophen (analgesic)
  - Gabapentin (antiepileptic)
- Nonpharmacological:
  - **Daily exercise**
  - Patient education
  - **Sleep hygiene**
  - CBT
  - Stress reduction
  - Acupuncture
  - Biofeedback
  - Scheduled visits

Complications

- Negative impact of social and occupational life
- Chronic pain

CHRONIC FATIGUE
- Primarily affects young-to middle-aged adults
- More common in women

CHRONIC FATIGUE SYNDROME

Definition/Diagnosis

- Diagnosis of exclusion
- Diagnosis requires the following:
  - Unexplained, persistent relapsing fatigue of new onset that is:
    - Not related to exertion
    - Not alleviated with rest
    - Results in dysfunction

PLUS four or more of following for >6 months:

- Change in short-term memory or concentration
- Sore throat
- Tender cervical or axillary nodes
- Headaches (new pattern/severity)
- Nonrejuvenating sleep
- Postexertional malaise ≥24 hours

Bibliography

Bono NA, Shflin DO. Fatigue. In: Ebell MH, Brown SR, Lindbloom E, eds. *Essential Evidence Plus.* 2011. https://www.essentialevidenceplus.com/content/eee/433 Accessed March 15, 2012.

Centers for Disease Control and Prevention. Chronic Fatigue Syndrome: A toolkit for providers. 2011. http://www.cdc.gov/cfs/toolkit/index.html. Accessed March 15, 2012.

Chen YA, Tran C. *Toronto Notes—Comprehensive Medical Reference & Review for MCCQE I and USMLE II.* Toronto, Canada: Toronto Notes for Medical Students Inc; 2011.

Craig T, Kakumanu S. Chronic fatigue syndrome: Evaluation and treatment. *Am Fam Phy.* 2002;15;65(6):1083-1091. http://www.aafp.org/afp/2002/0315/p1083.html. Accessed March 15, 2012.

Ebell MH. What is a reasonable initial approach to the patient with fatigue? In: Belden JL, ed. *Pepid. Primary Care Plus Platinum v. (12.1);* 2001.

Fosnocht KM, Ende J. Approach to the adult with fatigue. In: Fletcher RH, Sokol HN, eds. *Uptodate*; 2011. http://www.uptodateonline.com; http://www.uptodate.com/contents/approach-to-the-adult-patient-with-fatigue?source=search_result&search=fatigue&selectedTitle=1~150. Accessed March 15, 2012.

Gluckman SJ. Treatment of chronic fatigue syndrome. In: Weller PF, Thorner AR, eds. *Uptodate*; 2011. http://www.uptodateonline.com; http://www.uptodate.com/contents/treatment-of-chronic-fatigue-syndrome?source=search_result&search=fatigue&selectedTitle=3~150. Accessed March 15, 2012.

Goldberg DL. Treatment of fibromyalgia in adults. In: Schur PH, Roman PL, eds. *Uptodate*; 2011. http://www.uptodateonline.com; http://www.uptodate.com/contents/treatment-of-fibromyalgia-inadults?source=search_result&search=fibromyalgia&selectedTitle=1~134. Accessed March 15, 2012.

Sandore R. Approach to chronic fatigue syndrome. In: Rosenbloom M, ed. *Pepid. Primary Care Plus Platinum v. (12.1);* 2005.

CHAPTER 8

Preventative Medicine

Periodic Health Assessment
Priority Topic 72

DEFINITION

A dedicated appointment that incorporates evidence-based recommendations for adults from various professional bodies in several domains:

- Education/counselling
- Functional inquiry
- Physical examination
- Laboratory investigations
- Immunizations

PURPOSE

- Primary prevention—Identifies risk factors and implements strategies to prevent disease onset.
- Secondary prevention—Presymptomatic detection of disease so as to prevent disease progression and complications.
- Health promotion—Enables patients to increase control over and improve their health.
- Create and maintain an up-to-date patient profile—Optimizes both acute and chronic care (ie, current medications, allergies, hospitalizations).
- Enhance therapeutic relationship.

PROBLEMS AND CONTROVERSIES

- Low SES and minority group access
- High cost and demand on time (21.4 million half hour visits, $2 billion in costs)
- Debated-impact (effect on mortality and morbidity) of dedicated periodic health examination (PHE) versus appropriate case-finding manoeuvre during other visits (chronic disease management visits or symptom-based visits)

GUIDES AND CHECKLISTS

Checklists highlight best practices for average-risk populations, which include recommendations (those with good and fair evidence) from the CTFPH as well as other screening guidelines from various Canadian agencies.

FUNCTIONAL INQUIRY

"Screening" for depression is the only evidence-based manoeuvre (grade B evidence)
Over the past 2 weeks:

- Have you felt little pleasure in doing things?
- Have you felt down, depressed, or hopeless?

Other inquiry identifies and targets symptom-based problems for investigation, management, and discussion.

PHYSICAL EXAMINATION

Evidence is either **level A** or level B (Table 8-1).

TABLE 8-1	Preventative Health: Physical Examination Components	
MANOEUVRE	**INDICATION**	**COMMENT**
BP	**Treating to prevent stroke, CAD, and death** Screening for hypertension	General population <140/90; CKD or DM 2 <130/80
BMI	Prevention of obesity-related disease	For obese adults
Waist to hip ratio	Screening for abdominal obesity	High risk for more intensive screening
Waist circumference	Increased risk of DM 2, hypertension, and CAD	Men <102 cm Women <88 cm
Sensorium testing	In the elderly	Whispered test vs audiometry vs inquiry are all equivalent Snellen for visual acuity
Pap smear	Reduce the risk of invasive cervical cancer	Sexually active women based on provincial guidelines

CFPC Explanations, 2012.

LABS AND INVESTIGATIONS

Sexually Transmitted Infections

In high-risk populations (<30 years with two partners in past year, >16 at coitarche, prostitutes, sexual contact of known case)

- Syphilis serology
- Gonorrhea and chlamydia → Urethral/cervical swab or urine
- HIV serology
- HBV serology (HBsAg)

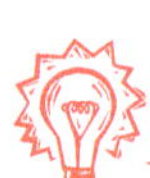

See Table 8-2 for management of abnormal PAP cytology.

Cancer Screening Manoeuvres

Cervical Cancer

- Provincial guidelines and screening programmes vary.
- Most are moving toward screening women >21 years of age or women who are >3 years from coitarche, whichever comes later.

TABLE 8-2	Management of Abnormal PAP Cytology
PAP RESULT	**RECOMMENDED MANAGEMENT**
Unsatisfactory	Repeat Pap test in 3 months
Atypical squamous cells of undetermined significance (ASC-US) and low-grade squamous intraepithelial lesion (LSIL)	Women 21 years and older: Repeat Pap test every 6 months for 1 year (two tests) *(tests must be at least 6 months apart)* • If all negative return to routine screening • If either result is ASC-US or greater refer for colposcopy Women <21 years: *(although routine cervical screening is not recommended)* Repeat Pap test every 12 months for 2 years (two tests): • At 12 months: Only high-grade lesions should be referred to colposcopy • At 24 months: Negative results return to routine screening ASC-US or greater refer to colposcopy
Atypical squamous cells–cannot exclude HSIL (ASC-H)	Refer for colposcopy
High-grade squamous intraepithelial lesion (HSIL)	Refer for colposcopy
Atypical glandular cells (AGC), adenocarcinoma in situ (AIS)	Refer for colposcopy
Squamous carcinoma, adenocarcinoma, other malignancy	Refer to specialist care
Endometrial cells	After the age of 40 should be managed or referred as appropriate

Source: Saskatchewan Cancer Agency.

- Pap smears should be done every 2 to 3 years, with changes in frequency depending on previous results.
- Repeated normal results warrant less frequent screening.
- Abnormal results warrant more frequent surveillance or screening, particularly among older women.
- Health status (ie, immunocompromised) intensifies screening frequency.

Breast Cancer (Canadian Task Force on Preventative Health, 2011)

- Provincial guidelines and screening programmes vary
- Discuss the risks and benefits of screening with all women, and ascertain individual preferences
  - Number needed to screen to prevent one breast cancer death is 720 every 2 to 3 years for 11 years.
  - In that time, 204 will have false-positive results on mammography, and 26 will have unnecessary biopsies.
- Screen average risk women between the ages of 50 and 74 with mammography every 2 to 3 years.
- Clinical breast examination is no longer recommended (weak recommendation; same strength of evidence as the above recommendation to screen with mammography).
- Advising women to perform self-breast examination is also not recommended.

Colorectal Cancer (Canadian Task Force on Preventative Health, 2016)

- Adults aged 50 to 59 years (weak recommendation; moderate-quality evidence)
  - Guaiac-based fecal occult blood test (FOBT) or more sensitive fecal immuno-chemical test (FIT) every 2 years
  - OR flexible sigmoidoscopy every 10 years

- Adults aged 60 to 74 (strong recommendation; moderate-quality evidence)
  - FOBT or FIT every 2 years
  - OR flexible sigmoidoscopy every 10 years
- Age 75 and above (weak recommendation; low-quality evidence)
  - Screening for colorectal cancer not recommended
- Higher risk groups (Canadian Association of Gastroenterology, 2010)
  - First-degree with diagnosis in relative <60 years → Every 5 years starting at age 40 or 10 years before relative's diagnosis
  - Genetic syndromes
    - Familial adenomatous polyposis → Annual colonoscopy starting at age 10 to 12
    - Hereditary nonpolyposis colorectal cancer → Colonoscopy every 1 to 2 years starting at age 20 or 10 years before earliest relative's diagnosis
  - Inflammatory bowel disease → Colonoscopy 8 years after diagnosis
  - Polyps on previous colonoscopy
    - One to two adenomas <1 cm → Repeat colonoscopy in 5 years
    - More than two adenomas → Repeat colonoscopy in 3 years

Prostate Cancer (Canadian Task Force on Preventative Health 2014)

See section on Men's GU Health

- Screening with prostate-specific antigen (PSA) is not recommended.
  - This applies to all med without a previous diagnosis of prostate cancer.
  - There is no trial data showing benefits/harms of screening differ in higher risk groups.
  - Clinicians may wish to discuss benefits and harms of screening with those at increased risk (family history of prostate cancer, black race).
- Canadian Urological Association still recommends offering yearly digital rectal examination.
  - Recommends discussing risks and benefits of PSA screening with all men.
  - Number needed to screen to prevent one prostate cancer death is 503.
  - Important health and psychological risks of over-diagnosis, biopsy, and treatment for cancers that may not have been clinically significant.
  - Recommends offering digital rectal examination (DRE) and PSA between ages 50 and 75.

Start at age 40 if risk factors (or 10 years before relative's diagnosis)

  - Do not screen men whose life expectancy is <10 years.

CHRONIC DISEASES

Diabetes Mellitus Type 2

See section on diabetes mellitus type 2.

- Fasting blood glucose and/or A1C every 3 years starting at age 40
- Earlier and more frequently in patients with the following comorbidities:
  - First-degree relative
  - Presence of complications associated with DM2
  - Hypertension or other vascular disease
  - Dyslipidemia
  - Overweight or abdominal obesity
  - High-risk population (Aboriginal, Hispanic, Asian, South Asian, African descent)

- History of impaired glucose tolerance, impaired fasting glucose, gestational diabetes mellitus, or macrosomic infant
- Other comorbidities: PCOS, schizophrenia, HIV, OSA

Osteoporosis

See section on osteoporosis (on page 202).

Bone mineral density (BMD) testing is indicated in the following groups:

- Everyone >65 years
- 50 to 64 years with risk factors:
  - Fragility fracture
  - High-risk medication: Prolonged glucocorticoid use (>3 months of >7.5 mg prednisone-equivalent/day, aromatase inhibitors, androgen deprivation therapy)
  - Parental hip fracture
  - Vertebral fracture or osteopenia on x-ray
  - Lifestyle: Current smoking, high alcohol intake
  - Low body weight (<60 kg) or major weight loss (>10% of weight at age 25 years)
  - Comorbidities: Rheumatoid arthritis, others (see osteoporosis section for full list)
- <50 with risk factors:
  - Fragility fracture
  - High-risk medications (same as above)
  - Hypogonadism or premature menopause
  - Malabsorption syndrome
  - Primary hyperparathyroidism
  - Other disorders strongly associated with rapid bone loss and/or fracture

Coronary Artery Disease

See Hyperlipidemia section (on page 167).

Canadian Family Physician Simplified Lipid Guidelines 2015

- Fasting lipid profile on all men ≥40 and all women ≥50
- May be considered earlier for patients with known CVD risk factors:
  - Chronic diseases: Diabetes, hypertension, inflammatory diseases (SLE, RA, psoriasis), CKD (eGFR <60), HIV on HAART
  - Risk factors: Current cigarette smoking, obesity
  - Family history of premature CAD (<60 years)
  - Evidence of atherosclerosis
  - Clinical manifestation of hyperlipidemia
  - Children with family history of hypercholesterolemia or chylomicronemia
- For patients not taking lipid-lowering therapy repeat lipid testing every 5 years
  - May be considered earlier if new risk factors develop in interim
- Stratify patients into low, medium, or high risk (based on Framingham criteria or other risk calculator)

IMMUNIZATIONS

Evidence: **Level A**, level B

Tetanus and Diphtheria (Td) +/− Pertussis (Tdap)

- Td booster every 10 years with one Tdap booster if not previously immunized.
- Primary series: Three doses at 0, 1 to 2, and 6 to 12 months (two doses Td, one dose Tdap).

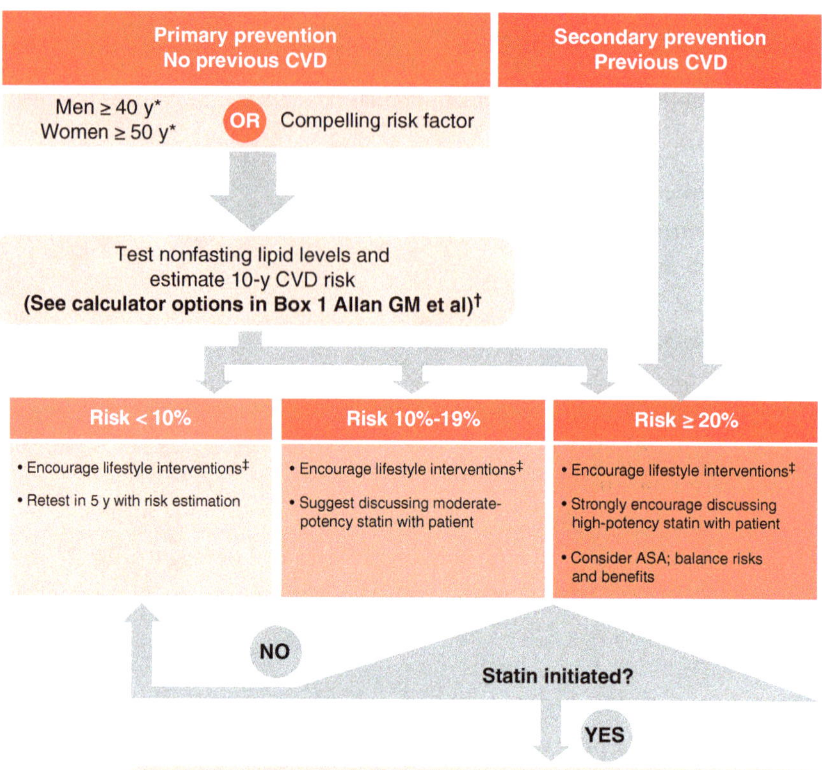

FIGURE 8-1:   Lipid algorithm: For primary or secondary prevention; excludes those with familial hypercholesterolemia. (*Source:* Allan GM, et al. Simplified lipid guidelines: Prevention and management of cardiovascular disease in primary care. *Can Fam Physician.* 2015;61(10):857-867.)

Pneumococcal

- Everyone >65 years
- All persons >5 years at high risk:
  - Common high-risk groups:
    - Immunosuppressed: Asplenia, HIV infection, sickle cell disease, lymphoma, Hodgkin disease, organ transplant recipients
    - Chronic diseases: Diabetes, cardiopulmonary disease (except asthma), kidney disease, cirrhosis, smokers
    - Marginalized populations (IVDUs, homeless)

Influenza A: Immunize Annually in the Autumn

- Those at high risk of influenza complications or those more likely to require hospitalization:
  - Cardiopulmonary diseases, metabolic diseases (including diabetes), kidney disease, anemia or hemoglobinopathies, nursing home residents
- Those >65 years and <23 months, healthy pregnant women
- Those capable of transmitting to those at high risk
  - Healthcare workers (HCWs), childcare workers, and household contacts of those above

Rubella

- One dose to nonpregnant women of child-bearing age unless evidence of immunity (records, serology)

Varicella:

- Determine status by history or serology
- Two doses at least 4 weeks apart to high-risk groups: HCWs, women of reproductive age who are not pregnant, teachers and daycare workers, newly arrived immigrants, household contact of immunocompromised

No A or B level evidence for the following.

HPV

- Recommended for females 9 to 13, indicated for women up to age 26
- Indicated for boys age 9 to 26 years, but not covered by any provincial vaccination programme currently

Pertussis

- Single dose to nonimmunized adults

Meningococcal

- To all high-risk groups:
  - Recent contacts of known cases
  - Occupational: Military recruits, lab workers exposed to meningitis
  - Travellers to endemic areas
  - Medical: Asplenia, deficiencies (factor D, complement, properdin)

Herpes Zoster

- Indicated for prevention of herpes zoster and its complications in >60 years but NNT = 91

Travel immunizations vary.

EDUCATION AND COUNSELLING

Evidence is either **level A** or level B for interventions listed (see Table 8-3).

TABLE 8-3	Preventative Health: Dietary Supplements	
INTERVENTION	**INDICATION**	**COMMENT**
Folic acid	Prevent neural tube defects in women of reproductive age	**Low risk: 0.4-0.8 mg/d for 1 month pre- and 3 months post-conception** **High risk: 4 mg/d for 3 months pre- and post-conception**
Calcium (B)	Prevent osteoporosis	OSC: 1000-1500 mg/d; >1200 mg/d for women >50 SOGC: 1500 mg/d if postmenopausal

TABLE 8-3	Preventative Health: Dietary Supplements (*Continued*)	
INTERVENTION	**INDICATION**	**COMMENT**
Vitamin D	Prevent osteoporosis (B) and hip fractures	OSC: 400-1000 IU/d; 800-1000 IU if >50 or moderate risk of vitamin D deficiency SOGC: 800 IU/d if postmenopausal
Diet (B)	Prevent CAD, colon cancer	Lower use of saturated and total fat; lower cholesterol; increase fibre intake Consider referral to nutritionist if at high risk
Physical activity (B)	Prevent hypertension and CAD Contribute to preventing DM 2 and osteoporosis	Moderate physical activity for 30 min/day on most days of the week
Sun exposure	Prevent skin cancer	Avoid excessive midday sun exposure with protective clothing
Safe sex	Prevent STI transmission	Abstinence Condoms
Obesity (BMI >30)		Multimodal strategy to achieve weight loss of 5%-10% at rate of 5-10 kg/week for 6 months
Smoking cessation	Prevent tobacco-caused diseases	**Counselling for smoking cessation** and use of nicotine replacement +/− bupropion Refer to cessation program
Oral hygiene	Prevent oral cancer and peri-odontal disease	Brushing and flossing with fluoride-containing toothpaste in areas where water is not fluoridated Smoking cessation to prevent oral cancer and periodontal disease
Alcohol	Prevent alcohol-related morbidities	Standardized inquiry (CAGE) Counsel for problem drinking (CAGE 2/4 is sensitive and specific for problem drinking) **At risk drinking: Women (>7 units/week or >3/occasion), Men (>14 units/week or >4/occasion)**
Elderly	**Cognitive decline** **Fall assessment**	When caregiver expresses concern with either
Personal safety	Various	Noise control protection or protection to prevent injures Seatbelts to prevent MVA-related injuries

Bibliography

Allan GM, Lindbald A, Comeau A, et al. Simplified lipid guidelines: Prevention and management of cardiovascular disease in primary care. *Can Fam Physician*. 2015;61(10):857-867.

Canadian Diabetes Association. Screening for Type 1 and Type 2 Diabetes. 2013. http://guidelines.diabetes.ca/fullguidelines. Accessed August 10, 2016.

Canadian Task Force on Preventative Health. Recommendations on screening for colorectal cancer in primary care. *CMAJ*. 2016;188(5):340-348.

Canadian Task Force on Preventive Health. Recommendations on screening for breast cancer in average risk women aged 40-74 years. *CMAJ*. 2010;183(17):1991-2001.

CFPC. Explanations for the Preventive Care Checklist Form. http://www.cfpc.ca/ProjectAssets/Templates/Resource.aspx?id=1184&langType=4105. Accessed November 11, 2012.

Genest J, et al. Canadian Cardiovascular Society guidelines for the diagnosis and treatment of dyslipidemia and prevention of cardiovascular disease in the adult—2009 recommendations. *Can J Cardiol*. 2009;25(10):567-579.

Howard-Tripp M. Should we abandon the periodic health examination? *Yes. Can Fam Phy.* 2011;57:159-160.

Leddin DJ, Enns R, Hilsden R, et al. Canadian Association of Gastroenterology position statement on screening individuals at average risk for developing colorectal cancer. *Can J Gastroenterol.* 2010;24(12):705-714.

Mavriplis C. Should we abandon the periodic health examination? No. *Can Fam Physician.* 2011;57:159-161.

National Advisory Committee on Immunization. Canadian Immunization Guide, 7th ed. 2006. http://www.phac-aspc.gc.ca/im/is-cv/index-eng.php#b. Accessed November 11, 2012.

Men's Genitourinary Health

Priority Topic 77

LOWER URINARY TRACT SYMPTOMS

Lower urinary tract symptoms (LUTS): Categorized as irritative or obstructive

- Irritative: Frequency, urgency, nocturia, and urge incontinence
- Obstructive: Hesitancy, poor flow, dribbling, incomplete voiding, and retention

Benign Prostatic Hyperplasia

Definition

- Benign, often progressive disorder due to prostate enlargement

Symptoms and Characteristics

- Most common, but not exclusive, cause of LUTS in men

Risk Factors

- Advancing age.
- BPH puts men at higher risk of sexual dysfunction.
- BPH is not a risk factor for prostate cancer.

Diagnosis

- Diagnosis is clinical, based on history, physical, and basic investigations.

Physical Examination

- May be normal.
- DRE may reveal symmetric, smooth, nonpainful, and enlarged prostate.
- Abdominal examination may reveal distended bladder.

Investigations

- Urinalysis and urine culture and sensitivity (C&S) to rule out infection.
- PSA if life expectancy >10 years and knowledge of prostate cancer would change management; if starting on 5-alpha reductase inhibitors (5-ARIs).
- Other investigations as indicated by presentation (postvoid residual, urine cytology, urodynamics, serum creatinine).

Management

- Use of a symptom inventory (International Prostate Scoring System) is helpful to assess "bother" (impact on patient), deciding on treatment, and in monitoring.
- Consider screening for sexual dysfunction.
- New focus on early treatment over watchful waiting.
  - Delay symptom progression
  - Prevent complications (surgery, acute urinary retention)

- Lifestyle:
  - Fluid restriction
  - Avoiding irritants
  - Timed voiding
  - Pelvic floor exercises
  - Medication review
- Pharmacotherapy:

Based on symptoms severity, bother, and patient preference

  - Alpha-blockers:
    - Nonselective (doxazosin, terazosin) → More side effects
    - Selective (tamsulosin) → Expensive
    - Choice based on patient comorbidities and tolerability
  - 5-Alpha reductase inhibitors (finasteride, dutasteride)
    - With documented large prostate (larger than 40 g)
    - Benefits: Limits prostate growth and prevents cancer, urinary retention, and need for surgery
    - Side-effects: Sexual dysfunction, gynecomastia, decreased libido
    - Monitor with PSA 6 months postinitiation → PSA must decrease by 50% or warrants urological referral
  - Either class alone or in combination is acceptable.

Consider alternative diagnosis, especially if no response to treatment:

- Prostatitis
- Urinary tract infections (UTIs)
- Overactive bladder

Key Points

- BPH is progressive—Early treatment may reduce complications
- Referral to urology if abnormal DRE
- PSA must be followed with 5-alpha reductase inhibitor use

Prostate Cancer

Definitions

- Informed screening:
  - Early detection and treatment of asymptomatic cancer to extend life
  - Requires accurate, reliable, easy-to-administer test that detects disease of clinical importance at a preclinical stage

Screening (see Table 8-4)

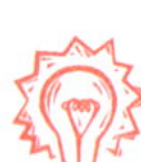

Both patient and clinician must understand that screening for prostate cancer with PSA or DRE does not fulfill many of these criteria.

TABLE 8-4	Prostate Cancer Screening Recommendations		
RECOMMENDATION FOR SCREENING	CANADIAN UROLOGICAL ASSOCIATION	AMERICAN UROLOGICAL ASSOCIATION	US PREVENTIVE SERVICES TASK FORCE
Age to offer	40 for high risk, otherwise age 50-75	40 for everyone	No one
Manoeuvre	DRE and PSA	DRE and PSA	None
Frequency	Yearly (do not screen if life expectancy <10 years)	Yearly	N/A

- Screening: Controversial
- Extremely large numbers needed to screen (to prevent 1 death = 503) (503 in ERSPC pooled and extrapolated data—*NEJM* article)
- Questionable impact on mortality versus financial cost to system and potential negative impacts on patient quality of life
- Risks of screening:
  - Worry → Cancer can exist with normal PSA and DRE
  - Risks of invasive investigations → Bleeding, pain, infection
- Risks of diagnosis:
  - Risks of therapies → Sexual, urinary, and bowel dysfunction
  - At least one-fourth of diagnoses are overdiagnosis → Cancer would not have become clinically significant
- Benefits of screening:
  - Small mortality benefit, unproven in RCTs
  - Relief and reassurance

Symptoms

- Frequently asymptomatic
- LUTS
- Hip or vertebral pain

Risk Factors

- Age >50 → 30% of those above 50 will have autopsy-proven cancer; 70% of more than 70
- Black → Higher incidence and more advanced stage at diagnosis
- Positive family history (first-degree relative <65) → Doubles risk

DRE does not cause elevated PSA.

Physical Examination

- Frequently normal
- Abnormal DRE → Nodular, firm, irregular, often peripheral zone affected

Differential Diagnosis of Elevated PSA

Inflammation, urinary retention, instrumentation, cancer, frequent/recent ejaculation, **not DRE!**

- PSA half-life is 2 to 3 days → Stays elevated for roughly 2 weeks (5½ lives).
- PSA variability is 20% (*CMAJ* article).

Workup (Figure 8-2)

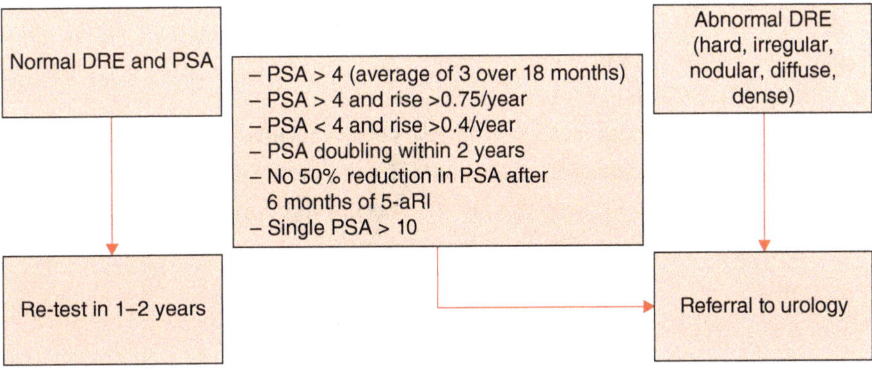

FIGURE 8-2:

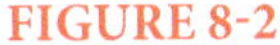

Diagnosis

- Requires transrectal ultrasound-guided biopsy

Treatment

Localized disease:

- Active surveillance for Gleason <6, locally confined
  - Trials underway
- Radical prostatectomy
  - Group I and II (all tumour confined to prostate).
  - Men >70 unlikely to be offered surgery as greatest benefit is in those <70 years.
- Radiation: Either external-beam radiation therapy (EBRT) or brachytherapy
  - EBRT → GI and GU side-effects; comparable to radical prostatectomy
  - Brachytherapy is comparable to EBRT with Gleason <6, PSA <10
  - Group 3 (includes some extra prostatic tumour): Either radical prostatectomy or radiation

Metastatic disease or local extension:

- Group 3: Either radical prostatectomy or radiation
- Group 4 (metastatic): Androgen deprivation therapy
- Chemotherapy for hormone-refractory tumours
  - Hormonal resistance occurs within 5 years, sometimes earlier

Follow-Up

- Local spread: Low back pain, hip pain, LUTS, well-being, appetite, lymphadenopathy
- Distant metastases: Bone, lung, liver, and adrenals
- Labs: CBC, liver enzymes and function, renal function, and PSA

Issues

- Fear of mortality and morbidity versus apprehension surrounding investigations and treatments
- A few comforting thoughts:
  - Roughly 20% of men will be diagnosed with prostate cancer.
  - Most die with it, few die from it.

Key Points

- Assessing patient values.
- Shared decision-making.
- Use of a decision aid for patients are all keys.

Guideline Summary

Canadian Urological Association

- Offer yearly DRE and PSA between 50 and 75.
- Start at age 40 with risk factors (or 10 years before relative's diagnosis).
- Do not screen men whose life expectancy is <10 years.

Canadian Taskforce on Preventative Health does not recommend yearly screening with PSA.

Prostatitis

There are three forms of clinically relevant prostatitis

- Acute prostatitis
- Chronic bacterial prostatitis
- Chronic prostatitis/pelvic pain syndrome

Acute Prostatitis

Definition

- Acute bacterial infection of the prostate gland

Symptoms

- Pain (rectal, perianal, low back, with ejaculation), LUTS, systemic (fever, chills)

Physical Examination

- Generally unwell and uncomfortable
- DRE → Boggy, very tender prostate

Investigations

- Urinalysis → bacteria, hematuria, pyuria
- Urine C+S → Positive for *Escherichia coli*, *Staphylococcus aureus*, Gram-negative bacilli
- Urine PCR for chlamydia and gonorrhea
- CBC → Increased WBCs
- No role for PSA
- Bladder ultrasound with severe obstructive symptoms

Treatment

- Severe illness may require admission
- Antibiotics for 2 to 4 weeks post resolution of symptoms
  - Severe: IV aminoglycoside + ampicillin *or* broad-spectrum penicillin + beta-lactamase inhibitor *or* third-generation cephalosporin
  - Mild-moderate: Oral fluoroquinolone

Chronic Bacterial Prostatitis

Definition

- Chronic bacterial infection, +/− symptoms, often the cause of recurrent UTI with consistent pathogen

Symptoms

- Presentation may be subtle or nonspecific (pain may or may not be present).
- Hematospermia may be present.
- Symptom scoring system is helpful (NIH—Chronic Prostatitis Symptom Index) in symptom evaluation and monitoring treatment.
- Suspect and treat if urogenital symptoms >3 months.

Physical Examination

- May be normal.

Investigations

Diagnosis

- Diagnosis is usually made through careful history.
- Sequential urine cultures before and after prostatic massage.

Treatment

Check susceptibility and treat for 6 to 12 weeks

- First-line: Ciprofloxacin 1 g daily or levofloxacin 500 mg daily
- Second-line: TMP-SMX 1 double-strength tab twice daily
- Consider urological referral if refractory to treatment

Chronic Prostatitis/Pelvic Pain Syndrome

Definition

- Chronic pelvic pain +/− voiding symptoms in the absence of UTI.

Physical Examination
- Extraprostatic pain is suggestive.

Workup
- Diagnosis of exclusion
- Urine cytology
- Postvoid residual volume
- Flow rate

Treatment
- No single modality has been shown to be effective on its own.
- Multimodal treatment plan targeted to improve symptoms:
  - Antibiotics for newly diagnosed or antimicrobial-naïve
  - Alpha-blockers for obstructive symptoms
  - Anti-inflammatories for short-term analgesia
  - Neuromodulating drugs (+/− muscle relaxants) and techniques (acupuncture, pudendal nerve modulation) for long-term analgesia
  - Phytotherapies (quercetin, pollen) for local tenderness
  - Other modalities: Physiotherapy, 5-alpha reductase inhibitors, electromagnetic stimulation, and psychotherapy

Key Points
- Chronic prostatitis/pelvic pain syndrome—Recurrent use of antibiotics for isolated pathogens only
- Individualize treatment—Target to symptoms and response

ACUTE SCROTAL PROBLEMS—SWELLING PREDOMINANT

Hydrocele

Definition

Filling of the tunica vaginalis' potential space (between parietal and visceral layers) with peritoneal fluid
- Communicating → Fluid flows through patent processus vaginalis from peritoneal cavity (with potential for other abdominal contents)
- Noncommunicating → Imbalance between absorption and resorption

Symptoms
- Swelling, dull pain may be present with large volume.

Physical Examination
- See Table 8-5. Increase in swelling at end of day or with Valsalva suggests communicating hydrocele.

TABLE 8-5   Differential Diagnosis and Physical Examination Findings of Scrotal Swelling

MASS	PALPATION	TRANSILLUMINATION	EFFECT OF VALSALVA
Tumour	*Firm*	No	Unchanged
Varicocele	Fluid filled	No	*Increase*
Hydrocele	Fluid filled	Yes	Unchanged
Spermatocele	Fluid filled	Yes	Unchanged

Spermatocele is superior to testicle, and should be isolatable, unlike a hydrocele.
Brenner and Aderonke, 2011.

Investigation

- Ultrasound may be necessary to rule out secondary or reactive hydrocele
  - May be secondary to neoplasm or torsion

Management

- Referral to urology if symptomatic, otherwise conservative
- Communicating hydrocele carries with it high risk of herniation and strangulation of bowel/mesentery → must be surgically corrected

Varicocele

Definition

- Dilation of pampiniform plexus or spermatic vein

Symptoms and Characteristics

- Typically left hemiscrotal swelling (due to increased pressure in left gonadal vein from the 90 degree angle made when draining to left renal vein).
- Dull pain may be present, worsens with straining.
- Testicular atrophy secondary to increased temperature.
- Ten to fifteen per cent present in the context of male infertility or subfertility.

Physical Examination

- See Table 8-5.
- Standing and supine examination.
- Persistence in supine position is a red flag for possible inferior vena cava (IVC) obstruction.

Investigations

- Semen analysis
- Doppler ultrasound if concerned about IVC obstruction

Management

- Patients with completed families → NSAIDs, scrotal supports
- Patients without completed families or fertility concerns → semen analysis
  - If normal, management may be supportive
  - If abnormal → refer for either surgical ligation or embolization
- Other criteria favouring intervention:
  - Reduced volume by 2 mL or 10%
  - Reduction with reduced sperm count
  - Symptomatic

Cystic Scrotal Swelling (spermatocele, epididymal Cyst)

Definition

- Fluid-filled (nonviable sperm) collection of the head of the epididymis >2 cm → spermatocele; <2 cm → epididymal cyst

Symptoms

- Painless swelling

Physical Examination

- See Table 8-5
- Cystic mass superior to and separate from body of testis

Testicular Cancer

Characteristics

- Most common solid tumour in men ages 18 to 40

Symptoms

- Typically painless mass or swelling

Risk Factors

- Cryptorchidism, personal or family history of testicular cancer, HIV, and testicular carcinoma in situ

Physical Examination

- See Table 8-5
- Typically nontender

Investigations

- Imaging: Ultrasound, or MRI if ultrasound is equivocal.
- Serum: Alpha-fetoprotein, beta-hCG (establishes risk).

Management

- Depends on specific diagnosis and risk profile

ACUTE SCROTAL PROBLEMS—PAIN PREDOMINANT

Pain-Predominant Scrotal Problems

Differential Diagnosis

Children and adolescents

- Torsion
- Torsion of appendage
- Strangulated inguinal hernia (testicle not tender)
- Trauma
- Orchitis (very rare)
- Henoch-Schonlein purpura

In adults, consider:

- Testicular cancer (pain an uncommon symptom)
- Fournier gangrene
- Postvasectomy

Epididymitis

Definition

- Infection (usually bacterial) of the epididymis

Symptoms

- Acute onset of unilateral testicular pain
- May have urethral discharge, dysuria, and fever

Risk Factors

- Sexually active males

Physical Examination

- See Table 8-6

TABLE 8-6	Differentiating Acute Scrotal Pain			
ETIOLOGY	DOPPLER U/S	CREMASTERIC REFLEX	AGE	FEATURE
Torsion	Decreased	Absent	12-18 years	Negative Prehn sign
Torsion of appendage		Present	Prepubertal	Blue dot sign
Epididymitis	Increased	Present	Sexually active	Positive Prehn sign

- Relief of pain with elevation of the testicle (Prehn sign) → Not reliable
- Unilateral swelling becoming generalized

- Exquisite tenderness
- Preserved cremasteric reflex

Investigations

- See Table 8-6
- Urinalysis and urine C + S → Often pyuria
- Urine PCR for chlamydia and gonorrhea

Prevention

- Safe sex

Treatment

For 10 to 14 days

- Age <35, likely organism chlamydia or gonorrhea → Cefixime and doxycycline
  - Treat sexual partner also
- Age >35, likely organism *E. coli*
- Oral fluoroquinolone to >35 years

Key Points

- Pubertal males, usually sexually transmitted
- Rule out other causes with history and physical
- Emergency referral to urology if any suspicion of torsion

Testicular Torsion

Definition

- Greater than 180 degree rotation of testis causing strangulation of blood supply.

Symptoms

- Severe scrotal pain
- Testicle may be swollen, erythematous, +/− induration, elevation
- Associated nausea and vomiting

Physical Examination

- See Table 8-6
- Testicle may be swollen, erythematous, +/− indurated, elevated

Investigations

- See Table 8-6

Treatment

- Emergency urological referral, ideally within 6 hours of onset

Key Points

- Ruling out torsion can be difficult as reliability of signs is examiner dependent →
  Referral to urology within 6 to 8 hours of onset if suspicious

Torsion of the Appendage of the Testicle

Definition

- Twisting of testicular/epididymal vestigial appendix

Symptoms

- Severe scrotal pain and swelling

Physical Examination

- See Table 8-6
- Less pain than torsion
- May have point tenderness over superior–posterior testicle

Treatment

- Analgesia as is self-limited within 1 week

Key Points

- Difficult to confidently exclude testicular torsion with acute presentation

Bibliography

Brenner JS, Aderonke O. Causes of scrotal swelling in children and adolescents. In: Basow DS, ed. *UptoDate*. Waltham, MA: UptoDate; 2011.

Canadian Taskforce on Preventative Health. Recommendations on screening for prostate cancer with the prostate-specific antigen test. *Can Med Asson J*. 2014;186(16):1225-1234.

Canadian Urological Association. Prostatitis guidelines (draft). 2011. http://www.cua.org/guidelines_e.asp.

Canadian Urological Association. Prostate cancer screening: Canadian guidelines 2011. 2011. http://www.cua.org/guidelines_e.asp.

Canadian Urological Association. 2010 Update: Guidelines for the management of benign prostatic hyperplasia. 2010. http://www.cua.org/guidelines_e.asp.

Eyre RC. Evaluation of the acute scrotum in adults. In: Basow DS (ed). *UptoDate*. Waltham, MA: UptoDate; 2012.

Hoffman RM. Screening for prostate cancer. *NEJM*. 2011;365:2013-2019.

Kantoff PW, Taplin M. Clinical presentation, diagnosis, and staging of prostate cancer. In: Basow DS, ed. *UptoDate*. Waltham, MA: UptoDate; 2012.

Osteoporosis

Priority Topic 69

Definitions

World Health Organization definition of postmenopausal osteoporosis in women without fragility fractures:

- T-score is bone density expressed as number of standard deviations (SD) above or below mean BMD value for a normal young adult, based on BMD measurement at spine, hip, or forearm by dual-energy x-ray absorptiometry (DEXA)
  - Normal is BMD within 1 SD of young adult mean (T-score at −1 and above).
  - Osteopenia is BMD within −1 SD and −2.5 SD below young adult mean (T-score between −1 and −2.5).
  - Osteoporosis is BMD ≤−2.5 SD below young adult mean (T-score at or below −2.5).
  - Clinical diagnosis of osteoporosis is fragility fracture regardless of T-score.

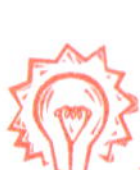

Fragility fracture is hip, vertebral, or extremity fracture sustained from fall from standing height.

Symptoms

Essentially asymptomatic until fragility fracture occurs

Characteristics

- Common: 40% lifetime risk (equivalent to cardiovascular disease), 80% will get a second fragility fracture
- Costly:
  - Financial: $1.9 billion are spent each year in Canada for treating osteoporosis and associated fractures.
  - Human: High mortality (23% with hip fractures at 1 year), high morbidity (60% will require help with activities of daily living and 40% will require mobility aids after hip fracture).
  - Gap in care: <20% of women and 10% of men with fragility fracture receive appropriate care.

Risk Factors

Focus since 2010 is on constellation of risk factors versus BMD score alone, with BMD being one among several independent risk factors.

All patients should get BMD testing if:
- Advancing age—Men and women at or over age 65
- Men and women at or over age 50 with risk factors:
  - Fragility fracture after age 40
  - High-risk medications
    - Corticosteroids (prednisone 7.5 mg daily for 3 months or equivalent)
    - Others (aromatase inhibitors, androgen deprivation therapy)
  - Parental hip fracture
  - Radiographic (vertebral fracture)
  - Current smoking
  - Alcohol (>3 drinks/day)
  - Low or loss of weight (<60 kg or loss of 10% of body weight from age 25)
  - Medical illnesses (rheumatoid arthritis, premature menopause, malabsorption, hypo gonadism, chronic liver disease, inflammatory bowel disease)

Physical Examination

Findings on PHE that may suggest osteoporosis:
- Loss of height of 2 cm/year or historical loss of 6 cm → Consider lateral spine x-ray to identify possible fracture
- Loss of iliocostal distance greater than two finger breadths
- Kyphosis >5 cm

Fall Assessment
- "Get up and go" screening test
- Assess and modify medications (polypharmacy, benzodiazepines, opioids, antihypertensives, TCAs, SSRIs)
- Home assessment
- Optimize vision, cardiovascular, neurological, and musculoskeletal conditions

Diagnosis

Made by fragility fracture, vertebral fracture (>25% loss of vertebral body height on lateral spine x-ray), or BMD of −2.5 or lower

Investigations
- To rule out secondary causes of osteoporosis once diagnosis has been made
- Corrected calcium, CBC, creatinine, ALP, TSH, S-PEP, and 25-OH vitamin D (initially and once after 3-4 months of supplementation)
- Frequent, repetitive BMD testing is an area of controversy:
  - Baseline BMD better than repeat BMD for predicting fracture risk over 8-year period
  - Repeat BMD in 1 to 3 years for high-risk patients to identify "early losers;" benefit from referral to rheumatology

Prevention

Optimize bone health with adequate calcium, vitamin D, smoking cessation, alcohol moderation, weight-bearing exercise as a young adult (bone density peaks at age 16 for women, 20 for men), and beyond

Treatment

Risk stratify with either tool
- CAROC → Requires BMD
- FRAX → Does not require BMD, but score improves with its addition
1. Low-risk/all groups:
   - 1200 mg of elemental calcium (supplement as needed, typically 500 mg daily)
   - 800 to 2000 IU of vitamin D_3 daily

- Fall prevention strategies
- Hip protectors for institutionalized patients
- Regular active weight-bearing exercise

2. Medium risk:
   - Consider pharmacotherapy. Patients with risk factors (steroid use, more than two falls in last 12 months, previous wrist fracture, or lumbar spine T-score significantly lower than femoral neck T-score) are more likely to benefit from pharmacotherapy

3. High risk:
   - Initiate pharmacotherapy

Pharmacotherapy

First line:

- Prevention of all fractures: Bisphosphonates
- Prevention of vertebral fractures: SERM (raloxifene) if breast cancer indication, HRT if indicated for vasomotor symptoms
- Bisphosphonates: Decrease bone resorption and turnover which increases BMD
  - Essentially all equivalent
  - Benefits
    - Vertebral fracture > nonvertebral (NNTs 13-50 vs NNTs of 91)
    - Alendronate
    - Risedronate: Monthly dosing available
    - Zoledronic acid: Yearly IV infusion possible (if covered)
    - Risks: Osteonecrosis of jaw (ONJ), atypical sub-trochanteric hip fractures, and esophagitis.
    - Treat for 5 years, then consider drug holiday.

Second line (if bisphosphonate-resistant or intolerant): Calcitonin or parathyroid hormone (teriparatide)

Guideline Summary

See Quick Reference Guide from Osteoporosis Canada (Figure 8-3).

Key Points

- Risk factor assessment is more important than BMD
- Ensure adequate calcium (1200 mg daily) and vitamin D (800-2000 IU daily) intake
- Treat high-risk patients with bisphosphonates
- ONJ, atypical sub-trochanteric hip fractures are important side effects of bisphosphonates

Bibliography

Journal Watch. Baseline BMD better than repeat BMD for predicting fracture risk over 8 year period. *Arch Intern Med.* 2007;167:155-160.

Osteoporosis Canada. Facts and statistics. 2011. http://www.osteoporosis.ca/index.php/ci_id/8867/la_id/1.htm. [Information page].

Rx Files. Potpourri of Q & As: osteoporosis, vitamin D, SMBG, & anti-infectives. 2010. http://www.rxfiles.ca/rxfiles/uploads/documents/QA-Remake.htm.

Rx Files. Osteoporosis treatment comparison chart. *Drug Comparison Charts.* 8th ed. 2010:72-73.

Scientific Advisory Council of Osteoporosis Canada. 2010 clinical practice guidelines for the diagnosis and management of osteoporosis in Canada: summary. *Can Med Assn J.* 2010;182(17):1864-1873.

SOGC. Menopause and osteoporosis update. *J Obst Gynecol Can.* 2009;31(1):S1-S3.

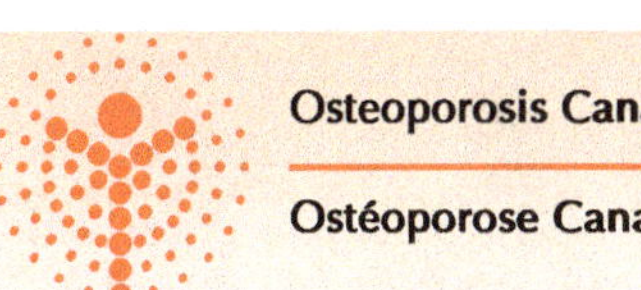

Osteoporosis Canada

Ostéoporose Canada

Quick Reference Guide

2010 Clinical Practice Guidelines for the Diagnosis and Management of Osteoporosis in Canada

This guide has been developed to provide healthcare professionals with a quick-reference summary of the most important recommendations from the **2010 Clinical Practice Guidelines for the Diagnosis and Management of Osteoporosis in Canada.** For more detailed information, consult the full guideline document at www.osteoporosis.ca.

Recommendations for Clinical Assessment

Assessment	Recommended Elements of Clinical Assessment
History	☐ Identify risk factors for low BMD, fractures and falls: ☐ Prior fragility fractures — ☐ High alcohol intake (≥3 units/day) ☐ Parental hip fracture — ☐ Rheumatoid arthritis ☐ Glucocorticoid use — ☐ Inquire about falls in the previous 12 months ☐ Current smoking — ☐ Inquire about gait and balance
Physical Examination	☐ Measure weight (weight loss of >10% since age 25 is significant) ☐ Measure height annually (prospective loss >2 cm) (historical height loss >6 cm) ⎱ Screening for ☐ Measure rib to pelvis distance ≤2 fingers' breadth ⎰ vertebral fractures ☐ Measure occiput-to-wall distance (for kyphosis) >5 cm ☐ Assess fall risk by using Get-Up-and-Go Test (ability to get out of chair without using arms, walk several steps and return)

Recommended Biochemical Tests for Patients Being Assessed for Osteoporosis

☐ Calcium, corrected for albumin
☐ Complete blood count
☐ Creatinine
☐ Alkaline phosphatase

☐ Thyroid stimulating hormone (TSH)
☐ Serum protein electrophoresis for patients with vertebral fractures
☐ 25-hydroxy vitamin D (25-OH-D)*

Should be measured after 3-4 months of adequate supplementation and should not be repeated if an optimal level ≥75 nmol/L is achieved.

Indications for BMD Testing

Older Adults (age ≥50 years)	Younger Adults (age <50 years)
• All women and men age ≥65 years • Menopausal women, and men aged 50-64 years with clinical risk factors for fracture: – Fragility fracture after age 40 – Prolonged glucocorticoid use[†] – Other high-risk medication use* – Parental hip fracture – Vertebral fracture or osteopenia identified on x-ray – Current smoking – High alcohol intake – Low body weight (<60 kg) or major weight loss (>10% of weight at age 25 years) – Rheumatoid arthritis – Other disorders strongly associated with osteoporosis such as primary hyperparathyroidism, type 1 diabetes, osteogenesis imperfecta, uncontrolled hyperthyroidism, hypogonadism or premature menopause (<45 years), Cushing's disease, chronic malnutrition or malabsorption, chronic liver disease, COPD and chronic inflammatory conditions (eg, inflammatory bowel disease)	• Fragility fracture • Prolonged use of glucocorticoids* • Use of other high-risk medications[†] • Hypogonadism or premature menopause • Malabsorption syndrome • Primary hyperparathyroidism • Other disorders strongly associated with rapid bone loss and/or fracture

[†] *≥ 3 months in the prior year at a prednisone equivalent dose ≥7.5 mg daily; *eg, aromatase inhibitors, androgen deprivation therapy.*

Assessment of Basal 10-year Fracture Risk: 2010 CAROC System

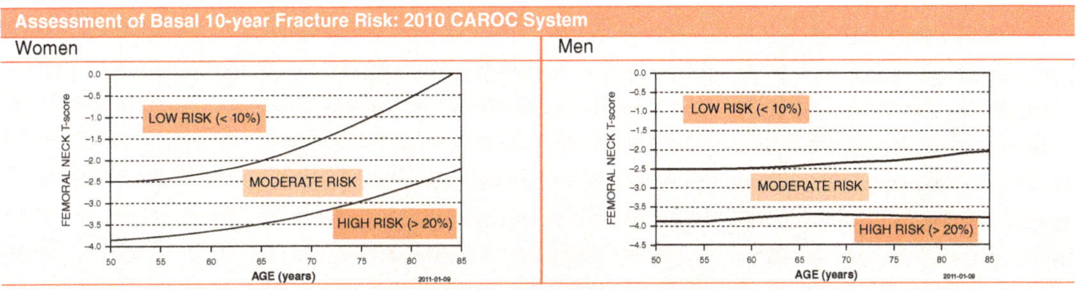

Note: (1) *Fragility fracture after age 40 or recent prolonged systemic glucocorticoid use increases 2010 CAROC basal risk by one category (ie, from low to moderate or moderate to high).*
(2) *Using this model in a patient on therapy only reflects the theoretical risk of a hypothetical patient who is treatment naïve and does not reflect the risk reduction associated with therapy.*
(3) *Femoral neck T-score should be derived from NHANES III Caucasian women reference database.*
(4) *Individuals with a fragility fracture of the vertebra or hip, or with more than one fragility fracture are at high fracture risk.*

Adapted from Papaioannou A et al. Clinical practice guidelines for the diagnosis and management of osteoporosis in Canada. CMAJ 2010 http://www.cmaj.ca/cgi/doi/10.1503/cmaj.100771. With permission from the publisher. © Osteoporosis Canada, October 2010. v-09-03-11.

FIGURE 8-3A: Quick reference guide from Osteoporosis Canada. (Adapted from Papaioannou A et al. 2010 clinical practice guidelines for the diagnosis and management of osteoporosis in Canada: summary. *CMAJ.* 2010;182(17):1864-1873. doi: 10.1503/cmaj.100771. http://www.cmaj.ca/content/182/17/1864.long.)

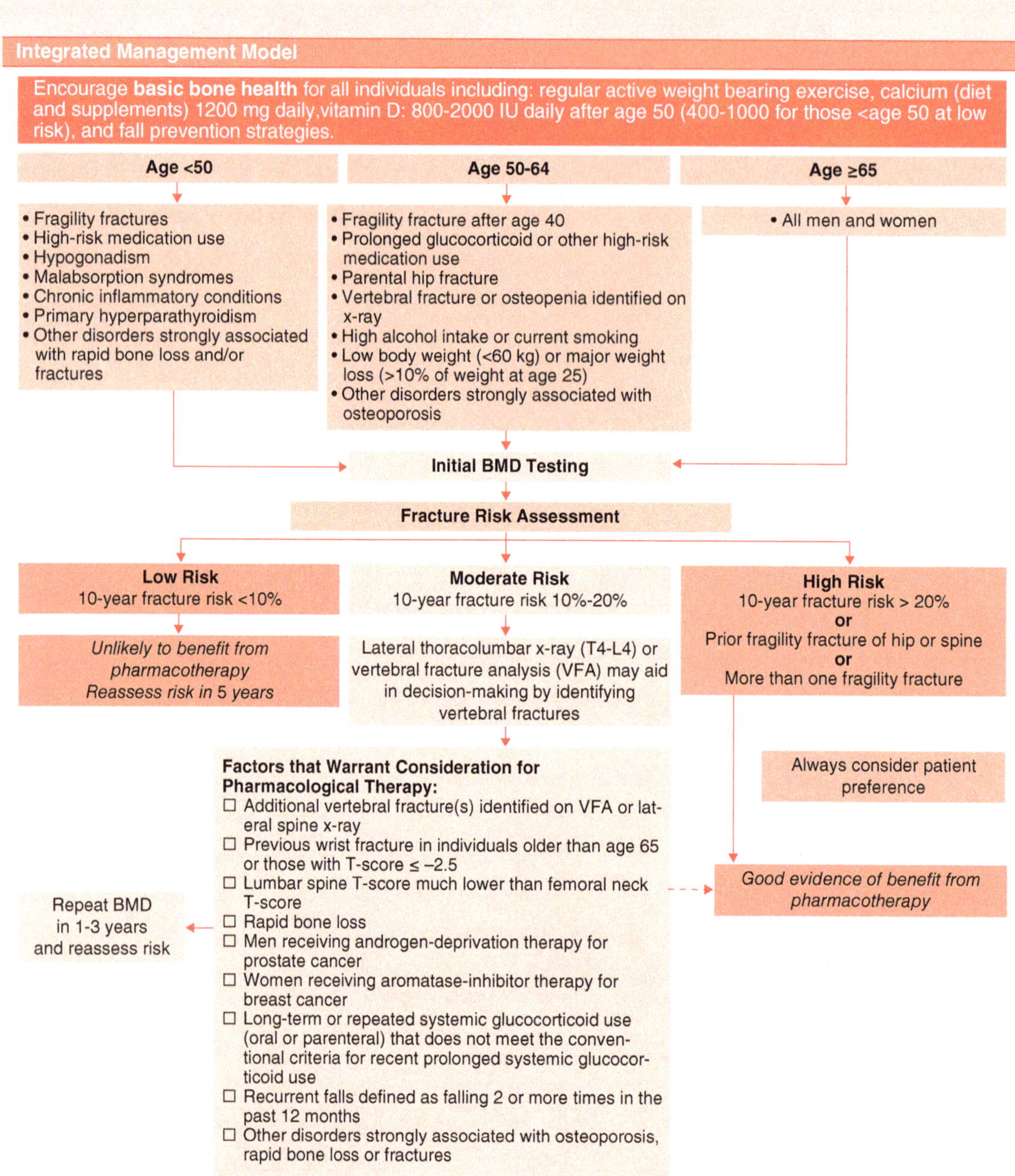

| Type of Fracture | Antiresorptive Therapy | | | | | | Bone Formation Therapy |
| | Bisphosphonates | | | Denosumab | Raloxifene | Estrogen** (Hormone Therapy) | Teriparatide |
	Alendronate	Risedronate	Zoledronic Acid				
Vertebral	✓	✓	✓	✓	✓	✓	✓
Hip	✓	✓	✓	✓	–	✓	–
Non-vertebral†	✓	✓	✓	✓	–	✓	✓

First Line Therapies with Evidence for Fracture Prevention in Postmenopausal Women*

†In Clinical trials, non-vertebral fractures are a composite endpoint including hip, femur, pelvis, tibia, humerus, radius, and clavicle.
*For postmenopausal women, ✓ indicates first line therapies and Grade A recommendation. For men requiring treatment, alendronate, risedronate, and zoledronic acid can be used as first-line therapies for prevention of fractures (Grade D).
**Hormone therapy (estrogen) can be used as first-line therapy in women with menopausal symptoms.

www.osteoporosis.ca

Adapted from Papaioannou A et al. Clinical practice guidelines for the diagnosis and management of osteoporosis in Canada. CMAJ 2010 http://www.cmaj.ca/cgi/doi/10.1503/cmaj.100771. With permission from the publisher. © Osteoporosis Canada, October 2010. v-09-03-11.

FIGURE 8-3B: Quick reference guide from Osteoporosis Canada. (Adapted from Papaioannou A et al. 2010 clinical practice guidelines for the diagnosis and management of osteoporosis in Canada: summary. *CMAJ.* 2010;182(17):1864-1873. doi: 10.1503/cmaj.100771. http://www.cmaj.ca/content/182/17/1864.long.

Smoking Cessation

Priority Topic 85

The five As: a brief intervention for smoking cessation

ASK AND ASSESS WILLINGNESS TO QUIT

Frequent starts and stops are common.

Review amount, habits, and previous quit attempts.

Assess willingness to quit using stages of change model (Table 8-7).

TABLE 8-7	Stages of Change
STAGE	**ACTION**
Precontemplation	Increase patient's awareness of risks in nonjudgmental manner, avoid resistance
Contemplation	Discuss pros and cons of quitting, understand ambivalence
Preparation	Offer practical advice and anticipate difficulties
Action	Support, reward, prevent relapse, review action plan
Maintenance	Address stressors and anticipate temptations

Patients unwilling to quit may benefit from multiple, short sessions using principles of motivational interviewing (the five Rs may be a helpful mnemonic):

Relevance to patient

Risks of smoking

Rewards of quitting

Roadblocks to quitting

Repetition at each visit

ADVISE TO QUIT

Brief advice from a physician increases cessation rate

Health benefits:

- Leading cause of preventable death
- Death an average of 6.5 to 9 years prematurely
- Reduced risk of mortality from myocardial infarction
- Reduced stroke risk
- Improvement in chronic lung disease
- Reduced number and severity of pulmonary infections
- Reduced cancer risk (bladder, cervical, stomach, oropharyngeal)
- Reduced risk of osteoporosis and fractures
- Reduced risk of peptic ulcer disease
- Improved healing
- Improved health of family/cohabitants

Improved quality of life:

- Less sexual dysfunction
- Financial gains (on average $3600/year)

ASSIST IN IMPLEMENTING A PLAN

Multistrategy approach may include some or all of the following:

- Establishing a quit day
- Prequit exercise program
- Alternative oral behaviours—gum, lozenges
- Anticipate obstacles such as withdrawal, weight gain, and triggers
- Support groups
- Counselling and cognitive behavioural therapy
- Hypnosis/acupuncture
- Repetition
- Pharmacotherapy (see Table 8-8)

TABLE 8-8	Pharmacotherapy	
DRUG (VS PLACEBO)	**BUPROPION**	**VARENICLINE**
NNT	8 vs placebo	8 vs placebo
SEs	Insomnia, headache, dizziness, tachycardia, xerostomia, weight loss, pharyngitis, nausea	Insomnia, h/a, abnormal dreams, GI upset
Tolerability	29% discontinued due to SEs	Better
Caution	ESRD, cirrhosis → Adjust dose Depression with suicide potential → Monitor mood	ESRD → Adjust dose Depression with suicide potential → Monitor mood Stable CAD → Currently under Health Canada and FDA review
Contraindication	Seizure disorder, eating disorder, MAO-I use, sedative withdrawal	None

- Nicotine replacement
  - Gum, patch, inhaler, nasal spray
- Bupropion
- Varenicline

ARRANGE FOLLOW-UP

- Peak withdrawal at 2 to 3 days
- Improvement in withdrawal at 2 to 3 weeks
- Highest relapse at 2 to 3 months

Bibliography

Lai DTC, Cahill K, Qin Y, Yang JL. Motivational interviewing for smoking cessation. *Cochrane Database Syst Rev.* 2010;(1):CD006936.

Mahoney MC, Cummings K. Chapter 57. Tobacco cessation. In: South-Paul JE, Matheny SC, Lewis EL, eds. *Current Diagnosis & Treatment in Family Medicine*, 3rd ed. 2011. http://www.accessmedicine.com/content.aspx?aID=8158522. Accessed November 12, 2012.

Rx Files. Tobacco/smoking cessation pharmacotherapy. *Drug Comparison Charts*. 8th ed. 2010:115.

Statistics Canada. Canadian Tobacco Use Monitoring Survey. 2003. http://www.hc-sc.gc.ca/hc-ps/tobac-tabac/research-recherche/stat/_ctums-esutc_fs-if/2003-smok-fum-eng.php. Accessed November 12, 2012.

Stead LF, Bergson G, Lancaster T. Physician advice for smoking cessation. *Cochrane Database Syst Rev.* 2008;(2):CD000165.

Tran, Christopher, Yingming A. (ed) The Toronto Notes 2011: Comprehensive Medical Reference and Review for the Medical Council of Canada Qualifying Exam Part 1 and the United States Medical Licensing Exam Step 2. Toronto: Toronto Notes for Medical Students, Inc, 2011. FM 8-9.

CHAPTER 9

Sexual Health

Gender-Specific Issues

Priority Topic 42

- Appreciate and anticipate that males and females may have different presentations of the same condition or disease.
- Be aware and consider the possibility of domestic violence in women with health concerns.
  - When/who to screen:
    - Assessment of new patients
    - Annual preventative visits
    - Prenatal patients
    - Symptoms/signs in keeping with abuse
  - WAST (Woman Abuse Screening Tool)
    - Validated, 90% sensitivity with first two questions
    - Part 1:
      1. In general, how would you describe your relationship?
         a. A lot of tension
         b. Some tension
         c. No tension
      2. Do you and your partner work out arguments with:
         a. Great difficulty
         b. Some difficulty
         c. No difficulty?
    - Positive WAST = A lot of tension, great difficulty
    - Part 2—If first part is positive
      1. Do arguments ever result in you feeling down or bad about yourself?
      2. Do arguments ever result in hitting or punching?
      3. Do you ever feel frightened by what your partner says or does?
      4. Does your partner ever abuse you physically?
      5. Does your partner ever abuse you emotionally?
      6. Does your partner ever abuse you sexually?

- Assess the possibility of role-balancing issues when presented with men or women experiencing stress-related health concerns.
- Ensure your office and practice provides comfort and choice, especially around sensitive examinations such as rectal or pelvic examinations.
- Be sure to interpret and use evidence-based medicine while being cognitive of the gender bias in clinical studies.

Bibliography

Cherniak D, Grant L, Mason R, et al. Intimate Partner Violence Consensus Statement. SOGC Clinical Practice Guideline. 157: April 2005.

The College of Family Physicians of Canada. http://www.cfpc.ca/uploadedFiles/Education/Priority%20 Topics%20and%20Key%20Features.pdf.

Family Practice Notebook. WAST Screen for Intimate Partner Violence. http://www.fpnotebook.com/ prevent/Exam/WstScrnFrIntmtPrtnrVlnc.htm.

Screening for Domestic Violence. Ontario College of Family Physicians. June 2004.

Infertility

Priority Topic 52

Definition

Failure to conceive after 1 year of regular, unprotected sex for women aged <35 years. Affects approximately 15% of couples, and one in five women.

- Primary infertility = No prior pregnancies
- Secondary infertility = Previous conception

Investigations

- When?
  - Women <35 years: After 1 year of trying to conceive
  - Women 35 to 40 years: After 6 months of trying to conceive
  - Women >40 years: Immediately
  - Sooner if history of:
    - PID
    - History of infertility
    - Prior pelvic surgery
    - Chemotherapy or radiation in either partner
    - Recurrent pregnancy loss
    - Moderate-to-severe endometriosis
- Who?
  - Both partners
    - Female factor approximately 30%
    - Male factor approximately 30%
    - Both male and female factors approximately 30%

Etiology

Female

- Ovulatory dysfunction
  - Polycystic ovarian syndrome (PCOS)
  - Premature ovarian failure

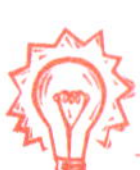

Sperm lives longer than eggs. Therefore, it is better to advise patients to have sex a few days prior to ovulation, rather than wait until the day they think they are ovulating.

Some recommend sex three times per week.

- Hypothalamic suppression
  - Intense exercise
  - Eating disorder
  - Stress
  - Hyperprolactinemia
- Thyroid disease
- Advanced maternal age
- Turner syndrome
- Medications
  - Contraceptives
  - Corticosteroids
  - Antidepressants/antipsychotics
  - Chemotherapy
- Tubular disease (Fallopian)
  - Pelvic inflammatory disease
  - Tubal blockage
  - Prior ectopic pregnancies
  - Endometriosis
  - Adhesions
- Uterine abnormalities
  - Fibroids
  - Asherman syndrome
  - Anatomic abnormalities
- Cervical abnormalities
  - Cervical stenosis

Male

- Idiopathic
- Testicular
  - History of cryptorchidism
  - Irradiation
  - Varicocele
  - Androgen insensitivity
  - Klinefelter syndrome
  - Infections
  - Chronic diseases
  - Drugs
    - Marijuana
    - Spironolactone
    - Ketoconazole
    - EtOH
- Altered sperm transport
  - Obstructed or absent vas deferens
  - Ejaculatory disorders
  - Epididymal dysfunction
- Hypothalamic–pituitary disorders
  - Hemochromatosis
  - Trauma/surgery
  - Medications

- Hormonal
- Chronic illness
- Eating disorders

Other factors

- Smoking
- BMI extremes
- Diet
- Environmental toxins
- Medical illnesses and treatments

Diagnosis

- History
  - **Female**
    - Menstrual cycle
      - Frequency and duration
      - Regular or irregular
      - Changing
      - Intermenstrual bleeding
    - Coitus
      - Frequency
      - Timing
    - PMHx
      - PID
      - Surgery
      - Systemic symptoms
      - Symptoms of PCOS
      - Nipple discharge/lactation
    - Gyne/obstetrical hx
    - Previous pregnancies
    - STIs
    - Pap smears
    - Family history of infertility/congenital issues
  - **Male**
    - Developmental history
      - Testicular descent, pubertal development
    - PMHx
      - Infections
      - Trauma/surgeries
      - Irradiation/chemo
    - Sexual hx
      - Libido
      - Previous pregnancies
    - Medications
    - EtOH/recreational drugs

Investigations

- Female
  - Day 3 FSH (test of ovarian reserve)
  - LH
  - TSH

- DHEA
- Testosterone
- Prolactin
- Day 21 to 23 serum progesterone (test of ovulation)
- Pelvic ultrasound
- Hysterosalpingography
- Laparoscopy
- Karyotype
- Male
  - Semen analysis
  - Free testosterone
    - If low, test for LH and FSH
  - Karyotyping

Treatment

- Lifestyle modifications
  - Weight loss
  - Smoking
  - EtOH/drugs
- Ovulation induction
  - Clomiphene citrate
  - Metformin
  - Tamoxifen
  - Laparoscopic ovarian drilling
- Tuboplasty
- Lysis of adhesions
- Artificial insemination
- IVF
- ICSI (intracytoplasmic sperm injection)
- IUI (intrauterine insemination)
- Sperm or ova donation
- Consider discussing adoption

POLYCYSTIC OVARIAN SYNDROME

Etiology

- Disorder of intraovarian androgen excess
- Most common in 15 to 35 years
- Most common cause for anovulation

Symptoms

- Hyperandrogenism
  - Acne
  - Hirsutism
- Infertility
- Insulin resistance
- Acanthosis nigricans
- Menstrual irregularity
- Obesity
- Menorrhagia

Diagnosis

Rotterdam Criteria 2003 needs two of the three:

1. Oligo-ovulation or anovulation
2. Hyperandrogenism (clinical or biochemical)
3. Polycystic ovaries on U/S

Investigations

- Transvaginal ultrasound
  - String of pearls—Polycystic ovaries
- LH:FSH > 2:1
- Fasting glucose
- Increased DHEAS
- Increased free testosterone

Treatment

- Cycle control
  - Weight loss
  - Increased exercise
  - Combined OCP
  - Metformin
  - Tranexamic acid for menorrhagia
- Infertility
  - Weight loss
  - Medical induction of ovulation
    - Clomiphene
    - Metformin
    - Letrozole
  - IVF
- Hirsutism
  - OCP +/− spironolactone for antiandrogen effect

Bibliography

Brander E, Hall J, McLean K, et al. *Infertility: Toronto Notes*, edited by Vojvodic M, Young A. Toronto, Toronto Notes for Medical Students, Inc; 2014. GY 22.

Chen YA, Tran C. *Toronto Notes—Comprehensive Medical Reference & Review for MCCQE I and USMLE II*. Toronto, Canada: Toronto Notes for Medical Students Inc; 2011.

Simon C, Everitt H, van Dorp F. *Oxford Handbook of General Practice*. Oxford, UK: Oxford University Press; 2010.

UpToDate. Causes of male infertility. https://www.uptodate.com/contents/causes-of-male-infertility.

UpToDate. Evaluation of female infertility. https://www.uptodate.com/contents/evaluation-of-female-infertility.

UpToDate. Evaluation of male infertility. https://www.uptodate.com/contents/evaluation-of-male-infertility.

UpToDate. Overview of infertility. https://www.uptodate.com/contents/overview-of-infertility.

UpToDate. Overview of treatment of female infertility. https://www.uptodate.com/contents/overview-of-treatment-of-female-infertility.

UpToDate. Treatment of male infertility. https://www.uptodate.com/contents/treatment-of-male-infertility.

UpToDate. Treatment of polycystic ovary syndrome in adults. https://www.uptodate.com/contents/treatment-of-polycystic-ovary-syndrome-in-adults.

Vojvodic M, Young A, eds. *Toronto Notes*, 30th ed. Toronto, ON: Toronto Notes for Medical Students Inc; 2014. FM3, GS55.

Sex

Priority Topic 82

Definitions

- Sexual minority
  - Variety of gender and sexual identities and expressions that differ from cultural norms, for example, lesbian, gay, bisexual, and transgender.
- Approach the topic of sexuality respectfully—don't lecture!
- Avoid assumptions!
- Just ask about sexual orientation.
- Ensure a safe and welcoming environment
  - Policy of openness and respect, ensure privacy and confidentiality
- SHEADDSSS psychosocial history
  - Strengths
  - Home
  - Education/employment
  - Activities
  - Drugs/tobacco
  - Depression
  - Suicidality
  - Safety
  - Sexuality

FEMALE SEXUAL DYSFUNCTION

Etiology

- Intrapsychic
- Relationship issues
- Physical/organic

Top Three Classifications of Female Sexual Dysfunction

1. Lack of desire (60%-70%)
2. Lack of arousal
3. Dyspareunia (vaginismus, vulvodynia, vulvar vestibulitis)

Treatment

- Rule out organic causes!
- Relationship therapy
- Self-exploration
- Kegel exercises
- Dilators
- Psychotherapy
- Lubricants
- Sexual position—Female on top (more control for female)
- Hormone replacement therapy if indicated

MALE SEXUAL DYSFUNCTION

Decreased Libido

- 5% to 15% prevalence in men
- Increases with age
- Frequently associated with other sexual disorders

Causes

- EtOH
- Depression
- Stress
- Fear/relationship issues
- Testosterone deficiency
- Systemic illness
  - Cancer
  - Lupus
  - DM
  - Renal failure
- Drugs
  - Recreational
  - SSRIs
  - Antiandrogens
  - Opioids
  - 5-α Reductase inhibitors

Treatment

- Treat underlying cause
- Testosterone replacement
  - Consider if patient has evidence of hypogonadism—signs/symptoms of hypogonadism *and* a decreased serum testosterone concentration
  - NOT useful in treating ED
  - Contraindications: Polycythemia, prostate hypertrophy, prostate/breast/testicular CA, severe OSA
  - Multiple formulations: Oral, transdermal gel/patch, injectable
  - Treat for 3 to 6 months or until improvement of symptoms/return of testosterone levels to normal range

Erectile Dysfunction

- Inability to obtain or maintain an adequate erection for sexual performance.

Impotence

Etiology

- Iatrogenic
  - Pelvic surgery
  - Pelvic radiation
- Mechanical
  - Peyronie disease
  - Postpriapism
- Psychological
  - Depression, stress, anxiety, PTSD, widower syndrome
- Occlusive vascular
  - HTN

- DM
- Smoking
- Hyperlipidemia
- PVD
- Trauma
  - Penile/pelvic
  - Bicycling
- Extra factors
  - Renal failure
  - Cirrhosis
  - COPD
  - Sleep apnea
  - Malnutrition
- Neurogenic
  - CNS (eg, Parkinson, MS, spinal cord injury, Guillain-Barré, spina bifida, stroke)
  - PNS (eg, DM, peripheral neuropathy)
- Chemical
  - Antihypertensives
  - Sedatives
  - Antidepressants
  - Antipsychotics
  - Anxiolytics
  - Anticholinergics
  - Antihistamines
  - Antiandrogens (including 5-α reductase inhibitors)
  - Statins
  - GnRH agonists
  - Illicit drugs
- Endocrine
  - DM
  - Hypogonadism
  - Hyperprolactinemia
  - Hypo/hyperthyroid

Diagnosis
- Generally self-reported but may require physician-directed inquiry to illicit symptoms
- ED Intensity Scale or ED Impact Scale can be used to assess the patient

Treatment
- Psychogenic causes
  - Counselling
- Organic causes
  - Lifestyle changes
    - Quit smoking
    - Decrease alcohol
- Medications
  - Phosphodiesterase-5 (PDE-5) inhibitors
    - Sildenafil (Viagra)
    - Tadalafil (Cialis)
    - Vardenafil (Levitra)

- Contraindications
  - Patient taking nitrates or α_1-blockers
- Side effects
  - Common: Flushing, headache, dyspepsia, and nasal congestion
  - Rare: MI, priapism (>4 h), and QT prolongation
- Other options include prostaglandins, vasodilators, implants, and vascular surgery.

Bibliography

Chen YA, Tran C. *Toronto Notes—Comprehensive Medical Reference & Review for MCCQE I and USMLE II*. Toronto, Canada: Toronto Notes for Medical Students Inc; 2011.

Rx Files. Erectile dysfunction comparison chart. *Drug Comparison Charts*. 10th ed. 2015;34,69.

UpToDate. Overview of male sexual dysfunction. https://www.uptodate.com/contents/overview-of-male-sexual-dysfunction

UpToDate. Sexual Minority Youth. https://www.uptodate.com/contents/sexual-minority-youth-overview-of-primary-care.

Sexually Transmitted Infections
Priority Topic 83

CHLAMYDIA

Most common reportable STI in Canada.

Etiology

- *Chlamydia trachomatis*

Symptoms

- May be asymptomatic (80% of women)
- Vaginal or urethral discharge
- UTI symptoms (frequency, urgency, dysuria)
- Pelvic pain
- Testicular pain
- Conjunctivitis
- Postcoital bleeding

Diagnosis

- Nucleic acid amplification test (NAAT) on "dirty" urine sample (no cleaning of genitalia prior, first catch)
- Throat swab for culture if oral sex

Prevention

- Condom use with every sexual contact

Complications

- Pelvic inflammatory disease
- Reactive arthritis (sterile arthritis, urethritis, conjunctivitis)
- Infertility
- Chronic pelvic pain
- Increased rate of ectopic pregnancy

Treatment

- Azithromycin 1 g po × 1
- Doxycycline 100 mg po bid × 7 days.
- **Always** treat for gonorrhea as well, as often coinfected.
- Consult local antibiograms for resistance patterns.

Key Points

- Reportable disease in most jurisdictions and must treat partners.
- In pregnant women, use azithromycin to avoid fetal bone and teeth effects.
- If treating during pregnancy, must retest patients 3 to 4 weeks after treatment to ensure cure.
- Abstain from sex until 7 days after completed treatment.

GONORRHEA

Etiology

Caused by *Neisseria gonorrhoeae*.

High-resistance patterns in some areas of Canada—consult local antibiograms for resistance patterns.

Symptoms

- May be asymptomatic (80% of women)
- Vaginal or urethral discharge
- UTI symptoms (frequency, urgency, dysuria)
- Pelvic pain
- Testicular pain
- Postcoital bleeding
- Pharyngeal infection
- Arthritis
- Rectal pain if prostatitis

Diagnosis

- NAAT on "dirty" urine sample (no cleaning of genitalia prior, first catch).
- Throat swab for culture if oral sex.
- In symptomatic males who have sex with males (MSM), nongenital infections, or exposure to known resistant gonorrhea, swab and culture is recommended.

Prevention

- Condom use with every sexual contact

Complications

- Same as for chlamydia.

Treatment

- Cefixime 800 mg po × 1.
- Ceftriaxone 250 mg IM × 1.
- Ciprofloxacin 500 mg po × 1 (only if contraindication to third-generation cephalosporins *and* susceptibility is demonstrated on culture *or* <5% local resistance rate *and* test for cure available).
- **Always** treat for chlamydia as well as often coinfected.

Key Points

- Reportable disease in most jurisdictions and must treat partners
- MSM—Ceftriaxone is the preferred treatment
- Pharyngeal infections—Ceftriaxone is the preferred treatment
- Test for cure in kids <14 years, in case of pregnancy, and if nongenital source

HUMAN PAPILLOMA VIRUS (HPV)

Most common nonreportable STI in Canada

Etiology

- Human papilloma virus (>100 subtypes)
  - 16 and 18—Oncogenic
  - 6 and 11—Warts

Symptoms

- Asymptomatic
- Warts (condyloma acuminate) visible or palpable on external genitalia
- Postcoital bleeding

Diagnosis

- Clinical
  - Visible, flesh-coloured papules causing pruritus and local bleeding.
- Pap smears
  - LSIL—Low-grade squamous intraepithelial lesions (CIN I, II)
  - HSIL—High-grade squamous intraepithelial lesions (CIN III-IV)

Prevention

- Abstinence
- Vaccination
  - Varies from province to province—Some offer to girls and boys, some only to girls
  - Timing of vaccination varies from grades 4 to 8
  - Three vaccine choices (note: There are no guidelines as to which vaccine to select)
    - Gardasil quadrivalent vaccine (vaccination for types 6, 11, 16, 18)
      - Girls age 9 to 26 years (official indication) but recommended for up to age 45
      - Boys age 9 to 26 years
    - Gardasil 9 vaccine (vaccination for types 6, 11, 16, 18, 31, 33, 45, 52, 58)
      - Girls age 9 to 26 years (official indication) but recommended for up to age 45
      - Boys age 9 to 26 years
    - Cervarix vaccine (bivalent—16, 18)
      - Girls age 9 to 26 years
- Condom use not shown to limit transmission

Complications

- Cervical cancer, vulvar and vaginal cancer, genital warts, anal cancer, pharyngeal cancer, and penile cancer

Treatment

Genital warts

- Imiquimod cream
  - Home treatment—Apply three times per week until clearance of warts (max 16 weeks of treatment)
  - Lower recurrence rates

- Trichloroacetic acid (80%-90%)
  - Physician applies treatment.
  - Applied every 1 to 2 weeks until lesions are gone.
  - Apply until lesion turns white.
  - Apply petroleum jelly to surrounding tissue for protection.
- Podophyllin (10%-25%)—Contraindicated in pregnancy
  - Physician applies treatment.
  - Repeated one or twice weekly.
  - Leave podophyllin for 1 to 4 hours then wash off.
- Podofilox (0.5%)
  - Home treatment
  - Applied with cotton swab bid for 3 consecutive days, repeat every week
- Cryotherapy—Generally safest in pregnancy
  - Physician applies treatment.
- Laser
- Surgery

Key Points

- Ensure regular cervical cancer screening
- MSM at higher risk of anal warts and anal cancer

HSV

Etiology

- Herpes simplex virus (I and II)
  - Type I: Oral, less likely genital.
  - Type II: Genital "traditionally."
  - Viral shedding can occur at any time but is increased during the prodrome and while lesions are present.

Symptoms

- Prodrome—Genital pruritus, tingling, burning, or pain
- Vesicles on an erythematous base leading to ulcerations
- Usually present with menstrual cycle, emotional stress, or illness
- Primary
  - Extensive painful ulcers
  - Systemic symptoms
  - Lymphadenopathy
  - Protracted course
- Nonprimary
  - Less extensive genital lesions
  - Systemic symptoms less likely

Diagnosis

- Primary infection
  - Usually clinical diagnosis, onset 2 to 21 days after exposure
- Viral swabs of vesicular fluid for culture
- Antigen testing
- PCR is most sensitive and 100% specific

Prevention

- Condoms can reduce transmission rate by approximately 50%
- Suppressive therapy for HSV-II-positive partner in a serodiscordant pair
  - Valacyclovir 500 mg daily seems to reduce transmission by 48%

Treatment

- First episode
  - Acyclovir 400 mg po tid × 7 to 10 days
  - Valacyclovir 1000 mg po bid × 7 to 10 days
- Subsequent episodes
  - Acyclovir 800 mg po tid × 2 days
  - Valacyclovir 1000 mg po daily × 3 days
- Suppressive therapy if more than six episodes per year
  - Acyclovir 400 mg po bid
  - Valacyclovir 1 g po daily

Key Points

- Primary outbreak can be severe, possibly with systemic flu-like symptoms.
- Possible to have HSV-I infection of genitalia or HSV-II infection of oral mucosa, but tend to be less severe.
- Can be treated with antivirals within 72 hours of prodromal symptoms or lesion presentation
- Offer suppressive therapy to pregnant women at 36 weeks and deliver via C-section if experiencing prodromal symptoms or active lesions at time of labour onset.

SYPHILIS

Etiology

- *Treponema pallidum*

Symptoms

- Primary syphilis: Painless papule or ulcer, lymphadenopathy
- Secondary syphilis: Rash and flu-like symptoms, condyloma lata, uveitis, retinitis, and mucous lesions
- Latent syphilis: Asymptomatic
- Tertiary syphilis: Neurologic, cardiovascular (aortic root dilatation), and tissue complications

Diagnosis

- RPR/VDRL reactive and treponemal test reaction (eg, TP-EIA) *or*
- Dark field microscopy positive *or*
- Direct fluorescent antibody positive

Prevention

- Consistent condom use

Treatment

- Primary: Benzathine penicillin G 2.4 million units IM × 1
- Secondary: Benzathine penicillin G 2.4 million units IM × 1

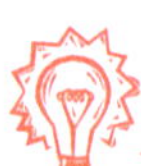

When diagnosing and treating primary syphilis, make sure to treat for chancroid (*Haemophilus ducreyi*) simultaneously. These lesions cannot be correctly distinguished from one another based on clinical assessment.

- Latent:
  - Early (<1 year from likely infection): Benzathine penicillin G 2.4 million units IM × 1
  - Late (>1 year from likely infection): Benzathine penicillin G 2.4 million units every week × 3 weeks
- Tertiary: Benzathine penicillin G 2.4 million units IM × every week × 3 weeks
  - Special case—Neurosyphilis: Penicillin G 3 to 4 million units IV q4H × 10 to 14 days

Key Points

- Latent syphilis is diagnosed in asymptomatic patients with reactive VDRL and TP-EIA; however, testing may also be reactive if they have had previously treated syphilis.
- After treatment, recheck VDRL and ensure at least fourfold decrease in titres; otherwise, consider reinfection.

VULVOVAGINITIS (SEE PRIORITY TOPIC 97)

Etiology

- Three most common infectious causes:
  - Bacterial vaginosis—**most common**
  - Vulvovaginal candidiasis
  - Trichomonas—sexually transmitted
- Noninfectious causes
  - Atrophic vaginitis
  - Foreign bodies
  - Allergic/irritant dermatitis
  - Lichen sclerosus—increases risk of vulvar cancer
  - Lichen planus

TABLE 9-1 Diagnostic Features and Manifestations of Vulvovaginitis

	BACTERIAL VAGINOSIS	CANDIDIASIS	TRICHOMONIASIS
Symptoms	• Vaginal discharge • Fishy odour • May be asymptomatic	• Vaginal discharge • Itch • Dysuria • +/− Dyspareunia	• Vaginal discharge • Itch • Dysuria • May be asymptomatic
Signs	• White/grey, thin discharge	• White, thick, curdy discharge • Erythema/edema of vulva	• Off white/yellow, frothy discharge • "Strawberry" cervix
Diagnosis	• Vaginal swab for microscopy	• Vaginal swab for microscopy	• Vaginal swab for microscopy
Vaginal pH	>4.5	<4.5	>4.5
Wet mount	Clue cells	Budding yeast Pseudohyphae	Motile flagellated protozoa
Whiff test	Positive	Negative	Negative
Treatment	Metronidazole 2 g single dose OR 500 mg bid × 7 days	Clotrimazole 1% topical cream 2-3 days (7-10 days for pregnancy) OR Fluconazole 150 mg po single dose	Metronidazole 2 g single dose *or* 500 mg bid × 7 days

PELVIC INFLAMMATORY DISEASE

Etiology

- Most common are chlamydia or gonorrhea
- May be GI organisms

Symptoms

- Fever
- Discharge
- Abdominal/pelvic pain
- Cervical motion tenderness
- Adnexal masses
- Asymptomatic (60%)

Diagnosis

- Clinical diagnosis
  - Sexually active young female who present with lower abdominal pain and evidence of cervical motion or adnexal tenderness on examination
- May also have the any (or none) of the following symptoms:
  - Temperature >38°C
  - Abnormal cervical/vaginal discharge
  - Documentation of chlamydial/gonococcal infection
  - Pelvic imaging (U/S or CT) with findings of thickened/fluid filled tubes or tubo-ovarian fluid collection

Treatment

- Mild/outpatient
  - Ceftriaxone 250 mg IM + doxycycline 100 mg PO bid × 14 days +/− Flagyl (if tubo-ovarian fluid collection found on imaging) 500 mg PO bid × 14 days
- Moderate-to-severe/inpatient
  - Ceftriaxone 1 to 2 g IV daily × 24 hours then switch to oral + doxycycline 100 mg IV/po bid × 14 days + Flagyl 500 mg PO bid × 14 days
  - Cefoxitin 2 g IV q6h × 24 hours + doxycycline 100 mg IV/PO bid × 14 days (switch to oral once clinical improved as above)
- Reassess in 48 hours

Key Points

- Do not remove IUD until after treatment.
- Treat partners regardless of symptoms/signs.

Bibliography

Canadian Cancer Society. HPV vaccines. http://www.cancer.ca/en/prevention-and-screening/be-aware/viruses-and-bacteria/human-papillomavirus-hpv/hpv-vaccines. Accessed January 9, 2017.

DynaMed. Chlamydia Genital Infection. Ipswich, MA: EBSCO Publishing; 2012, February 12. http://search.ebscohost.com/login.aspx?direct=true&site=DynaMed&id=113862; http://web.ebscohost.com.cyber.usask.ca/dynamed/detail?vid=9&hid=21&sid=f693f962-f812-4ab7-bdf3-40973d062e32%40sessionmgr14&bdata=JnNpdGU9ZHluYW1lZC1saXZlJnNjb3BlPXNpdGU%3d#db=dme&AN=114223.

DynaMed. Herpes Genitalis. Ipswich, MA: EBSCO Publishing. 2012, March 22. http://search.ebscohost.com/login.aspx?direct=true&site=DynaMed&id=113862; http://web.ebscohost.com.cyber.usask.ca/dynamed/detail?vid=3&hid=21&sid=2e1251fa-304f-48b9-ab96-202194d757cf%40sessionmgr14&bdata=JnNpdGU9ZHluYW1lZC1saXZlJnNjb3BlPXNpdGU%3d#db=dme&AN=114875&anchor=suppressive.

Health Canada, Healthy Living. Human papilloma virus (HPV). 2010. http://www.hc-sc.gc.ca/hl-vs/iyh-vsv/diseases-maladies/hpv-vph-eng.php.

Health Canada. Public Health Agency—Canadian guidelines on sexually transmitted infections. Public Health Agency of Canada Issued Important Notice on gonococcal infection; 2011. http://www.phac-aspc.gc.ca/std-mts/sti-its/alert/2011/alert-gono-eng.php.

Hick C. Diagnostic testing for syphilis. In UpToDate: Rose B, ed. *UpToDate*. 2012. http://www.uptodate.com/contents/diagnostic-testing-for-syphilis?source=search_result&search=syphilis+treatment&selectedTitle=4~150.

Lee M, Jensen B, Regier L, et al. Common Infections. *RxFiles drug comparison charts*. 10th ed. Saskatoon, SK: Saskatoon Health Region; 2015:81.

Merck. Prescribing Information: Gardasil & Gardasil9. https://www.merckvaccines.com/Products/Pages/vaccine-Prescribing-Information. Jan 2017.

Sparling F, Hicks C. Pathogenesis, clinical manifestations, and treatment of late syphilis. In: Rose B, ed. *UpToDate*. 2012. http://www.uptodate.com/contents/pathogenesis-clinical-manifestations-and-treatment-of-late-syphilis?source=search_result&search=syphilis+treatment&selectedTitle=2~150#H22.

Wald A. Prevention of genital herpes virus infections. In UpToDate: Rose B, ed. *UpToDate*. 2012. http://www.uptodate.com/contents/prevention-of-genital-herpes-virus-infections?source=search_result&search=prevention+of+hsv&selectedTitle=5~150.

Wong T, Kropp R, Mann J, et al. Canadian Guidelines on Sexually Transmitted Infections. Public Health Agency of Canada. 2006.

Breast Lump

Priority Topic 11

Definition

- Any lump or mass noted on clinical examination or noted by patient

Physical Examination

- Findings suggestive of benign breast disease
  - Smooth
  - Rubbery
  - Discrete
  - Mobile
  - Well circumscribed
  - Hormone-dependent (cyclic)
  - No skin or nipple changes
  - Young age
- Findings concerning for breast cancer
  - Firm
  - Indistinct/not well circumscribed
  - Skin or nipple changes (retraction)
  - Peau d'orange
  - Fixed
  - Increasing size

Risk Factors for Breast Cancer

- Female
- Age >40
- Prior history of breast cancer
- Prior breast biopsy (regardless of pathology results)
- First-degree relative with breast cancer
- Menarche before age 12
- Menopause after 55

- Nulliparity
- First pregnancy after age 30
- Radiation
- HRT for >5 years duration
- OCP use*
- Alcohol*
- Sedentary lifestyle*
- Obesity*

(*modifiable risk factors)

** Note—Decreased risk of breast cancer with breastfeeding, early menopause, and early childbirth**

Investigations

- Imaging
  - Women <30 years: Ultrasound is investigation of choice due to denser breasts
  - Women >30 years: Diagnostic mammography (may require U/S for more information)
  - Possible MRI—Case-by-case basis, especially if dense breasts
- Tissue sample
  - Fine needle aspiration
  - Core biopsy
  - Surgical excision

Screening

- Breast cancer screening for average-risk women
  - Women 50 to 74: Routine screening mammography q2 to 3 years.
  - No routine screening for women <50 years old or >74 years old.
  - No routine clinical breast examination alone or in conjunction with mammography.
  - Do not advise women to perform routine breast self-examinations as there is no benefit and possible harm due to increased benign biopsies and no increased survival rates.
- Breast cancer screening for high risk
  - Consider earlier/more frequent for women with strong family history of breast cancer or *BRCA 1 or 2* positive or prior chest wall radiation
- Diagnostic mammograms required when:
  - Postsurgical biopsy
  - Post benign core biopsy
  - Breast implants
  - Pregnant or breastfeeding
  - Breast cancer survivors
  - Women <40 years

Treatment of Breast Cancer

- Lumpectomy + radiation
- Mastectomy
- Sentinel node biopsy
- Node dissection
- Hormone therapy
- Chemotherapy

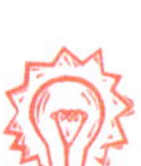

BRCA 1 and *2* are tumour suppressor genes.

If inherited, a mutation in these genes increases a women's risk of breast, ovarian, colon, cervical, and uterine cancer.

Men who inherit a harmful *BRCA 1* mutation also have an increased risk of breast cancer.

- Metastases
  - Nodal status is the most important prognostic factor.
  - Bone >lung >pleura >liver >brain.
  - Monitor for symptoms of metastases in cases of known breast cancer.

Complications of Breast Cancer

- Lymphedema possibly from nodal metastases or after node dissection
- Generalized aches and pains
- Side effects from radiation and chemotherapy

Differential Diagnosis

Benign Breast Lumps

- Fibrocystic changes
  - Age 30 years to menopause
  - Focal areas of nodularity or cysts
  - A normal variant, but does increase baseline risk of breast cancer slightly
- Fibroadenoma
  - Age <30 years
  - Most common breast lump in young women
  - Solid
  - Most often in upper-outer quadrant of breast
  - Cannot differentiate from cancer on physical examination or on U/S
  - Will need biopsy to ensure not cancerous
- Fat necrosis
  - Due to trauma
  - Firm
  - Ill-defined mass
  - Skin or nipple retraction possible
- Abscess
  - Hot, firm, erythematous overlying skin
  - Common during breastfeeding due to blockage of ducts causing mastitis
  - Most common pathogen is *Staphylococcus aureus*
  - Fever and leukocytosis usually present
  - Must consider inflammatory breast cancer
- Intraductal papilloma
  - Solitary
  - Intraductal
  - Benign polyp
  - Unilateral bloody nipple discharge
  - 10% risk of transformation to DCIS

Inflammatory Breast Cancer

- Aggressive cancer defined by dermal lymphatic invasion
- May or may not be associated with a mass
- Skin hot, red, painful, peau d'orange
- Generally have normal WBC and no fever
- If concerned, arrange for urgent mammography and obtain at least two skin punch biopsies

Bibliography

Chen YA, Tran C. *Toronto Notes—Comprehensive Medical Reference & Review for MCCQE I and USMLE II.* Toronto, Canada: Toronto Notes for Medical Students Inc; 2011.

Michel J, Gabriela L. Recommendations on screening for breast cancer in average-risk women age 40–74 years. *CMAJ.* 2011;183(18):2146-2146. DOI: 10.1503/cmaj.111–2101.

Taghian A, El-Ghamry M, Merajver S. Inflammatory breast cancer: clinical features and treatment. In UpToDate: Rose B, ed. *UpToDate.* 2011. Available from http://www.uptodateonline.com. http://www.uptodate.com/contents/inflammatory-breast-cancer-clinical-features-and-treatment?source=search_result&search=inflammatory+breast+cancer&selectedTitle=1~34.

Vojvodic M, Young A, eds. *Toronto Notes.* 30th ed. Toronto, ON: Toronto Notes for Medical Students Inc; 2014. FM3, GS55.

10
Women's Health

Contraception
Priority Topic 16

LOW-DOSE ESTROGEN <35 µg

1. **Contraindications (CI) to OCP**
   - Active or past VTE
   - Undiagnosed vaginal bleeding
   - Smoking >35 years and >15 cigarettes/day
   - Known/suspected breast cancer
   - Hypertension
   - Heart disease
   - Diabetes with retinopathy, nephropathy, or neuropathy
   - Stroke
   - Less than 6 weeks postpartum (coagulation/fibrinolysis normalizes 3 weeks postpartum)
   - Known/suspected pregnancy
   - Liver cirrhosis or tumour
   - Migraine with aura

2. **Relative contraindications to OCPs**
   - HTN if controlled
   - Migraine and age >35
   - History of or OCP-related cholestasis or active cholecystitis
   - Older age (>35) and obese ($\uparrow$ DVT risk)
   - Bariatric surgery (may $\downarrow$ absorption)

3. **Risks of OCP use**
   - VTE
   - MI/stroke (arterial clot)
   - Increased cervical cancer in women with persistent HPV (decreased ovarian cancer and endometrial cancer)
   - Gallbladder disease (theoretical)

4. **Signs/symptoms**

   Estrogen deficiency
   - Early spotting (days 1-9)
   - Continuous bleeding
   - Vasomotor symptoms (hot flush, sweats, flushing)
   - Amenorrhea

   Estrogen excess
   - Hypermenorrhea
   - Dysmenorrhea
   - Breast tenderness ($\uparrow$ size)
   - VTE
   - UTI
   - HTN

   Progesterone deficiency
   - Late spotting (days 10-21)
   - Late withdrawal bleeding

   Excess progestin
   - Fatigue
   - Depression
   - Breast tenderness
   - Weight gain
   - $\uparrow$ Appetite
   - $\downarrow$ Libido
   - Dizziness

5. **Reduced OCP efficacy with**
   - Poor compliance (theoretical failure rate 0.3%, typical use failure 3%-8%)
   - Many antiepileptics which increase OCP metabolism
   - Some antibiotics (rifampin and possibly other antibiotics decrease OCP efficacy)
   - Vomiting or malabsorption (bariatric surgery)

6. **Other options**

   Progestin injection q12 weeks
   - $\downarrow$ Endometrial cancer risk
   - $\downarrow$ Drug interactions with anticonvulsant medications

   CI: Pregnancy, unexplained vaginal bleeding, current breast cancer, current thrombophlebitis, or venous thromboembolic disorders (DVT, PE)

   Adverse effects: Weight gain, $\downarrow$ bone density (affect on peak BMD unknown), delayed recovery of fertility (2-12 months)

   Good option for patients with the following:
   - Poor compliance/reliability on OCP
   - Migraine
   - Breastfeeding
   - CI to estrogen
   - Smoker age $\geq$35
   - Sickle cell anemia
   - Anticonvulsant
   - $\uparrow$ VTE risk

   Theoretical failure 0.3%; typical use failure = 3% to 6%

   Progestin-only pill (Micronor)
   - Similar adverse effects and CI as injection
   - Decreased efficacy, therefore scheduled adherence important
   - Theoretical failure 0.5% typical use failure 5% to 10%

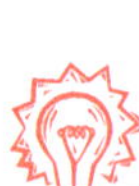

Generally try a pill for 3 months before considering switching to a new pill.

If late in taking Micronor by >3 hours, backup contraception is required.

Patch (Evra patch) and ring (NuvaRing)

- Similar CI as OCP.
- Patch ↓ effective in women >90 kg.
- Theoretical failure: 0.3% to 0.8%, typical use failure = 8%.

IUD: Types include copper IUD and levonorgestrel-releasing IUD (Mirena and Jaydess)

- Most effective method of reversible contraception and equally effective to other permanent contraceptive methods.
- Effective for 5 years (copper IUD and Mirena) and 3 years (Jaydess).
- Do NOT increase the rate of infertility.
- Both copper and levonorgestrel-releasing IUDs significantly reduce the risk of endometrial carcinoma.
- Higher continuation rates if inserted postpartum (10 minutes postplacental to 48 hours), post-Caesarean section, or post abortion.

Risks of IUD use

- Uterine perforation—0.3 to 2.6 per 1000 insertions; risk decreased with inserter experience but increased in postpartum and breastfeeding women.
- Increased risk of pelvic inflammatory disease (PID) within the first month of insertion but overall low absolute risk.
- Device expulsion most common under 3 months to 1 year of use—risk factors include heavy menstrual bleeding, dysmenorrhea, young age, atypical uterine shape, leiomyoma, and previous expulsion.
  - Nulliparity is NOT a risk factor for expulsion.

Contraindications

- Active pelvic infection (STI, endometritis) (may consider leaving IUD in place for treatment of pelvic infections)
- Known or suspected pregnancy
- Unexplained vaginal bleeding

TABLE 10-1	Pregnancy Rate of Contraceptives Within the First Year of Use	
METHOD	**TYPICAL USE (%)**	**CORRECT USE (%)**
Most Effective		
Intrauterine Device (IUD): Copper or Hormonal	<1	<1
Female sterilization	<1	<1
Vasectomy	<1	<1
Effective		
Depo Provera Injection	6	<1
Contraceptive Patch	9	<1
Oral Contraceptive Pill (OCP) Combined or Progestin-only	9	<1
Contraceptive Vaginal Ring	9	<1
Diaphragm	12	6
Least Effective		
Condom	Male 18; Female 21	Male: 2; Female: 5
Spermicides	28	18
Coitus interruptus	22	4
No method	85	85

Adapted from Trussell J. *Contraception*. 2011; 83(5): 397–404 and Martin KA, Barbieri RL. Overview of the use of estrogen-progestin contraceptives. *Up to Date*. 2016. https://www.uptodate.com/contents/overview-of-the-use-of-estrogen-progestin-contraceptives?source=search_result&search=overview%20of%20contraception&selected Title=1~150. Accessed July 1, 2017.

- Anatomic abnormalities (bicornuate uterus/fibroids)
- Current breast cancer (only for levonorgestrel-releasing IUD)
- Cervical or endometrial cancer
- Wilson disease or copper allergy (copper IUD) (Dean and Goldberg, 2012)
  - May be inserted immediately following abortion
    - At the time of TOP, providing long-acting reversible contraception, especially with IUD, is associated with a reduction of repeat abortion over the next 2 years
    - Failure (copper): 0.06% perfect use and 0.8% typical use
    - Failure (IUD-LNG): 0.2% perfect and typical use

7. **Emergency contraception**
   - General: Use if unprotected sex, failure of barrier method, ↓ efficacy of usual contraceptive
     - No physical examination or pregnancy test is required to provide this medication.
     - No medical CI to this therapy.
     - Confirm that intercourse was consensual.
     - Advise patients to take antiemetic prior to oral method of emergency contraception (Yuzpe method only).
   - Copper IUD
     - Can be used up to 7 days postcoital
     - Most effective method of emergency contraception
   - Plan B (levonorgestrel 1.5 mg po × 1)
     - Works best if <72 hours postcoital, but may be given up to 120 hours (less effective as time increases). Less side effects than Yuzpe method and is available without prescription
     - 75% effective if taken within 72 hours
   - Yuzpe (200 mg estradiol + 1 mg levonorgestrel). Generally no longer used due to side effects of nausea and vomiting.
     - Works best <72 hours postcoital but again may be given up to 120 hours

8. **Approach to contraceptive selection**
   - Assess absolute and relative CI to contraceptive use
   - Assess for STI exposure
   - Assess barriers to selected method of oral contraception (personal, financial, or cultural)
   - Discuss/manage common side effects (breakthrough bleeding, breast tenderness, nausea, weight gain, acne, headache, and chloasma)
   - Obtain BP and BMI
   - Advise about risks of ↓ efficacy (medications, bariatric surgery, late initiation) and availability of emergency contraception

9. **Approach to missed OCP**
   - Ovulation rarely occurs after 7 days of combined oral contraceptive use
   - To prevent unintended pregnancy, the hormone-free period should not extend beyond 7 days in combined oral contraceptive users
   - If the hormone-free interval >7 days, consider emergency contraception to prevent unintended pregnancy + back up × 7 days
   - Miss one pill in <24 hours in week 2 or 3 take ASAP. No back up required.
   - Miss, more than two pills, use back up or quit and start a new cycle after breakthrough bleed

10. **Therapeutic Abortion**
    - Common and legal medical procedure experienced by 31% of Canadian women during their reproductive lifetime.

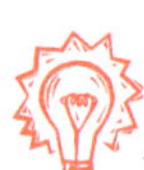

Always advise that condoms should be used in addition to OCP, to decrease STI risk.

Important to review missed dose guidelines for all contraceptive forms, in order to counsel patients correctly.

- Nonjudgmental counselling for unplanned unwanted pregnancy
- Surgical abortion: Suction D&C to 14 weeks gestation
- Medical abortion:

    Regimens: 1. Methotrexate/Misoprostol—highly effective up to 49 days post-LMP

    2. Mifepristone/Misoprostol (Mifegymiso)—95% effective up to 63 days post-LMP; recently approved by Health Canada but not effective in ectopic pregnancy
- Use a reliable method to confirm pregnancy is intrauterine and of appropriate GA
- Either ultrasound and/or serial serum β-hCG measurements provide definitive evidence of pregnancy termination (80% drop)

Bibliography

Black A, Guilbert E, Costescu D, et al. SOGC clinical practice guideline: Canadian contraception consensus Part 1. *Obstet Gynaecol Can.* 2015;37(10):S1-S28.

Black A, Guilbert E, Costescu D, et al. SOGC clinical practice guideline: Canadian contraception consensus Part 2. *J Obstet Gynaecol Can.* 2015;37(11):S1-S39.

Black A, Guilbert E, Costescu D, et al. SOGC clinical practice guideline: Canadian contraception consensus Part 3, Chapter 7 – Intrauterine Contraception. *Obstet Gynaecol Can.* 2016;38(2):182-222.

Black A, Guilbert E, Costescu D, et al. SOGC clinical practice guideline: Canadian contraception consensus Part 3, Chapter 8 – Progestin-Only Contraception. *Obstet Gynaecol Can.* 2016;38(3):279-300.

Costescu D, Guilbert, E, Bernardin J, et al. SOGC clinical practice guideline: Medical abortion. *J Obstet Gynaecol Can.* 2016;38(4):366-89.

Dean G, Goldberg AB. Overview of intrauterine contraception. *Up to Date.* 2012. http://www.uptodate.com/contents/overview-of-intrauterine-contraception?source=preview&anchor=H23833369#H23833369.

Jensen B, Regier LD (eds). *Rx Files: Drug Comparison Charts.* 10th ed. Saskatoon, SK: Saskatoon Health Region; Oct 2014. Available from www.RxFiles.ca.

Rose SB, Lawton BA. Impact of long-acting reversible contraception on return for repeat abortion. *Am J Obstet Gynecol.* 2012;206(1):37.e1-37.e6.

Zieman M. Overview of contraception. *Up to Date.* 2012. http://www.uptodate.com/contents/overview-of-contraception?source=preview&anchor=H31#H31.

Pregnancy

Priority Topic 77

General Definitions

1. Trimesters:
    a. T1: 0 to 12 weeks
    b. T2: 12 to 28 weeks
    c. T3: 28 to 40 weeks
2. Normal pregnancy: 37 to 42 weeks
3. Active labour: Regular contractions that result in cervical change and descent of the presenting part of the fetus.

Investigations

1. Confirm pregnancy with urine or serum pregnancy test
2. Establish desirability of pregnancy
3. Establish accurate dates and maternal risk factors (medical and social)
4. In high-risk patients, rescreen for HIV at 28 to 36 weeks; intrapartum rapid point-of-care testing if available
5. Complete appropriate prenatal screening and visits. See Prenatal Care Flow sheet (Table 10-2) for all prenatal visit information.

TABLE 10-2 Prenatal Care Flow Sheet: Page 1

At least 2-3 months preconception *Ref: Joint SOGC-Motherisk Guideline Dec 2007.* *(Modified 2016)*		• Start **folic acid 0.4-1 mg od** in women without risk factors • **Folic acid 5 mg od** for hx of previous baby with defect (NTD, facial cleft, heart/urinary tract/limb defect), family hx NTD, DM, smoking, obesity, poor diet, substance abuse, epileptics on valproic acid or carbamazepine, or if forgets to take vitamins regularly
<12 weeks	Visits q monthly until 28 weeks	**Obstetrical ultrasound** for dating may be offered to all women; should be obtained for accurate dating if last menstrual dates uncertain or unknown
12 weeks		Start listening for fetal heart with handheld Doppler
8-14 weeks		• **Routine prenatal blood work**: *ABO blood group, Rh and Ab, CBC, HIV, rubella, syphilis, HepB sAg, U/A, Hep C Ab, NAAT for GC/Chlamydia* • ***Consider:*** *VZV Ab (if no history of varicella), A1c/FBG for high risk of DM* • Physical examination • **Pap smear** if regular screening indicated • Fill out prenatal forms, refer if needed
9-10 weeks		• Cell-free fetal DNA (cffDNA) testing for Trisomy 13, 18, and 21 which may be considered prior to invasive diagnostic testing (amniocentesis or chorionic villus sampling) • Second-tier test, should not replace conventional serum screening; may perform up until delivery • Does NOT screen for neutral tube defects • 83% PPV in high-risk populations (>35 years of age, U/S abnormality or positive 1st/2nd trimester screen, previous baby with chromosomal disorder) • 33% PPV in general population
11-13 weeks + 6 days	**CVS** done at 11-13 wks 6 days, risk of loss 1%, allows for earlier diagnosis than amniocentesis	**1st trim. integrated serum screen**[a] (part 1 of 2) offered to all women (preferred option) for Trisomy 18, 21 **and** if indicated, NT ultrasound (see reverse for indications for NT U/S)
16 weeks		Gestation at which **therapeutic abortion** is not available in all provinces
15-17 weeks		**Amniocentesis** routinely offered to all women >40 years and >35 years with multiple gestation (results take 10-14 days) loss risk 1:400
15-20 weeks + 6 days Best at 16-18 weeks		**2nd trim. serum screen**[a] (part 2 of 2) (85% detection) or **quad screen** done *without 1st trim.* *Serum screen in late presenters (77% detection, false positive 5.2%) (for trisomy 19, 21, and ONTDs)*
18-24 weeks		**Routine ultrasound** for dates/anomalies *Note: **Earliest** ultrasound establishes dates, **not** the most recent ultrasound.*
20 weeks		Start measuring **SFH** routinely
26-28 weeks	**BG targets:** Fasting 3.8-5.2 1 hour PP 5.5-7.7 2 hours PP 5.0-6.6	Screen for **gestational diabetes: 50 g nonfasting GCT**

For the 26-28 week gestational diabetes screening results:

<7.8 = normal **7.8-10.2** requires 75 g OGTT **≥10.3** = GDM	**75 g OGTT** results: **≥5.3/10.6/8.9** at 0,1,2 h 1 of 3 = IGT; 2 of 3 = GDM

28 weeks	Visits q 2 weeks 28-36 weeks	• Repeat **CBC** or Hg by fingerpoke • **Rh neg**: Repeat type and screen for alloantibodies before administering **Rhlg (WinRho) 300 mcg IM** • **Rh Pos**: Repeat **type and screen** for alloantibodies; however, this is *not* necessary if there are two previous results on file
30-32 weeks		**Ultrasound** to rule out **IUGR** in women with initial weight >90 kg or BMI>30.0 (obese)
28-36 weeks		Repeat **HIV, GC/Chlamydia, syphilis** testing if at risk Consider Tdap vaccine if no history of adult immunization (age >18) or during periods of regional pertussis outbreak
35-37 weeks		**GBS swab** (results valid for 5 weeks), *send results to delivering hospital*
38+ weeks	Visits q 1 week until term	• Consider **cervical examination** at prenatal visit • May offer **sweeping of membranes** to prevent postterm gestation
41-42 weeks		**Induction** to prevent postterm gestation vs **expectant management** (requires fetal monitoring with NST and AFI twice weekly) *Ref: SOGC Guideline Sept 2008*
DELIVERY		• **Rh negative mother:** WinRho 300 mcg IM within 72 h of delivery if infant Rh+ • **Rubella** immunization to nonimmune women (Public Health) • **BCG** for baby, routinely offered to high-risk populations, mother must have negative HIV result

PRENATAL CARE FLOWSHEET: PAGE 2

Indications for nuchal translucency ultrasound[a]	Indications for first trimester ultrasound[a] *Ref: SOGC Guideline Oct 2003 (reaffirmed Dec 2008)*
Multiple gestation HIV positive Maternal age ≥ 40 at EDD Personal or family history of Down syndrome, trisomy 18, or trisomy 13 Age >35 years with ≥ 3 miscarriages	Threatened abortion, incomplete abortion Prior to termination Suspected multiple gestation, ectopic pregnancy, molar pregnancy, and suspected pelvic masses Increased risk of major fetal congenital malformations Very uncertain dates

[a]Use of diagnostic imaging is not limited to these indications.

Gestational diabetes screening in pregnancy: *Ref: SOGC guideline Nov 2002, Can Diabetes Assoc. 2008*		
Test	Standard screen is **1 h 50 g** nonfasting glucose challenge test at **24 to 28 weeks**	
Early testing	Start screening in first trimester if multiple risk factors present, **and repeat in subsequent trimesters**	
Risk factors	• Aboriginal, Hispanic, South Asian, Asian, African • Previous history of GDM or glucose intolerance • Previous macrosomia (>4000 g) • Previous unexplained stillbirth • Previous neonatal hypoglycemia, hypocalcemia, or hyperbilirubinemia	• Advanced maternal age (≥ 35 years) • Obesity • Repeated glucosuria in pregnancy • Polyhydramnios • Suspected macrosomia • PCOS • Acanthosis nigricans • Corticosteroid use
Postpartum	If GDM is diagnosed in pregnancy, a **75 g OGTT** should be done at **6-12 weeks postpartum** to screen for persistent DM or impaired glucose tolerance.	

Group B Streptococcus Screening: *Ref: Prevention of Perinatal Group B Streptococcal Disease, CDC guidelines, August 16, 2002:*

Vaginal and rectal GBS screening cultures at **35-37 weeks** in **all** pregnant women (unless patient had GBS bacteriuria during the current pregnancy or previous infant with GBS disease).

Intrapartum prophylaxis indicated:	Intrapartum prophylaxis not indicated:
• Previous infant with invasive GBS disease • GBS bacteriuria during current pregnancy • Positive GBS screening culture in current pregnancy • Unknown GBS status and (1) delivery at <37 weeks or (2) ROM >18 hours or (3) intrapartum temp >38°C *(if amnionitis suspected, use broad-spectrum antibiotic instead)*	• Previous pregnancy with positive GBS culture (unless culture also positive in current pregnancy) • Planned cesarean delivery in absence of ROM or labour • Negative GBS culture in current pregnancy, regardless of intrapartum risk factors

Recommended antibiotics for intrapartum prophylaxis:

Recommended:	**Penicillin G**, **5 million units IV** initial dose, then **2.5 million units IV q 4 h** until delivery
Alternative:	**Ampicillin**, **2 g IV** initial dose, then **1 g IV q 4 h** until delivery (broader spectrum, better for amnionitis, but potential for increased antibiotic-associated adverse effects)
If penicillin allergic:	**Not at high risk for anaphylaxis:** • **Cefazolin**, 3 g IV initial dose, then 1 g IV q 8 h until delivery. **High risk for anaphylaxis:** • **Clindamycin**, 900 mg IV q 8 h until delivery, or (must do susceptibility testing anenatally) • **Erythromycin**, 500 mg IV q 6 h until delivery (must do susceptibility antenatally) **GBS resistant to clindamycin or erythromycin or susceptibility unknown:** • **Vancomycin**, 1 g IV q 12 h until delivery

BV in Pregnancy *Ref: SOGC Guideline Aug 2008*	**UTI and asymptomatic bacteriuria in pregnancy**
Do not routinely screen for and treat BV in asymptomatic women **not** at increased risk of preterm birth. If at increased risk of preterm birth, treatment may reduce risk of low birth weight. **Risks of BV in pregnancy:** preterm birth, PPROM, spontaneous abortion, chorioamnionitis, postpartum endometritis, C-section wound infection. **Treatment:** (SOGC Aug 2008) • **Metronidazole** 500 mg bid × 7 days or • **Clindamycin 300 mg bid × 7 days** (topical agents not recommended, since not associated with risk reduction)	Treat both **asymptomatic bacteriuria** (midstream culture positive >10⁵ cfu/mL) and **symptomatic UTI** (symptoms + midstream culture positive >10² cfu/mL) to reduce risks. Repeat culture 1-2 weeks after treatment. **Treatment options:** • **Nitrofurantoin (Macrobid)** 100 mg bid × 7days *(avoid at labour and delivery because of hemolytic anemia)* • **TMP-SMX** 1 DS tab bid × 3 days *(avoid in first trimester and near term)* • **TMP** 100 mg bid × 7 days *(avoid in first trimester)* • **Amoxicillin** 500 mg tid × 7 days *or* **Ampicillin** 250 mg tid × 7 days • **Amoxicillin-clavulanate** 500 mg bid × 7 days • **Cephalexin** 250 mg qid × 7 days **Effective for GBS in urine:** amoxicillin, ampicillin, nitrofurantoin, TMP, TMP/SMX

Courtesy of Lisa Friesen, MD, CCFP.

HELLP SYNDROME
Hemolysis
Elevated Liver Enzymes
Low Platelets

COMMON MEDICAL CONDITIONS IN PREGNANCY

Hypertensive Disorders in Pregnancy

Definitions

1. Gestational hypertension (GHTN): SBP >140 mm Hg or DBP >90 mm Hg occurring after 20 weeks gestation confirmed by two measurements, at least 15 min apart.
   - Severe hypertension if SBP >160 mm Hg or DBP >110 mm Hg confirmed by two measurements, at least 15 min apart
2. HELLP syndrome: Gestational hypertension may progress to HELLP syndrome. The syndrome includes hemolysis, elevated liver enzymes, and low platelets in the setting of gestational hypertension.

Symptoms

1. RUQ pain
2. Headache
3. ↓ Urine output
4. Nausea +/− vomiting
5. Visual disturbance
6. Hyperreflexia

Risk Factors

1. Primigravid
2. Medical history or family history of GHTN
3. First child with new partner
4. DM
5. Extremes of age (<18 or >35)
6. IUGR
7. Oligohydramnios
8. Twin gestation

Investigations

- Hb, platelets, coags, ALT, AST, LDH, U/A (proteinuria)

Treatment

1. If nonsevere with no comorbid conditions: Treat with labetalol, nifedipine, or methyldopa until term. Target SBP <130 to 155 mm Hg and DBP <80 to 105 mm Hg. Monitor growth and placental flow by Doppler U/S

   If comorbid conditions: Target SBP <140 mm Hg and DBP <90 mm Hg

   If severe: Target SBP <160 mm Hg and DBP <110 mm Hg (consider inpatient admission with severe hypertension or preeclampsia.)

   Treatment options:

   a. Labetalol 20 mg IV, then 40 mg IV, then 80 mg IV × 2 q 30 min until achieve target BP (max dose 220 mg/day)
   b. Hydralazine 5 mg IV, repeat 5 to 10 mg IV q 30 min until BP controlled (max dose 20 mg/day)
   c. Nifedipine 10 mg po and repeat with 20 mg in 30 minutes
2. Pregnancy less <34 weeks GA or unstable mother should be managed by obstetrician
3. Hb and platelets
4. Start IV
5. Assess status of fetus
6. Laboratory work including blood type, crossmatch
7. Urgent delivery and ICU postpartum may be needed

Gestational Diabetes

Definition

Onset of DM 2 during pregnancy

Complications

1. Maternal
   a. HTN
   b. Polyhydramnios
   c. Retinopathy
   d. Hypoglycemia
   e. Pyelonephritis/UTI
2. Fetal
   a. Macrosomia
   b. IUGR
   c. Hypoglycemia
   d. Polycythemia
   e. Fetal lung immaturity

Risk Factors

1. Obesity
2. Previous pregnancy with gestational DM 2 or IGT
3. Family history of DM

Diagnosis

1. If risk factors for diabetes II, conduct fasting glucose at initial prenatal visit.
2. If low risk of DM II, screen for GDM at 24 to 28 weeks GA with 50 g OGTT.
3. Screening at 24 to 28 weeks GA
   a. 1-hour 50 g OGCT
      i. <7.8 mmol/L is normal
      ii. 7.8 to 10.2 mmol/L → Indication for a 2-hour 75 g OGTT
      iii. ≥ 10.3 = GDM
   b. A 2-hour 75 g OGTT
      i. FPG ≥5.3 mmol/L
      ii. At 1 hour ≥10.6 mmol/L
      iii. At 2 hours ≥8.9 mmol/L
   c. Impaired glucose tolerance
      i. Fasting: 6.1 to 6.9 mmol/L
      ii. 75 g OGTT: 7.5 to 11.0 mmol/L

Treatment

1. Blood glucose targets for GDM (see Table 10-3)
2. Induce by 40 weeks gestation
3. Blood sugars hourly during labour
4. Follow-up 75 g OGTT 6 weeks to 6 months postpartum as gestational DM mothers have 50% increased risk of developing DM 2
5. Dietary advice
6. Pharmacotherapy, insulin, metformin, and/or glyburide
7. Consider serial ultrasound for growth parameters to monitor insulin therapy

TABLE 10-3 Glucose Targets	DM	GDM
A1C	≤7	≤6
FPG (mmol/L)	4-7	3.8-5.2
2-h PPG (mmol/L)	5-10	5.0-6.6

Intrahepatic Cholestasis of Pregnancy—ICP

Definition

- Onset of pruritus (hands and soles) associated with elevated serum bile acids and/or transaminases in the absence of any other cause for symptoms.
- Occurs in the second and third trimesters and carries an increased risk of fetal complications, most seriously sudden fetal death.
- 60% to 70% recurrence in subsequent pregnancies.

Complications

- Increased risk of:
  1. Prematurity
  2. Meconium staining
  3. Neonatal respiratory distress
  4. Preeclampsia.
  5. Stillbirth (with higher bile acid levels and advancing gestational age, although no test reliably predicts risk of fetal demise)

Diagnosis

- Clinical diagnosis aided by serum bile acid testing (which may take several days to perform, making it is an impractical tool for immediate risk stratification)

Treatment

- Rx focuses on reducing symptoms of pruritus and preventing maternal and fetal complications
- Ursodeoxycholic acid (UCDA/ursodiol) is most useful (15 mg/kg/day)
- Increases bile flow relieving pruritus and improves LFTs
- Early delivery—at 36 weeks or upon diagnosis of ICP > 37 weeks.

Popular Pruritus of Pregnancy—PUPP

Diagnosis

- Most common dermatosis of pregnancy.
- Usually presents as pruritic erythematous papules within abdominal striae and spreads to extremities or coalesces to form urticarial plaques.
- Face, palms, and soles usually spared.
- Usually begins later in third trimester but may develop postpartum or worsen immediately after delivery.
- Unknown etiology and no associated lab abnormalities or increased risk of fetal or maternal morbidity.
- Differential: Early gestational pemphigus or erythema multiforme.

Treatment

Relief of symptoms, nonsedating antihistamines, low potency topical steroids, and early delivery if necessary

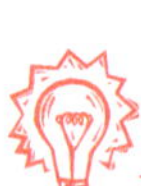

ALARMER (MNEMONIC) THINGS TO CONSIDER IN SHOULDER DISTOCIA

Ask for help
Legs flexed (McRoberts)
Apply suprapubic pressure
Release posterior shoulder
Manual Corkscrew
Episiotomy
Rollover (hands and knees)

COMMON PROBLEMS ENCOUNTERED DURING LABOUR

Dystocia

Definitions

1. Labour dystocia is prolongation of labour. Consider three Ps (Power, Passage, Passenger). Clinical definitions:
   a. >4 hours of <0.5 cm/h dilation or
   b. >1 hour of no descent with active pushing
2. Shoulder dystocia: Impaction of the anterior shoulder of fetus against symphysis after fetal head has been delivered. **This is a life-threatening emergency**.

Risk Factors for Shoulder Dystocia

1. Obesity
2. DM
3. Macrosomia
4. Instrument delivery (currently or previously)
5. Most women with shoulder dystocia have no identifiable risk factors.
   Be prepared.

Uterine Rupture

Definition

Potentially catastrophic complication of pregnancy whereby the uterus tears during labour.

Symptoms

1. Shock
2. Acute onset of abdominal pain
3. Acute change in station
4. Abnormal fetal heart rate (FHR)
5. Vaginal bleeding

Risk Factors

1. Uterine scar
2. Hyperstimulation (usually from pharmacological agents for IOL)
3. Grand multiparity

Diagnosis

1. Stable patients can usually be evaluated with ultrasound to confirm diagnosis.
2. Unstable patients usually warrant emergent delivery.

Treatment

1. Rule out placenta abruption
2. Maternal stabilization
3. Emergent delivery

Placental Abruption

Definition

Potentially catastrophic complication of pregnancy where the placenta prematurely separates from the uterine wall.

Symptoms

1. Painful vaginal bleeding
2. ↑ Uterine tonicity/contractions
3. +/− Fetal distress

Risk Factors

1. Abdominal trauma
2. Cocaine abuse
3. Polyhydramnios
4. Hypertension (essential, pregnancy induced, preeclampsia)
5. Premature rupture of membranes (PROM)
6. Chorioamnionitis
7. Thrombophilia
8. Previous abruption
9. Maternal age

10. Smoking during pregnancy

11. Parity

Diagnosis

Clinical diagnosis as ultrasound not sensitive

Investigations/Management

1. Establish IV access
2. WBC, Hb, platelets, blood type and Rh status, C&M, coagulation studies, and Kleihauer-Betke test
3. Abdominal U/S
4. Foley catheter to monitor urine output
5. Continuous EFM

Treatment

1. Delivery indicated (if GA >34 weeks) or watchful waiting if maternal and fetal stability confirmed.
2. Cesarean section indicated if nonreassuring FHR or ongoing maternal blood loss.
3. If stable, vaginal delivery is a reasonable option, induce, and augment.

Chorioamnionitis

Definition

Infection of the chorion or amniotic fluid from ascending organism

Symptoms

1. Maternal fever
2. Maternal/fetal ↑ HR
3. Foul/purulent discharge
4. Uterine tenderness

Risk Factors

1. Prolonged rupture of membranes
2. Prolonged labour
3. Multiple vaginal examinations
4. Bacterial vaginosis, STI, GBS
5. Intrauterine or fetal monitoring devices

Diagnosis

Clinical

Treatment

1. IV ampicillin 2 g q 6 hours and gentamycin 1.5 mg/kg q 8 hours in patients with normal renal function
2. Expedient delivery
3. Higher risk of PPH

Rupture of Membranes

Definitions

1. PROM: Rupture of membranes before the onset of labour
2. Preterm PROM (PPROM) ≤37 weeks GA (may require steroids if <34 weeks GA)
3. Prolonged rupture of membranes: Rupture of membranes >18 hours

Symptoms

1. Gush clear or yellow fluid from the vagina
2. Intermittent constant leakage of fluid from the vagina
3. Overdiagnosed based on history of per vaginum (PV) fluid

Diagnosis/PE Findings

1. Sterile speculum and fluid pooling in vaginal vault
2. Positive nitrazine
3. Ferning on microscopic examination
4. U/S for AFI and BPP

Differential Diagnosis

1. Urinary incontinence
2. Vaginal discharge
3. Perspiration

Management/Treatment

1. If <34 weeks gestation, betamethasone 12 mg IM q 24 hours × 2
2. Consider expert consultation (OBS, NICU)
3. Admit with vitals q 4 hours daily BPP and WBC count
4. Cultures for STI and GBS
5. Consider antibiotics
6. Emergent delivery if fetal distress

Endometritis

Definition

Endometrial infection (may be intrapartum, postpartum, or following TOP).

Symptoms

1. Rising fever
2. Uterine tenderness postpartum day 2 to 3

Risk Factors

1. Prolonged labour, prolonged ROM (>18 hours), amnionitis
2. Meconium-stained amniotic fluid
3. Maternal age <17
4. Manual placental removal
5. Bacterial vaginosis during pregnancy

Diagnosis

Rule out other causes of postoperative fever

Treatment

1. Provide anaerobic coverage (clindamycin 900 mg IV q 8 hours + gentamicin 5 mg/kg q 24 hours)
2. Give cefazolin prophylactically after C/S

Postpartum Hemorrhage

Definition

Loss of >500 mL of blood after SVD or 1000 mL after C/S. Early PPH occurs within 24 hours of delivery, and late PPH occurs after 24 hours and within 6 weeks of delivery.

Etiology (four Ts)

1. Tone: Uterine atony secondary to prolonged/augmented labour, infection, GHTN, grand multiparity, macrosomia, and polyhydramnios
2. Tissue: Retained placenta
3. Trauma: Vaginal, cervix, or uterus
4. Thrombin: Coagulopathy

FOUR Ts OF POSTPARTUM HEMORRHAGE

Tone

Tissue

Trauma

Thrombin

Risk Factors

1. May occur in women without any risk factors
2. History of postpartum hemorrhage
3. Preeclampsia
4. Placenta previa
5. Multiple gestation
6. Obesity
7. Macrosomia
8. Induced labour and other intrapartum interventions
9. Chorioamnionitis
10. Prolonged labour

Blood loss estimates for PPH are notoriously incorrect

Diagnosis

1. Based on blood volume lost
2. Decline in postpartum hematocrit >10%

Prevention

Active management in the third stage of labour (oxytocin with delivery of the anterior shoulder, controlled cord traction to deliver placenta, and uterine massage)

Treatment

1. Stepwise approach is required
2. Labs: Cross match, CBC, Coags
3. Uterine massage
4. Pharmacotherapy (uterotonics)
   a. Oxytocin 10 units IM or add 40 units to 1 L NS and run IV until bleeding controlled
   b. Carboprost 0.25 mg IM q 15 to 90 minutes (maximum eight doses)
   c. Misoprostol 800 to 1000 μg sublingual or rectally
   d. Methylergonovine 0.2 mg IM or intrauterine. May repeat at 2 to 4 hour intervals (avoid if hypertensive, Raynaud syndrome, or scleroderma)
5. If bleeding not controlled following use of uterotonics, consider the following:
   a. Foley catheter (full bladder may prevent uterine contraction)
   b. R/O genital tract lesion/trauma
   c. Examine placenta for missing parts
   d. If under shock, consider hematoma, uterine rupture, partial inversion
   e. Uterine tamponade
6. Obtain expert consult for manual removal of retained placenta or exploratory laparotomy or hysterectomy

Retained Placenta

Definition

Placenta not delivered within 30 minutes of delivery

Types

1. Trapped placenta—Placenta caught behind a closed cervix
2. Placenta adherens—Easily removed manually from the uterine wall
3. Placenta accreta—Placenta pathologically invading into the myometrium

Symptoms

1. No lengthening of the umbilical cord
2. No gush of blood from the vagina (no separation)
3. Failure of the fundus to contract

Risk Factors

1. Prior manual removal
2. Infection
3. Placenta previa
4. Uterine scar

Diagnosis

1. Usually a clinical diagnosis.
2. Ultrasound may be used to differentiate between placenta adherens and accrete but is rarely used.

Treatment

1. Treat for postpartum hemorrhage as patient may bleed.
2. +/− manual removal or D&C.

COMMON PROBLEMS POSTPARTUM

Postpartum Blues and Postpartum Depression

Definitions

1. Postpartum blues: Onset day 3 to 10 postpartum characterized by increased anxiety, irritability, weariness, ↓ concentration, and sleep disturbance. Self-limited and does not last >2 weeks. Normal secondary to hormonal changes.
2. Postpartum depression (PPD): Major depressive episode within 1 month of childbirth. Suspect if blues last >2 weeks or severe in first 2 weeks. Psychosis can occur within in the first month postpartum.

Symptoms

1. Tearfulness
2. Fatigue
3. Irritability
4. Mood liability
5. ↓ Affect
6. Sensitive to criticism
7. Occasional homicidal/infanticidal ideation

Risk Factors

1. History of depression
2. Family history of depression
3. Inadequate social support
4. Psychosocial stress
5. Pregnancy loss

Treatment

1. SSRI
2. Psychotherapy
3. Supportive care
4. ECT

FETAL HEART RATE MONITORING

Definitions

1. Normal FHR baseline: 110 to 160 bpm. High baseline (maternal/fetal/placental etiologies): Fever, hyperthyroid, anemia, hypoxia.
2. Variability (normal 5-25 bpm). If ↓ or absent for >40 minutes, fetal wellbeing must be assessed. There is ↓ variability with maternal dehydration or infection.

Early decels are benign.

3. FHR Accelerations (accels): Increase of ≥15 bpm lasting ≥15 seconds in response to fetal movement of uterine contractions.

4. FHR decelerations (Decels):

   a. Early: Uniform in shape with onset early in contraction and returns to baseline by the end of the contraction. Due to vagal response to head compression.

   b. Variables: Most common. Variable in shape, onset, and duration. Secondary to cord compression or forceful pushing. Complicated variables = rule of 60s: decels <60 bpm, >60 bpm below baseline, >60 seconds in duration with slow return to baseline.

   c. Late: Uniform in shape with late onset in contraction, return to baseline after end of contraction. Must see three in a row to define as late decels. Abrupt decrease in FHR secondary to fetal hypoxia, academia, maternal hypotension, uterine hypertonus, or uteroplacental insufficiency.

5. Normal FHR: At least two accelerations of FHR >15 bpm from baseline lasting >15 seconds in a 40-minute strip.

Management

1. Decelerations:

   a. Call for help

   b. Roll to LLDP

   c. 100% O_2 to mother via nonrebreather mask

   d. Stop oxytocin

   e. Fetal scalp electrode

   f. Vaginal examination to r/o prolapse

   g. C/S if needed

Bibliography

Anath CV, Kinzler WL. Clinical features and diagnosis of placental abruption. *Up to Date*. http://www .uptodate.com/contents/clinical-features-and-diagnosis-of-placental-abruption?source=preview& anchor=H4#H8. Accessed March 16, 2012.

DynaMed. Metritis (postpartum). 2011. http://web.ebscohost.com/dynamed/detail?sid=1f5fe243-c64d-4d09-9738-7f312e001a51%40sessionmgr12&vid=4&hid=21&bdata=JnNpdGU9ZHluYW1lZC1saXZl JnNjb3BlPXNpdGU%3d#db=dme&AN=113859. Accessed March 17, 2012.

DynaMed. Postpartum hemorrhage. 2011. http://web.ebscohost.com/dynamed/detail?vid=6&hid=21&sid =1f5fe243-c64d-4d09-9738-7f312e001a51%40sessionmgr12&bdata=JnNpdGU9ZHluYW1lZC1saXZl JnNjb3BlPXNpdGU%3d#db=dme&AN=114247. Accessed March 17, 2012.

Lindor K, Lee, R. Intrahepatic cholestasis of pregnancy. *Up to Date*. 2016. https://www.uptodate.com/ contents/intrahepatic-cholestasis-of-pregnancy. Accessed October 12, 2016.

Magee LA, Pels A, Helewa M, et al. SOGC clinical practice guideline: Diagnosis, evaluation, and management of the hypertensive disorders of pregnancy: Executive summary. *J Obstet Gynaecol Can*. 2014;36(5):416-438.

Pomeranz, MK. Dermatoses of pregnancy. *Up to Date*. 2016. https://www.uptodate.com/contents/ dermatoses-of-pregnancy. Accessed October 12, 2016.

Weeks A. Diagnosis and management of retained placenta after vaginal birth. *Up to Date*. 2011. http:// www.uptodate.com/contents/diagnosis-and-management-of-retained-placenta-after-vaginal-birth? source=search_result&search=retained+placenta&selectedTitle=1~24. Accessed March 15, 2012.

Vaginal Bleeding

Priority Topic 96

Always rule out pregnancy first

Factors to consider with vaginal bleeding:

- Pregnancy status
- Age

- Timing (cycle, acute vs chronic)
- Systemic disease
- Medications (hormones)

If pregnant and bleeding always consider: Ectopic pregnancy, placental abruption, abortion, trophoblastic disease, and treat hemodynamic instability.

Definitions

1. Normal menses: Average menses lasts 7 days, approximately 35 mL of blood loss, wide range of normal
2. Menorrhagia—Excessive bleeding during menses
3. Metrorrhagia—Uterine bleeding at irregular intervals
4. Oligomenorrhea—Menses occurring at intervals >35 days

Never conduct a pelvic examination on a woman with PV bleeding in the second or third trimester without r/o vasa or placenta previa.

TABLE 10-4	Causes and Treatment of Vaginal Bleeding		
	ETIOLOGIES	SYMPTOMS	TREATMENT/MGMT
Ovulatory	Anatomic: • Cervix (polyp, inflammation, PID, IUD) • Uterus (fibroid, cancer)	Menorrhagia	Treat specific etiology
	Concurrent disease: Coagulopathy, thyroid, renal, hepatic	Menorrhagia and/or metrorrhagia	Treat specific etiology
	Foreign body	Foul odour	Removal of foreign body
	Medications: Anticoagulation, antipsychotic, corticosteroids, SSRI, tamoxifen, ginseng, ginkgo, soy	Metrorrhagia	Correct coagulopathy, change contraceptive delivery, discontinue offending medication/product.
Anovulatory	OCP: Inadequate estrogen or poor adherence(compliance)	Metrorrhagia	Trial of OCP with higher estrogen
	Hypothalamic: PCOS, ↓ thyroid, excess androgen, ↑ cortisol or prolactin, stress, WT loss, puberty, perimenopause	Menorrhagia, oligomenorrhea, or amenorrhea Spotting	Treat specific etiology
Postmenopause (age > 40)	Vaginal: Atrophic Cervix: Polyps, erosion, cancer Uterus: Polyp, fibroid, endometrial cancer	Spotting or menorrhagia (postmenopausal)	Considered to be endometrial cancer until proven otherwise. Evaluate endometrium before treatment.

NONPREGNANT VAGINAL BLEEDING

Management

1. Stabilize ABC
2. r/o pregnancy
3. Laboratory investigations: β-hCG, CBC (Hg, WBC, platelets), INR, PTT, TSH, prolactin, glucose, PAP smear, G+C urine PCR, (signs of androgen excess? → DHEA, free testosterone)
4. Endometrial assessment—Biopsy indications
   a. Age > 40
   b. Bleeding not responsive to medical therapy

   c. Consider in young women with risk factors for endometrial cancer (BMI >30 kg/m^2, nulliparity, PCOS, diabetes, hereditary nonpolyposis colorectal cancer)

   d. Consider in women with infrequent menses suggestive of anovulation

5. Imaging:

   a. Transvaginal ultrasound (detect pregnancy with quantitative β-hCG of 1500 mIU/mL and in experienced hands detect placenta previa)

   b. Hysteroscopy—If unresponsive to treatment

   c. CT pelvis

Treatment

1. Treat hemodynamic instability

2. Acute heavy bleeding with hypovolemia or Hg <70 units

   a. High dose of oral estrogen (OCP tid × 7 days) or IV estrogen

   b. Tranexamic acid 1300 mg po tid for 5 days during menstruation

   c. Ferrous gluconate 325 mg tid duration (reevaluate in 6 weeks)

   d. If bleeding continues—IV DDAVP +/− D&C, hysteroscopy

   e. Consider transfusion if severe hemorrhage or medical comorbidities

3. Chronic frequent or heavy bleeding

   a. Treat underlying cause

   b. Nonhormonal treatments: NSAIDs (promote platelet aggregation) and tranexamic acid (antifibrinolytic)

   Hormonal treatments: Combined oral contraceptive, oral/injected progestin, levonorgestrel IUD

   c. Severe/refractory—Consider ablation/hysterectomy

   d. Postmenopausal

     i. Hyperplasia and not cancer/atypia—IM medroxyprogesterone and repeat endometrial evaluation q 3 to 6 months for hyperplasia

     ii. Atypical hyperplasia—D&C or hysterectomy

     iii. Atrophic—Consider OCP or HRT

ENDOMETRIAL CANCER

Etiology

Estrogen (↑ unopposed estrogen → hyperplasia → cancer)

Types

Adenocarcinoma ≥80% of endometrial cancers

Risk Factors

1. Obesity
2. DM
3. HTN
4. HRT with unopposed estrogen
5. Tamoxifen >5 years
6. Nulliparous
7. Early menarche/late menopause
8. Pelvic radiation
9. Family history of breast or ovarian cancer
10. Family history of HNPCC

Symptoms

1. Abnormal uterine bleeding
2. Vaginal discharge
3. Rarely, bladder symptoms due to pressure, back pain radiating anteriorly, increased abdominal girth, and dyspareunia

Diagnosis

1. Invasive approaches:
   - D&C
   - Endometrial biopsy
   - Hysteroscopy and directed biopsy
2. Noninvasive approach includes ultrasonography (Brand et al, 2000)

Treatment

Obtain transvaginal U/S and office endometrial biopsy if capable. Based on biopsy results:

1. Unsatisfactory or unable to obtain biopsy—High risk of cancer → D&C if low risk, consider hysteroscopy with directed biopsy
2. Negative biopsy but ongoing symptoms → Repeat biopsy or consider hysteroscopy with directed biopsy
3. Hyperplasia with no atypia
   a. IM medroxyprogesterone
   b. Repeat biopsy in 3 months (if follow-up biopsy unchanged, hysterectomy or IM medroxyprogesterone q 6-12 months)
4. Atypical hyperplasia—Hysterectomy (D&C or ablation are also options but they are not recommended if unwell or comorbidities)
5. Atrophic—Consider OCP or HRT
6. Cancer—Hysterectomy + node sampling + peritoneal sampling
   a. Radiation if stage 1B (chemotherapy for palliative cases only as endometrial cancer not very responsive)

Guideline Summary (SOGC—Renaud et al, 2013)

1. In a patient with suspected endometrial cancer, a complete history and physical examination should elicit details about potential factors for excess estrogen stimulation, including history of anovulation, obesity, menstrual irregularity, or long-term use of exogenous estrogen. Consider family history and genetic counselling in appropriate individuals.
2. In perimenopausal and postmenopausal women presenting with vaginal bleeding, rule out endometrial cancer.
3. Office endometrial biopsy and transvaginal ultrasound are preferred modalities of initial investigation in patients with suspected endometrial cancer.
4. Histologic investigation (office biopsy, D&C, hysteroscopy with direct sampling) should be performed in all patients with suspected endometrial cancer. In patients with persistent uterine bleeding, consider hysteroscopy with previously benign or insufficient endometrial sampling.
5. Tumour serum markers and other imaging should not be used routinely.

VAGINAL BLEEDING IN PREGNANCY

Always consider ectopic pregnancy, abruption, and abortion (see Table 10-5).

TABLE 10-5	**Vaginal Bleeding in Pregnancy**		
	ETIOLOGIES	SYMPTOMS	[a]MGMT/TREATMENT
First trimester	Ectopic pregnancy	Abdominal/pelvic pain Vaginal bleeding Missed period	See separate topic below
	Spontaneous abortion	Vaginal bleeding Complete passage of products of conception Open cervix	No D&C Expectant management
	Threatened abortion	Vaginal bleeding +/− cramping Cervix closed	US viable fetus <5% abort Watch and wait
	Inevitable abortion	Vaginal bleeding Cramping +/− ROM Cervix closed until products expelled	Watch and wait Misoprostol 400-800 mg PO/PV D&C
	Molar pregnancy	Vaginal bleeding Enlarged uterus Hyperthyroidism	Abnormally elevated β-hCG U/S suggestive of molar pregnancy Expert consult: • Evacuation of molar pregnancy • Serial β-hCG until 3 weekly normal values
Second or third trimester	Placenta abruption	See topic under pregnancy	
	Vasa previa	Vaginal bleeding Sonographic or clinical evidence of vasa previa	Emergent C/S
	Placental previa	Painless vaginal bleeding	ABCs r/o abruption Determine placental location with transvaginal US Expert consult <34 weeks GA: Consider hospitalization, steroids, and decide on delivery method at 36 weeks GA Low lying (>2 cm from cervical os) may be candidates for vaginal delivery
	Bloody show	Term or near-term gestation Vaginal bleeding +/− contractions +/− cervical changes	Prepare for delivery
	Cervical: neoplasia, infection, polyps	See specific topics	

[a]If Rh negative, give Rh (D) immune globulin 300 mcg IV/IM.

ECTOPIC PREGNANCY

Fertilized ovum implanted outside the endometrium

Symptoms

1. Pelvic pain
2. PV bleeding
3. Amenorrhea

Risk Factors

1. Previous ectopic pregnancy
2. IUD (overall fewer number of ectopic pregnancies, but between 15% and 50% of pregnancies with an IUD are ectopic)
3. Damaged fallopian tubes (STI history, PID, tubal surgery)
4. DES exposure in utero

PE Findings

1. One-third women have no physical signs
2. Pelvic examination may reveal adnexal mass

Diagnosis

Positive β-hCG with abnormal doubling time

Imaging

Visualization of ectopic pregnancy on ultrasound or surgery (intrauterine pregnancy visible on abdominal U/S when β-hCG >2000)

Treatment

1. If hemodynamically unstable, stabilize and prepare for surgery
2. Methotrexate therapy is an option for stable patients if fetal pole <3 cm on U/S. Follow with serial β-hCG
   - Methotrexate 50 mg/m^2 IM × 1
   - Measure serum β-hCG levels on days 4 and 7
   - If needed repeat dose on day 7
3. Surgery
4. Rh D immunoglobulin if indicated

Guideline Summary (Ectopic Pregnancy)

1. There is no difference between methotrexate therapy and tube sparing laparoscopic surgery in overall tube preservation, recurrence of ectopic pregnancy, or future pregnancy.
2. An increase in serum β-hCG of <53% in 48 hours confirms abnormal pregnancy.
3. In patients with β-hCG >5000 mIU/mL, multiple or higher doses of methotrexate may be appropriate.
4. Methotrexate can be used in women with confirmed or highly suspected to have ectopic pregnancy, who are stable with an unruptured mass.
5. If β-hCG does not fall by at ≥15% from day 4 to day 7 of methotrexate therapy, this is considered a treatment failure and repeat methotrexate therapy or surgery is warranted.
6. Posttreatment β-hCG levels should be monitored until a nonpregnancy level is reached.
7. In initial β-hCG levels <200 mIU/mL, 88% resolve spontaneously (ACOG, 2008).

Bibliography

American College of Obstetricians and Gynecologists (ACOG). *Medical Management of Ectopic Pregnancy*. Washington (DC): American College of Obstetricians and Gynecologists (ACOG); 2008 Jun. 7: ACOG practice bulletin; no. 94

Barnhart KT. Clinical practice. Ectopic pregnancy. *N Engl J Med*. 2009;361(4):379-387. Review.

DynaMed. Ectopic pregnancy. 2012. http://web.ebscohost.com/dynamed/detail?vid=3&hid=127&sid=b8 65201a-68c5-480e-a862-f82f04138595%40sessionmgr111&bdata=JnNpdGU9ZHluYW1lZC1saXZlJn Njb3BlPXNpdGU%3d#db=dme&AN=115772&anchor=other-medications.

Renaud MC, Le T. Joint SOGC-GOC-SCC clinical practice guideline: Epidemiology and investigations for suspected endometrial cancer. *J Obstet Gynaecol Can*. 2013;35(4 eSuppl C):S1-S9.

Vaginitis

Priority Topic 97

Definition

Nonspecific symptom complex of inflammation of the vagina often associated with pruritus, discharge, and/or pain

Symptoms

Include the following irrespective of etiology

- Burning
- Pruritus

- Erythema
- Increase in quantity, colour, and odour of vaginal discharge
- Dyspareunia
- Irritation
- Foul odour
- Dysuria (when urine comes in contact with inflamed areas)

Types

Usual causes are inflammation or infection; however, symptoms are similar despite etiology.

1. Vulvar lesions
2. Vaginal atrophy
3. Infectious (increased vaginal discharge)
4. Inflammation (bubble baths, chemical irritants, allergies)

Develop an age-based approach to vaginitis.

VAGINAL DISCHARGE

Testing for the causes of vaginitis (see Table 10-6) is important as they account for over 90% of all causes of vaginitis in premenopausal women.

TABLE 10-6	Vaginal Discharge			
	CANDIDIASIS	**BACTERIAL VAGINOSIS**	**TRICHOMONIASIS**	**PHYSIOLOGIC**
Organism	*Candida albicans* (90%)	*Gardnerella vaginalis*	*Trichomonas vaginalis*	Lactobacillus
Vaginal discharge	Whitish, "cottage cheese," minimal	Thin, grey, "dish water"	Yellow-green, malodorous	White or transparent, thick or thin, mostly odourless
Signs/symptoms	1/5 asymptomatic Pruritus Inflamed/swollen vulva Vulvar burning, dysuria, dyspareunia	Up to ¾ asymptomatic Fishy odour Absence of vulva/vaginal irritation	¼ asymptomatic Petechiae on vagina/cervix Occasional irritated/tender vulva Dysuria, frequency	None or mild/transient Normal quantity of discharge 1 = 4 mL/24 h
Vaginal pH	4.0-4.5	>4.5	5.0-6.0	4.0-4.5 (premenopause) ≥ 4.7 (premenarche and postmenopausal)
Saline wet mount	Hyphae Budding yeast (non albicans)	>20% clue cells + Whiff test	Motile, flagellated, trichomonads	PMN rare, squamous cells
Treatment	• Clotrimazole, butoconazole, miconazole, terconazole, nystatin of various durations • Fluconazole 150 mg orally × 1 • Usually topical treatment in pregnancy • Consider topical boric acid suppression for recurrent infections (avoid in first 4 months of pregnancy) • Treat only if symptomatic. No adverse outcome for untreated woman in pregnancy (Cotch et al, 1998)	• If pregnant, always treat (vaginal route not recommended) If not pregnant, treatment recommended if symptomatic • **Oral:** Metronidazole 500 mg po bid × 7 days Clindamycin 300 mg po bid × 7 days • **Vaginally:** Metronidazole gel 0.75% 5 g PV daily × 5 days Clindamycin 2% 5 g PV qhs × 7 days	• Always treat • Metronidazole 2 g po single dose or 500 mg po bid × 7 days • Pregnant: Metronidazole 2 g po single dose • Co-treat partners	• Rule out pathologic causes • If investigations normal, advise patient that discharge is normal to reduce anxiety and discourage multiple consults • Advise patient that changes in sexual activity, diet, hormone levels, and medications can affect quantity of discharge

Baxter S, McSheffrey G. *The Toronto Notes for Medical Students*, 2010, p. 25; Sobel, 2012.

VAGINAL ATROPHY

Vestibule thin, dry, pale, or mildly erythematous on physical examination

- Occurs with menopause, anorexia, or prolonged breastfeeding.
- For dyspareunia and vaginal dryness, a trial of nonhormonal vaginal lubricants and moisturizers is recommended (Replens or KY jelly).
- If nonhormonal treatment fails in those treated for vaginal atrophy (with menopause), low-dose vaginal estrogen therapy is recommended:
  - Premarin 0.625 mg conjugated estrogen/g of cream, 0.5 g of cream intravaginally twice weekly.
  - Vagifem 10 μg estradiol/tablet, one tablet intravaginally daily for 2 weeks followed by twice weekly.
  - Estring 7.5 μg of estradiol released daily over 90 days.
  - Estrace 100 μg estradiol/g of cream, 2 to 4 g daily for 1 to 2 weeks, then gradually half dose over similar time frame. Maintenance dose of 1 g intravaginally one to three times per week.
  - In women using local estrogen therapy for vaginal atrophy, progestin co-therapy is not routinely recommended in women who are postmenopausal and have no abnormal vaginal bleeding. (SOGC managing menopause.)
  - Use caution in patients with breast cancer.
- Progressive mechanical vaginal dilatation (vaginal dilators) can also be used for treatment.

VULVOVAGINITIS

Rule out vaginal lesions

- Lichen sclerosis—Bluish–white papula → White plaque. Thin parchment-like skin (subepithelial fat is diminished → thin atrophic labia). Usually occurs in postmenopausal women. Diagnosis is confirmed by biopsy and treatment is with potent topical steroids (0.05% clobetasol ointment daily at night for 6 to 12 weeks then one to three times per week for maintenance).
- Vulvar cancer—Average age is >65 years. Three types: squamous cell (associated with HPV), Paget disease (red lesion, postmenopausal white women, associated with cancer of the GI, GU, and breast), and melanoma. Diagnosis is confirmed by biopsy and treatment is vulvectomy with node excision.

KEY POINTS—VAGINAL DISCHARGE

1. In patients with no alarm features on history, physical examination, and negative test, make the diagnosis of physiologic discharge and communicate this to the patient to avoid recurrent presentation and unnecessary treatment and investigation in the future.
2. In children with vaginal discharge, rule out sexually transmitted diseases and foreign bodies. If candida infection is diagnosed, look for underlying illness such as diabetes or other immunocompromised state.
3. In nonpregnant, asymptomatic patients, electing not to treat BV/candida is appropriate.

Bibliography

Bachmann G, Santen RJ. Treatment of vaginal atrophy. *Up to Date*. 2011. http://www.uptodate.com/contents/treatment-of-vaginal-atrophy?source=search_result&search=vaginal+atrophy&selectedTitle=1~62#H16.

Chen YA, Tran C. *Toronto Notes—Comprehensive medical Reference & Review for MCCQE I and USMLE II*. Toronto, Canada: Toronto Notes for Medical Students Inc; 2008.

Cotch MF, Hillier SL, Gibbs RS, Eschenbach DA. Epidemiology and outcomes associated with moderate to heavy Candida colonization during pregnancy. Vaginal Infections and Prematurity Study Group. *Am J Obstet Gynecol*. 1998;178(2):374-380.

Martin KA, Barbieria RL. Preparations of postmenopausal therapy. *Up to Date*. 2011. http://www.uptodate .com/contents/preparations-for-postmenopausal-hormone-therapy?source=preview&anchor=H5#H18.

Priestley CJ, Jones BM, Dhar J, Goodwin L. What is normal vaginal flora? *Genitourinary Medicine*. 1997. http://www.ncbi.nlm.nih.gov/pmc/articles/PMC1195755/pdf/genitmed00001-0030.pdf.

Sobel JD. Evaluation of Women with Symptoms of Vaginitis. *Up to Date*. 2012. http://www.uptodate.com/ contents/evaluation-of-women-with-symptoms-of-vaginitis?source=search_result&search=vaginitis &selectedTitle=1~150.

van Schalkwik J, Yudin MH, et al. Vulvovaginitis: SOGC clinical practice guidelines: Screening for and management of trichomoniasis, vulvovaginal candidiasis, and bacterial vaginosis. *J Obstet Gynaecol Can*. 2015;37(3):266-274.

Menopause

Priority Topic 64

Definition

One year after the last menstrual period

Types

1. Physiologic: Average age 52 (Canada)
2. Premature ovarian failure: Occurs before 40 years of age
3. Iatrogenic (surgical/radiation/chemotherapy)

Symptoms

1. Vasomotor instability: Hot flashes, night sweats, nausea, sleep disturbance
2. Urogenital atrophy: Vaginal, urethral, bladder; leading to dyspareunia, itch, vaginal dryness, bleeding, urinary frequency, urgency, and incontinence
3. Skeletal: Osteoporosis, joint, and muscle pain
4. Skin and soft tissue: ↓ Breast size, skin thinning
5. Psychological: Mood disturbance, ↓ libido, fatigue, irritability, and memory loss

Diagnosis

- This is a clinical diagnosis that does not require laboratory testing.
- Alternative diagnosis should be considered if atypical symptoms occur.

Treatment

1. Vasomotor symptoms: Hormone therapy (HRT), SSRI, venlafaxine (Effexor), gabapentin, and propranolol
2. Vaginal atrophy: Oral or vaginal estrogens or vaginal moisturizers
3. Assess, prevent, and treat osteoporosis: Calcium and vitamin D, smoking cessation, exercise, SERM, and bisphosphonate
4. ↓ Libido: Vaginal lubrication, counselling, testosterone (cream or oral/systemic)
5. Specifically inquire regarding use of alternative therapies: Black cohosh (hot flushes), soy (hot flushes), St. John Wort (mood), gingko biloba (memory loss), valerian (sleep), evening primrose oil, ginseng, and dong quai

No evidence for alternative therapies in treatment of menopausal symptoms and some drug interactions exist, especially with St. John Wort

6. HRT CI (remember ABCD):
   a. **A**ctive liver disease
   b. **B**leeding (undiagnosed vaginal bleed)
   c. **C**ancer (hormone sensitive)
   d. **D**VT

HRT CI (REMEMBER ABCD)

A—**A**ctive liver disease

B—**B**leeding (undiagnosed vaginal bleed)

C—**C**ancer (hormone sensitive), Coronary Heart Disease, Clot (Past Stroke)

D—**D**VT

7. HRT considerations:
   a. Establish the risks and benefits of HRT.
   b. No risk of breast cancer if used <5 years, after 5 years ↑ by 2% year. Within 5 years of stopping risk returns to baseline.
   c. Benefits of HRT: ↓ Colon cancer, ↓ osteoporosis.
   d. Risks of HRT: ↑ Coronary disease, stroke, DVT, and breast cancer.
   e. HRT should not be initiated for prevention of cardiovascular disease; indicated only for treatment of menopausal symptoms (primarily vasomotor).
   f. Women with uteruses must treat all systemic HRT with progestogens (estrogen creams may also require progesterone therapy).
   g. Vaginal moisturizers are good alternatives (use three times per week) for HRT-contraindicated women.

Guideline Summary

1. The primary indication for HRT should be for the management of moderate-to-severe menopausal symptoms.
2. HRT should not be prescribed for the prevention of dementia or primary or secondary prevention of cardiovascular disease.
3. For vulvovaginal symptoms alone, topical HRT alone is recommended.
4. Nonhormonal prescriptions such as gabapentin and antidepressants can be prescribed as alternatives to HRT for vasomotor symptoms.
5. Any vaginal bleeding that occurs after 12 months of amenorrhea is considered postmenopausal bleeding and should be investigated.
6. If prescribing HRT to older postmenopausal women, ultra-low or low dosing regimens should be used.
7. Routine progesterone co-therapy is not required for endometrial protection in woman receiving vaginal estrogen in **appropriate doses.**
8. HRT should be offered to premature ovarian failure patients and those with early menopause and is recommended until the normal age of menopause.
9. Health care providers may prescribe HRT to patients with DM to relieve menopausal symptoms.
10. All unscheduled bleeding should be investigated as no HRT therapy is entirely protective against endometrial carcinoma.
11. Health care providers may prescribe HRT therapy to women at increased cancer risk of menopausal symptoms provided they have received adequate counselling and surveillance.

Bibliography

Chen YA, Tran C. Comprehensive medical reference & review for MCCQE I and USMLE II. *Toronto Notes*. Toronto, Canada: Toronto Notes for Medical Students Inc; 2008.

Henneber E. Canadian Consensus Conference on Menopause, 2006. SOGC Clinical Practice Guidelines. http://www.sogc.org/guidelines/public/171E-CONS-February2006.pdf.

Reid R, Abramson B, Blake J, et al. SOGC clinical practice guideline: Managing menopause. *Obstet Gynaecol Can.* 2014;36(9 eSuppl A):S1-S80.

CHAPTER 11

Musculoskeletal Medicine

Fractures

Priority Topic 40

1. One must **ALWAYS** be aware that if someone has incurred enough injury to break a bone, they may well have a ruptured spleen, or a perforated bowel, or a bleed in their head. Performing the ATLS protocol appropriately is crucial, and saves lives. Fractures rarely kill people in the first few hours following trauma. They are distracting, and shocking, but they are rarely life threatening.

Life-Threatening Fractures
- Pelvic fracture (in particular open book or vertical shear)
- Massive long bone fracture (usually femur)
- Traumatic amputations

Limb-Threatening Fractures
- Crush injuries
- Vascular injury at or above the knee or elbow
- Open fracture
- Dislocation knee
- Compartment syndrome

COMMON INJURIES/CONDITIONS

Open Fracture

- **ANY** communication between fracture site and external surface of skin
- Risk of osteomyelitis
- Important steps (other than 1, not necessarily in order):
  1. Recognition
  2. Reduction of fracture
  3. Irrigation, debridement, and dressing
  4. Appropriate antibiotics
  5. Tetanus prophylaxis
  6. Communication with on-call orthopedic or plastic surgeon

Anterior talofibular ligament is the most common ligament injured in inversion ankle sprain.

Shoulder Dislocation

- Anterior dislocation is most common.
- Occasionally risk injury to axillary and musculocutaneous nerve—hence importance of prompt reduction.
- Posterior dislocation secondary to seizures and risks damaging radial artery. Often missed due to inappropriate faith being place in the trans-axial ("Y") view, instead of the appropriate axillary lateral view.

Colles Fracture

- An extra-articular fracture of the distal radius with posterior comminution and apex volar angulation. Named after Dr. Abraham Colles.
- Often caused by fall on outstretched hands (FOOSH).
- "Dinner fork" deformity.

Scaphoid Fracture

- Anatomical snuff box tenderness.
- X-ray may be normal initially. If clinical suspicion is high, place in thumb spica cast and repeat x-ray in 1 to 2 weeks.

Compartment Syndrome

- Increased interstitial pressure in anatomical compartment (forearm, calf) resulting in decreased perfusion, muscle and/or nerve ischemia, and finally necrosis.
- **Excessive** pain: Very resistant to analgesia (such as renal colic, or childbirth), worse with stretching of involved muscles
- Five, six, and seven Ps have been described: **P**allor, **p**ain (out of proportion), **p**aralysis, **p**aresthesia, **p**ulse discrepancy/**p**ulselessness, **p**ressure, and **p**oikilothermia
  - In reality, pain, paresthesias, and pressure are the only Ps of utility. If you are finding pulselessness, or pallor, or a cold limb, you're likely too late. *Pain* is as described, *paresthesia* is often a guide to what compartment is involved, and *pressure* refers to the "tight," shiny appearance of the skin over the involved compartment.
- Treatment: Early suspicion, recognition, and acknowledgement. These things *DO* happen. Removal of any and all constrictive casts or dressings and seek help. Emergent surgical consult—fasciotomy will likely be required emergently.

THE POSSIBLE Ps OF COMPARTMENT SYNDROME

Pallor

Pain out of proportion

Paralysis

Paresthesia

Pulselessness/**p**ulse discrepancy

Poikilothermia

Pressure

GUIDELINES TO INVESTIGATION

Follow Ottawa x-ray rules when deciding whether to x-ray a patient

- Ottawa knee rules: X-ray if one or more of following:
  - Age ≥55
  - Tenderness at head of fibula
  - Isolated tenderness of patella
  - Inability to flex to 90 degrees
  - Inability to bear weight both immediately and in ER
- Ottawa ankle rules (see Figure 11-1)
- Ottawa foot rules (see Figure 11-1)
- If x-ray is normal and have suspicion of fracture (scaphoid fracture, stress fracture, fracture in elderly, growth plate fracture) consider casting and repeating x-ray in 1 to 2 weeks, or CT/bone scan to confirm diagnosis, but only if result may change management.

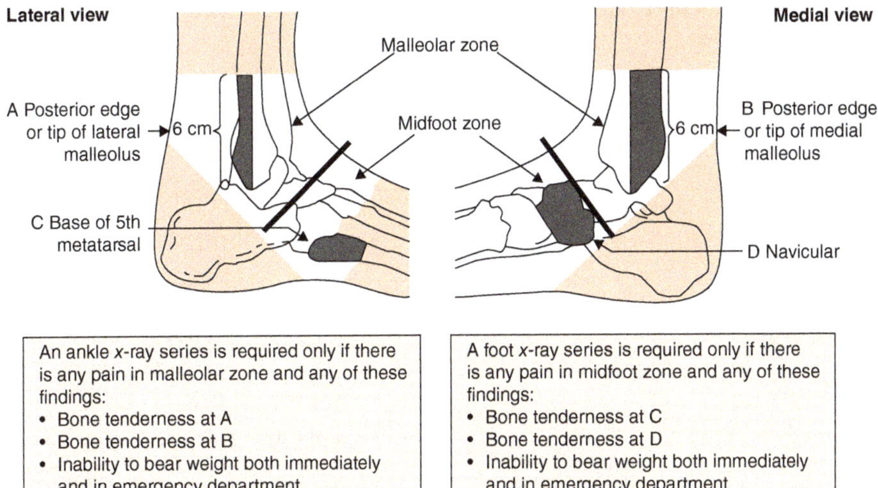

FIGURE 11-1: Ottawa ankle and foot x-ray rules. Stiell IG, et al. A study to develop clinical decision rules for the use of radiography in acute ankle injuries. *Ann Emerg Med.* 21(4);384-390. Reprinted with permission from Elsevier.

MANAGEMENT

- Dependent on fracture type, location, displacement of fragment
- Immobilize in splint or cast and refer to orthopedics if unsure

Bibliography

Brukner P, Khan K. *Clinical Sports Medicine.* 3rd ed. New York, NY: McGraw-Hill; 2009.

Chen YA. *Toronto Notes 2011: Comprehensive Medical Reference Review for MCCQE I USMLE II.* 27th ed. Toronto, ON: Toronto Review; 2008.

Stiell IG, Greenberg GH, Wells GA, et al. Derivation of a decision rule for the use of radiography in acute knee injuries. *Ann Emerg Med.* 1995;26:405-413.

Stiell I, Wells G, Laupacis A, et al. A multicentre trial to introduce clinical decision rules for the use of radiography in acute ankle injuries. *BMJ.* 1995;311:594-597.

Joint Disorders

Priority Topic 55

OSTEOARTHRITIS

Definition

- "Wear and tear," nonimmunologic arthritis

Risk Factors

- Family history
- Advanced age (80% of 85-year olds have osteoarthritis of some kind)
- Female >male
- Obesity

Signs/Symptoms

- Asymmetric joint pain relieved with rest and worse with activity.
- Functional joint pseudoinstability secondary to pain, and pseudoinstability on examination due to asymmetric wear of joint.

- Short duration of stiffness (<10 minutes) following a period of immobility.
- Loss of function.
- Crepitus with ROM.
- Insidious onset of pain that is gradually progressive.

Most Common Sites

- Knee
- Hips
- Hands (DIP = Heberden nodes, PIP = Bouchard nodes, first MCP)
- Spine (L4-5, L5-S1)

Investigations

- Blood work not needed unless concerned about diagnosis of other arthropathies (eg, RA)
- X-ray: Joint space narrowing, subchondral sclerosis, subchondral cyst formation, osteophytes

Treatment

- Conservative:
  - Weight loss (minimum 5%-10% of current body weight), rest, physiotherapy, and low-impact exercise programs
  - Unloader braces for knees
  - Walking aids—Cane
- Medications:
  - Acetaminophen
  - NSAIDs
  - Glucosamine—Some evidence for effectiveness, low cost, no known risks
  - Topical NSAIDs/capsaicin
  - Corticosteroid joint injections
  - Hyaluronate injections (Neovisc, Synvisc, Durolane)
- Surgical: Joint replacement

SEPTIC JOINT

Definition

- Invasion of a joint space by an infectious agent
- Most common organisms: *Staphylococcus* and *Streptococcus*
  - Consider gonorrhea in the sexually active people
- Cause: Hematogenous spread; rarely direct contamination from either trauma or injection
  - Higher risk in immunocompromised, diabetics, IV drug users, HIV, patients with prosthetic joints, etc.
- **Always consider sepsis in a patient with a joint replacement**
  - Can have a very low grade, innocuous presentation

Symptoms

- Severe pain
- Erythema
- Warmth
- Swelling
- Inability to bear weight

- Joint will be held in position that provides largest volume of joint capsule, patient **very** unwilling to move from that position
  - Knee—Flexed ~30 degrees
  - Hip—Flexed ~30 degrees, externally rotated ~30 degrees, and abducted ~30 degrees
- Fever, but not always

Investigations

- X-ray
- ESR, CRP, WBC, and blood cultures
  - CRP + ESR are extremely sensitive markers, but poor in specificity.
- Joint aspirate absolutely essential—**must aspirate joint before giving antibiotics**
  - Knees, elbows, wrists, and ankles can be done in ER by primary care physicians.
  - Hips and shoulders require fluoroscopic guidance by radiologist.
  - Observe the fluid for:
    - Colour
      - Bright yellow—Gout
      - Murky white with stringy material—Pus
    - Homogeneity
      - Very homogenous—Gout
      - Inhomogeneous—Pus
  - Send for:
    - Cell count—General rule <50,000 white cells, not bacterial sepsis
    - Gram stain
    - Crystal analysis—To differentiate from gout/calcium pyrophosphate dehydrate (CPPD)
    - Culture and sensitivity
- Using the data from the questions above, a decision **must** be made based on story, examination, observing fluid, ESR, CRP, cell count, Gram stain, and crystal analysis
- Septic arthritis is a **surgical emergency** and requires appropriate *incision and drainage* as soon as possible. One **must not** wait for the culture and sensitivity to come back.

Treatment

- Orthopedic consultation is **mandatory**; debridement is needed.
- IV antibiotics **only** after aspirate has been attained.

RHEUMATOID ARTHRITIS

Definition

- Symmetric, erosive, immunologic-based polyarthritis of unknown origin affecting mainly peripheral joints

Age of onset typically 20 to 40 years

Signs/Symptoms

- Morning stiffness >1 hour
- Pain aggravated by rest and improved with use (whereas OA is worse with use and better with rest)
- Joint instability, crepitus

All acute monoarticular arthritides require an aspiration!!!
"Aspirate or litigate"

Monoarticular septic arthritis + migrating polyarthralgia + rash + tendon pain = disseminated *Neisseria gonorrhoea*

- Typical deformities: Swan neck, boutonniere, radial deviation of wrist, ulnar deviation of MCP, hammer toe, mallet toe, claw toe, flexor contractures
- Constitutional symptoms often present: Fatigue, myalgias, rash

Risk Factors

- Females >males (3:1)
- Genetic predisposition (HLA-DR4/DR1)

Investigations

- +RF (**only** 80% sensitive)
- Elevated ESR/CRP, low specificity
  Anti-CCP (high specificity can help identify patients who are likely to have more sever disease)
- X-ray: Loss of joint space, synovial inflammation

Treatment

- Rheumatologist consultation
- Conservative:
  - Education, PT, OT, vocational counselling
- Medications:
  - NSAIDs, acetaminophen, local/systemic corticosteroids for symptom relief (do not alter disease progression "non-DMARDS")
  - Disease modifying antirheumatic drugs (DMARDs)—Standard of care
    - Start DMARDS within 3 months of diagnosis
    - Nonbiologics (eg, methotrexate [gold standard], hydroxychloroquine, sulfasalazine)
    - Biologics (infliximab, etanercept)
- Surgical: Synovectomy, joint replacement/reconstruction/fusion

SYSTEMIC LUPUS ERYTHEMATOSUS

Definition

- Chronic inflammatory multisystem disease
- Characterized by production of autoantibodies

Symptoms

- Diagnosis is with +ANA plus three symptoms from "MD SOAP BRAIN" mnemonic

Risk Factors

- Genetics/family history
- Female >male (10:1)
- Age
- Race (African American, Hispanic, Asian)

Investigations

- +ANA (98% sensitive)
- Anti-dsDNA (95%-99% specific)
- C_3/C_4 (to monitor treatment response, lowered in SLE)

Treatment

- Rheumatology consultation.
- Patient education (avoid UV light, use sunscreen).

Felty syndrome: Arthritis, splenomegaly, neutropenia

SLE Symptoms (MD SOAP BRAIN)
Malar rash ("butterfly" rash on face—sparing of nasolabial folds)
Discoid rash (may cause scarring)
Serositis (pleuritis leuritic/pericarditis)
Oral ulcers (aphthous—usually painless)
ANA (+)
Photosensitivity
Blood (hemolytic anemia, thrombocytopenia)
Renal (nephrotic glomerulonephritis)
Arthritis (two joints, nonerosive)
Immune (antiphospholipid, anti-Ro, anti-DS DNA, anti-Smith)
Neurologic (seizures, psychosis)

- Treat early and avoid long-term steroid use.
- Treatment is highly varied and tailored to organ system involvement.

REACTIVE ARTHRITIS (REITER SYNDROME)

Definition
- Noninfectious, immunologic arthritis following an infection (typically 1-4 weeks postinfection)—Usually GI (*Shigella*, *Salmonella*, *Campylobacter*, *Yersinia*) or GU (*Chlamydia*, *Mycoplasma*)

Symptoms
- Triad of arthritis, conjunctivitis, urethritis = 99% specific
- May also have skin and/or mucosal membrane (GI), as well as possible tendon ligament involvement

Treatment
- Antibiotics for nonarticular infections
- NSAIDs
- Physiotherapy, exercise

SLIPPED CAPITAL FEMORAL EPIPHYSIS (SCFE)

Definition
- Slipped capital femoral epiphysis (SCFE) is a common childhood/adolescent hip disorder.
- Failure/slip of the growth plate (the physis) in the femoral head during the period of physeal closure, resulting in slippage of the epiphysis on the metaphysis.

Risk Factors
- Almost exclusively obsess males
- Usually **not** traumatic in nature

SCFE Symptoms
- Sudden, severe pain with limp
- Restricted ROM (inability to internally rotate femur)

Investigations
- AP/lateral/**frog-leg lateral** x-ray. Will show disconnect in cortical alignment from metaphysis to epiphysis
  - **Lateral view is most telling**—Look for apex anterior "buckling" of the physis

Treatment
- Restrict weight bearing **immediately** (wheelchair if needed) to limit any further slip.
- Surgical consultation and management required.

LEGG-CALVE-PERTHES

Definition
- Self-limited avascular necrosis and (partial) reformation of the femoral head
- Usually occurs in kids 4 to 10 years of age

Reiter syndrome triad—"Can't pee, can't see, can't climb a tree"
Arthritis
Conjunctivitis/uveitis
Urethritis/cervicitis

Guide to pediatric hip disorders by age of presentation
Dysplasia—Birth
Septic hip—Toddler
Transient tenosynovitis—3 to 6 years
Legg-Calve-Perthes—4 to 10 years (boys >girls)
SCFE—Obese 12 to 14 years (boys >girls)

Pediatric bone tumours
Osteogenic sarcoma
- Location: Around knee
- X-ray: Sunburst pattern
- Age: 10 to 25 years (male >female)
Ewing
- Location: Diaphysis of long bones
- X-ray: Onion skinning
- Age: 5 to 15 years

SCFE can lead to irreversible changes to the morphology of the hip joint, and in turn early degenerative changes, if not treated promptly and accurately.

Risk Factors

- Family history
- Low birth weight
- History of hip trauma

Symptoms

- Spontaneous hip pain and/or limp
- Flexion contracture/decreased internal rotation of hip

Diagnosis

- X-ray: Collapse of femoral head is diagnostic
- X-ray can often be normal early in disease progression

Treatment

- Conservative = physiotherapy, ROM exercise, bracing
- Surgical = femoral or pelvic osteotomy

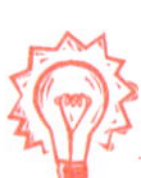

The new onset of pain or limp in a child **always** warrants pediatric orthopedic consultation.

SCOLIOSIS

Definition

- A three-dimensional deformity of the spine lateral bending but also twisting
- 90% idiopathic, occasionally with a structural cause (ie, hemivertebra), and rarely tumour or neurogenic

Symptoms

- Back pain usually not present
- Asymmetric shoulder height when bent over for Adam's forward bend test
- Positive Adam's test = rib hump when bent forward
- Apparent leg length discrepancy

Investigations

- Standing, full length, spine x-ray

Treatment

- Pediatric orthopedic consultation
- Depends on degree of curvature
- Observe if <20 degrees
- Bracing if >20 degrees
- Consider surgery if >40 degrees or respiratory compromise

15% of patients with PMR develop temporal arteritis.

POLYMYALGIA RHEUMATICA

Definition

- PMR results in pain and stiffness in girdle area.

Diagnostic PMR Criteria

1. Age >50
2. Bilateral aching/morning stiffness >1 month
3. Elevated ESR (>40)
4. Prompt response to low-dose corticosteroids (within 48 hours of treatment)

Symptoms/Investigations

- Symmetrical morning stiffness of proximal muscles
- May have constitutional symptoms (fever, malaise)
- Elevated ESR and CRP

Treatment

- Rheumatology consultation
- Low-dose steroids (15-20 mg po daily)
- Often need to treat for 2 years or longer (50% relapse rate once off treatment)

Bibliography

Brukner P, Khan K. *Clinical Sports Medicine*. 3rd ed. New York, NY: McGraw-Hill; 2009.

Chen AY, Tran C. *Toronto Notes*. Toronto, ON: Type & Graphics Inc; 2011.

Simon C, Everitt H, van Dorp F. *Oxford Handbook of General Practice*. Oxford, UK: Oxford University Press; 2010.

PMR vs polymyositis

PMR

- Pain, stiff in girdle area
- ESR >40

Polymyositis

- Symmetric, proximal muscle weakness
- **Increased CK** and ESR

Low Back Pain

Priority Topic 61

GENERAL

- Acute back pain is <12 weeks
- Chronic back pain is >12 weeks

RED FLAGS

1. Cancer: Night pain, weight loss, past history of cancer, age >50
2. Compression fracture: Acute bony tenderness, osteoporosis, history of fall or trauma
3. Osteomyelitis or discitis: Fever, chills, sweats, IV drug use
4. Spinal cord compression: Neurological symptoms (motor/sensory)
5. Cauda equina (**Emergency**): Loss of sphincter tone, fecal incontinence, perineal numbness, leg weakness, change in sexual function, acute urinary retention, or overflow incontinence
6. Other: Worsening symptoms

DIFFERENTIAL DIAGNOSIS OF BACK PAIN

- Pyelonephritis
- Ruptured AAA
- Cancer
- Cauda equine syndrome
- Compression fracture
- Osteomyelitis
- Mechanical/MSK back pain
- Spondylosis/spondylolisthesis
- Disc herniation
- Spinal stenosis

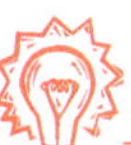

Lower limb movements and myotomes

- L2 = Hip flexion
- L3 = Knee extension
- L4 = Ankle dorsiflexion
- L5 = Great toe extension
- S1 = Ankle plantar flexion
- S2 = Knee flexion

Sciatica refers to pain, and/or numbness, and/or leg weakness caused by pressure on one of the roots that comprise the sciatic nerve (L4-S3). Multiple diagnoses should be considered when a patient presents with sciatica type symptoms.

COMMON CAUSES OF BACK PAIN

- Herniated disc:
  - Protrusion of nucleus pulposus
  - Most common secondary to flexion/lifting injury
  - Pain can be back dominant (central herniation) or leg dominant (lateral herniation)
  - Abrupt onset of pain
  - Worse with coughing, flexion
  - Numbness/weakness may be present in nerve root distribution
- Lumbar spinal stenosis: Neurogenic claudication
  - Narrowing of spinal canal → Compression of the roots or entire cauda equina
  - Age >60 is risk factor
  - Pain is:
    - Radicular +/− back pain
    - Progresses proximal to distal
    - Gradual onset
    - Aggravated by extension
    - Poor walking/standing tolerance
    - Leg pain often subsides with lying/sitting
- Mechanical back pain:
  - Most common causes of mechanical back pain are degenerative disc or facet joints, and muscle- or ligament-related injuries.
  - Generally investigations are not needed in the absence of any red flags.
  - Most improve within 3 months with conservative treatment.

TREATMENT OF MECHANICAL BACK PAIN

Acute

- Educate (most resolve in 2-3 weeks)
- Self-care strategies and attitudes
- Early return to work/activity
- Analgesia—Avoiding narcotics if at all possible
- Physio/chiro/massage

Chronic

- Multidisciplinary approach (physio, chiro, massage, etc)
- +/− Physiatrist referral
- Analgesia—Avoiding narcotics if at all possible
- Referral to spine surgeon if appropriate

Analgesia

Acute

Acetaminophen
NSAIDs
Muscle relaxant (short course)
Short-acting opioids if course of NSAIDs and Tylenol is maximized and fails.

Chronic

Acetaminophen
NSAIDs
Low-dose TCA
Muscle relaxants (ie, Cyclobenzaprine)
Opioids if course of NSAIDs plus Tylenol is maximized, yet fails.

INVESTIGATIONS

Indications for lumbar spine x-ray:

1. No improvement within 1 month
2. Fever
3. Weight loss
4. History of cancer
5. Prolonged steroid use
6. Significant trauma
7. Progressive deficits
8. Other red flags

Consider CT/MRI if neurological deficits or differential diagnosis includes infection or cancer.

TABLE 11-1	Low Back Pain Memory Cues/Key Findings
DIAGNOSIS	**SIGNS**
Compression #	• Local pain (spinal) • No pain radiation
Herniated disc	• Positive straight leg raise • Worse with flexion
Spinal stenosis	• Worse with extension
Vascular claudication	• Worse with walking set distance • Better when stop walking (<2 minutes) • Muscular cramping pain
Neurogenic claudication	• Worse with walking or standing (distance variable) • Better when change position (>10 minutes)
Mechanical back pain	• Resolves in 2-3 weeks • No red flags • Often paraspinal pain

Bibliography

Brukner P, Khan K. *Clinical Sports Medicine*. 3rd ed. New York, NY: McGraw-Hill; 2009.

Chen YA. *Toronto Notes 2011: Comprehensive Medical Reference Review for MCCQE I USMLE II*. 27th ed. Toronto, ON: Toronto Review Notes; 2008.

Neck Pain

Priority Topic 66

APPROACH TO PATIENT WITH NECK PAIN

1. History
2. Inspect
3. Palpate
4. ROM
5. Strength
6. Reflexes
7. Special tests

Neck pain strength and motor innervation

Motor testing	Nerve root
Neck flexion	C1, C2
Side flexion	C3
Shoulder elevation	C4
Shoulder abduction	C5
Elbow/wrist flexion	C5
Elbow/wrist extension	C7
Thumb extension	C8
Intrinsics of the hand	T1

Spinal cord compression

Increased pain with recumbency, movement, and Valsalva

Patient will have neurological symptoms (sensory +/− motor)

Risk factors—Cancer, osteoporosis

Diagnosis with history, physical examination, and MRI

Differential Diagnosis of Neck Pain

- Carotid dissection (most common cause of stroke in young adults)
- Referred pain from ACS
- Retropharangeal abscess, epiglottitis (infection)
- Spinal stenosis/spinal cord compression
- Disc herniation
- Nerve impingement
- Whiplash
- Lymphoma
- Pseudotumour cerebri (referred pain from idiopathic intracranial HTN)
- Muscular neck pain (posture, stress, etc.)

INVESTIGATIONS

- Follow C-spine rules (see Figure 11-2) to determine if x-ray is needed.
- Complete AP, lateral, and odontoid views.
- X-ray: Ensure visualization of C1-T1 vertebrae before clearing C-spine. Repeat x-ray with swimmer view, pull-down view, or CT scan if C7/T1 is poorly visualized.
- Consider MRI if neurological symptoms are present.

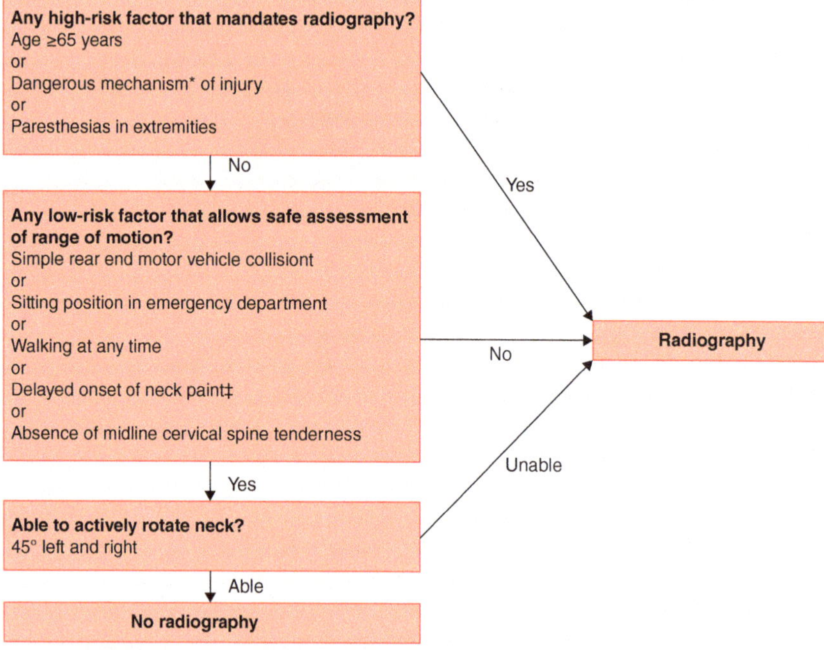

FIGURE 11-2:   Canadian C-spine rule. Reprinted from Stiell IG, et al. *BMJ*. 2009; 339:b4146.

MANAGEMENT

- Dependent on diagnosis
- Use multidisciplinary, conservative approach for chronic neck pain secondary to muscular issues or degenerative disc disease

Bibliography

Brukner P, Khan K. *Clinical Sports Medicine*. 3rd ed. New York, NY: McGraw-Hill; 2009.

Chen YA. *Toronto Notes 2011: Comprehensive Medical Reference Review for MCCQE I USMLE II*. 27th ed. Toronto, ON: Toronto Review Notes; 2011.

Filate W, Ng D, Leung R, Sinyor M. *Essentials of Clinical Examination Handbook*. 5th ed. University of Toronto: The Medical Society Faculty of Medicine; 2005.

Stiell IG, Clement CM, Grimshaw J, et al. Implementation of the Canadian C-Spine Rule: a prospective 12-centre cluster randomized trial. *BMJ*. 2009;339:b41-b46.

Lifestyle

Priority Topic 58

- Always ask about lifestyle behaviours that affect health at every visit (ie, diet, exercise, EtOH/substance use, safe sex, injury prevention).
- Ensure that you know if your patient is ready to make appropriate lifestyle modifications.
- Explore your patient's context (ie, financial, cultural, family) to guide lifestyle recommendations, so as to avoid making recommendations that your patient cannot comply with (unaffordable, etc).
- Review lifestyle modifications at each encounter, understanding that behaviours may change over time.
- Reinforce positive behaviour modifications, and demonstrate how they have improved health (ie, improved blood pressure, glucose management, lipids, renal function, stroke risk, etc).
- Recommend 30 minutes of activity daily.

Bibliography

Working Group on the Certification Process. Priority topics and key features with corresponding skill dimensions and phases of the encounter. The College of Family Physicians of Canada; 2010. http://www.cfpc.ca/uploadedFiles/Education/Certification_in_Family_Medicine_Examination/Definition%20of%20Competence%20Complete%20Document%20with%20skills%20and%20phases.pdf.

Obesity

- **BMI = weight (kg)/height (m)^2**
  - Normal BMI (adults) = 18.8 to 25
  - Overweight = 25 to 29
  - Obese = 30 to 39
  - Morbidly obese = 40 to 49
  - Children (>2 years): BMI >95th percentile for age and gender = obese
- Obesity is associated with:
  - Increased risks of CV death and overall mortality
  - Increased morbidity for hypertension, CAD, stroke, diabetes mellitus, hyperlipidemia, sleep apnea, gallbladder disease, GERD, knee osteoarthritis, low back pain, and neoplastic diseases (colon, renal, gallbladder)

If caloric intake is reduced by 500 to 1000 kcal/day, it will result in 1 to 2 lb weight loss/week (assuming the same total daily energy expenditure).

Treatment

1. Counselling and behaviour interventions can change eating patterns and increase exercise
   - Five As:
     - **Ask**   Determine patient's understanding, awareness of obesity
     - **Assess** Determine patient's readiness to make necessary changes to lose weight
     - **Advise** Appropriate dietary, exercise, support measures
     - **Assist** Facilitate patient resources as needed
     - **Arrange** Discuss progress and readjust plan according to patient needs
2. Medications (orlistat, SSRIs, sympathomimetics) only if diet and exercise have failed and patient has significant comorbidities. Used for short-term management only
3. Surgery (gastric bypass/banding): Consider if BMI >40 or >35 + significant comorbidities

Lifestyle modification, prevention of DM 2 and CVD

Bibliography

Working Group on the Certification Process. Priority topics and key features with corresponding skill dimensions and phases of the encounter. The College of Family Physicians of Canada; 2010. http://www.cfpc.ca/uploadedFiles/Education/Certification_in_Family_Medicine_Examination/Definition%20of%20Competence%20Complete%20Document%20with%20skills%20and%20phases.pdf.

GOUT

Definition

Monosodium urate crystals infiltrating joints, soft tissue, or renal tissues

Signs/Symptoms

Abrupt onset, excruciating pain, localized erythema/warmth/swelling, recurrent, +/− loss of joint mobility, tophi (urate deposits from previous attacks), renal calculi/nephropathy

Typical joints: First MIP, ankle, knee

Four stages of gouty arthritis:

1. Asymptomatic hyperuricemia
2. Acute gouty arthritis
3. Intercritical gout
4. Chronic tophaceous gout (tophi—erosions—nephropathy/calculi)

Risk Factors

Males>females, high purine diet, obesity, family history of hyperuricemia, CKD, HTN, hyperlipidemia

Precipitants

Medications = **FACT: F**urosemide, **A**SA/EtOH, **C**ytotoxic drugs, **T**hiazide (and loop) diuretics/Theophylline

Foods = **SALTS: S**hellfish, **A**nchovies, **L**iver, **T**urkey, **S**ardines

Investigations

Definitive: Joint aspartate yielding, needle-shaped, negatively birefringent monosodium urate crystals

Presumptive: Acute monoarthropathy + hyperuricemia + dramatic response to NSAID/colchicine

Treatment

Acute attack

1. NSAIDs (first line)
2. Colchicine (antigout agent)
3. Intra-articular steroid injection
4. Short-term systemic glucocorticoid

Maintenance/prophylaxis

1. First attack—Lifestyle changes and remove precipitating drugs
2. Treat if one of the following:
   a. Serum uric acid >800 umol/L
   b. Three or more attacks per year
   c. Chemotherapy
   d. Advanced disease
3. Medication choices:
   a. Allopurinol (xanthine oxidase inhibitor)—(first line, though)—do not start or adjust during an acute attack
   b. Colchicine (low dose, <0.6 mg) + probenecid

PSEUDOGOUT (CHONDROCALCINOSIS)

Definition

- Acute inflammatory arthritis due to phagocytosis if IgG-coated CPPD crystals—inflammatory mediated release

Risk Factors

- Females = males, advanced age, advanced osteoarthritis, neuropathic joints, diabetes mellitus, hypothyroidism, hemochromatosis, elevated PTH, decreased magnesium, and decreased phosphate

Triggers

- Dehydration, illness, surgery, trauma

Signs/Symptoms

- Polyarticular > monoarticular, slower onset (than gout), self-limited (up to 3 weeks)

Typical Joints

- Knee, wrist, MCP, first MTP

Investigations

- Aspirate to rule out septic arthritis or acute gout—positively birefringent, rhomboid-shaped crystals
- X-ray: Chondrocalcinosis

Treatment

- NSAIDs
- Colchicine—Controversial for prophylaxis
- Intra-articular steroids

Bibliography

Chen AY, Tran C. *Toronto Notes*. Toronto, ON: Type & Graphics Inc; 2011.

Longmore M, Wilkinson I, Davidson E, Foulkes A, Mafi A. *Oxford Handbook of Clinical Medicine*. 8th ed. Oxford, UK: Oxford University Press; 2010.

CHAPTER 12

Care of the Elderly

Elderly

Priority Topic 35

- Avoid medication side effects in the elderly:
  - Avoid polypharmacy when possible.
  - Review medication list periodically; every time a new medication is added, consider interactions.
  - Avoid medications and over the counter (OTC)/herbals known to have increased risk. This includes prescription and nonprescription medications.
  - Be aware of the need for dose adjustments based on kidney function.
  - Ensure reliable pill taking (eg, bubble pack from pharmacy).
  - Inquire about nonprescription medication use (eg, herbal medicines, cough drops, OTC drugs, vitamins).
- Promote safety and prolong independence: Screen for modifiable risk factors (eg, visual disturbance, impaired hearing, falls).
- Assess functional status: Allow for timely discussion of changes in living arrangements and social supports available.
- Consider age, life expectancy, and frailty. This will help guide the recommendations toward preventive care and management plans. A useful tool for this assessment is the Clinical Frailty Scale (developed from the Canadian Study of Health and Aging).
  - Preventive care considerations include CCFP (**C**ancer, **C**ardiovascular Disease, **F**alls and Osteoporosis, and **P**reventive immunizations).
- Fall prevention.
- Consider atypical presentations of disease in the elderly patient
  - Infection—Frequently does not present with fever.
  - Pain—Can present as restlessness, confusion, etc.
  - Depression—Often presents as somatic complaints (changes in weight, sleep, energy) or anxiety symptoms, poor performance on cognitive tests (because patient is giving up trying to answer).
  - Myocardial infarction—Less classic chest pain presentation, may have dyspnea or fatigue as main symptom.
  - Acute abdomen—Often has fewer symptoms, less pain for given pathology, less rebound tenderness, less fever.

Bibliography

The American Geriatrics Society 2015 Beers Criteria Update Expert Panel. American geriatrics society updated beers criteria for potentially inappropriate medication use in older adults. *J Am Geriat Soc.* 2015;63:2227-2246.

MacKay M. Financial and personal competence in the elderly: the position of the Canadian Psychiatric Association. *Can J Psy.* 1989;34:829.

Priority topics and key features with corresponding skill dimensions and phases of the encounter. 2010. Available from: http://www.cfpc.ca/uploadedFiles/Education/Priority%20Topics%20and%20Key%20Features.pdf.

Tazkarhi B, Lam R, Lee S. Approach to preventive care in the elderly. *Can Fam Physician.* 2016;62:717-721.

Multiple Medical Problems

Priority Topic 65

- Clarify the primary reason(s) for the visit and prioritize problems through negotiation with the patient.
- Consider depression, anxiety, or abuse (including physical, medication, or drug abuse) in the differential along with organic pathology.
- Set limits for the frequency and duration of visits in patients with multiple visits with unchanging symptoms.
- Screen periodically for depression due to higher risk if multiple chronic medical conditions are present.
- Review periodically the management of patients with multiple conditions with goal to:
  - Simplify management (pharmacologic and nonpharmacologic).
  - Limit polypharmacy and eliminate medications that are no longer necessary/recommended.
  - Minimize possible drug interactions through review of medication list including OTCs and herbals.
  - Update management based on new scientific evidence.
- Reassess the patient's condition and situation for possible change, which will affect management.
- Assist the patient with multiple medical problems (and potentially seeing many specialists) with coordination of care and management.

Bibliography

The American Geriatrics Society 2015 Beers Criteria Update Expert Panel. American geriatrics society updated beers criteria for potentially inappropriate medication use in older adults. *J Am Geriat Soc.* 2015;63:2227-2246.

Canadian Task Force on Preventive Health Care. Recommendations on screening for cognitive impairment in older adults. *CMAJ.* 2015;188(1):37-46.

Priority topics and key features with corresponding skill dimensions and phases of the encounter. 2010. Available from: http://www.cfpc.ca/uploadedFiles/Education/Priority%20Topics%20and%20Key%20Features.pdf.

Dementia

Priority Topic 23

DEFINITION

Acquired disorder characterized by multiple diffuse cognitive deficits that interfere with daily function. Dementia is manifested by memory impairment and substantial decline from previous cognitive functioning plus one of the following:

- Aphasia
- Apraxia

- Agnosia
- Disturbance in executive function (eg, planning, organizing, abstracting)

INCIDENCE AND PREVALENCE

- Incidence in Canada of 43 per 1000 population in 65 to 79 years; this increases with age (212 per 1000 among those over 85).
- 9.9% to 35.2 % among adults over 70 years.
- Most common is Alzheimer of mixed Alzheimer disease (AD) patients.
- Other types of dementia include vascular, frontotemporal, Parkinson, Lewy body.

DIAGNOSIS

- Dementia is a clinical diagnosis.
- Brief cognitive tests (Montreal Cognitive Assessment [MoCA], Mini Mental Status Exam [MMSE]) can help discriminate between dementia and normal state.
- For cognitive testing, keep in mind other factors that may affect performance such as language barrier/advanced age/low education. Testing is most helpful when repeated over time. There is no benefit in screening asymptomatic patients over 65 years.
- MoCA (www.mocatest.org) is for mild impairment (sensitivity 89%, specificity 75%).
- MMSE: A score of 25 means mild, 19 to 10 means moderate, 9 to 0 means severe dementia (sensitivity 81%, specificity 89%).
- Laboratory testing is recommended to rule out causes of chronic metabolic encephalopathy.
  - CBC, TSH, electrolytes, calcium, fasting glucose, vitamin B_{12} (consider folate in patients with celiac or inadequate diet).
  - CT scan can be used to rule in concomitant cerebrovascular disease that can affect management, rule out other conditions (eg, normal pressure hydrocephalus, bleeding, malignancy) or in specific situations including patients under age 60, rapid decline in cognition (within 1-2 months) and new onset of neurologic deficit symptoms.
  - Genetic testing: Consider in appropriately selected patients (eg, family with young onset disease).

DIFFERENTIAL DIAGNOSIS

- Delirium and depression (see Table 12-1).
- Brain pathology: Vascular insult, infectious, metabolic insult, paraneoplastic syndrome, tumour, epilepsia, hydrocephalus.

TABLE 12-1	Comparison of Dementia, Delirium, and Depression		
	DEMENTIA	**DELIRIUM**	**DEPRESSION**
Onset	Insidious	Acute	Gradual with life changes
Duration	Months to years	Hours	At least 2 weeks
Course	Stepwise	Fluctuates, more at night	Diurnal, worse in morning
Alertness	Normal	Fluctuates	Normal
Orientation	Normal or mild impairment	Always impaired	Normal
Perception	Normal	Disoriented and hallucinations	Normal
Tests	MMSE	CAM (Confusion Assessment Method)	GDS (Geriatric Depression Scale)

- Mild cognitive impairment.
  Delirium differential diagnosis—**I WATCH DEATH SOB**
    Infection
    Withdrawal from drugs
    Acute metabolic disorder
    Trauma
    CNS pathology
    Hypoxia
    Deficiencies in vitamins
    Endocrinopathies
    Acute vascular
    Toxins
    Heavy metals
    Sleep
    Ouch (pain)
    Bowel (constipation)

RISK FACTORS AND PRECIPITATING FACTORS

- Risk factors: Age over 65, male, impaired cognition, impaired functional status, sensory impairment, poor nutritional status, medications (psychoactive, anticholinergic), alcohol abuse, medical comorbidities, systolic hypertension, elevated cholesterol, head injury with loss of consciousness, low education level.
- Precipitating factors: Drugs (sedative hypnotic, narcotic, anticholinergic, polypharmacy, alcohol or drug withdrawal), primary neurologic disease, current illness, surgery, ICU, physical restraints, bladder catheter, pain, emotional stress, prolonged sleep deprivation.

TYPES OF DEMENTIA

- **Alzheimer dementia:** Progressive worsening of cognitive function (months to years). Memory impairment is the most common presentation but may not be found as primary cognitive deficit.
- **Frontotemporal dementia:** In middle-aged patients, gradual-onset and prominent behavioural changes (eg, disinhibition) or prominent language impairment.
- **Parkinson dementia:** Have idiopathic Parkinson disease for 1+ year prior to onset of dementia (motor parkinsonian symptoms), may have visual hallucinations and fluctuation in disease course.
- **Lewy body dementia:** Begins with cognitive and behavioural disorder that can have concurrent parkinsonian features, may have visual hallucinations and fluctuation in disease course.
- **Vascular dementia:** Typically stepwise decline, focal neurologic features often found in course, dys-executive syndrome.
- **Mixed AD and vascular dementia:** Most common type of dementia. Abilities decline gradually, associated with vascular disease.
- **Rapid progressive dementia:** Dementia that develops within 12 months after appearance of first cognitive symptoms or patients with AD and decline in 3 points of MMSE within 6 months (exclusion of delirium and other conditions). Includes Creutzfeldt-Jakob disease (mandatory reportable condition). Prompt referral is needed.
- **Early-onset dementia:** Diagnosed before age 65.

MILD COGNITIVE IMPAIRMENT (MCI)

- Definition: Impairment in memory but no significant decrease in function and do not meet criteria for dementia.
- Diagnosis: Clinical—decline from previous level of functioning, gradual in onset and duration of >6 months, not due to depression/delirium/other psychiatric disorder.
- Screening with MoCA helps demonstrate objective cognitive loss, monitor closely since high risk for progressing to dementia.
- Treatment includes managing vascular risk factors, increased cognitive and physical activity, assessing and treating sleep disorders.

MANAGEMENT OF DEMENTIA

Note: Cognition-enhancing medications are not part of CCFP objectives and will not be discussed here.

1. Primary prevention

- Control systolic hypertension (>160 mm Hg).
- Treatment of specific medical conditions solely for dementia primary prevention is not indicated (statins, ASA, correction of carotid artery stenosis, antithrombotic therapy).
- Lifestyle factors: Assess potential fall risks to reduce risk of head injury, smoking cessation, reduce alcohol consumption, increase physical and mental activity.
- Medications: None indicated for primary prevention, estrogen not indicated for prevention of dementia.

2. Mild to moderate

Disclosure of diagnosis: Respect patient's autonomy/confidentiality/safety

Medical

- Treat comorbid medical conditions.
- Start management with nonpharmacological treatment with behavioural or environment modifications.
- Although limited improvement, cholinesterase inhibitors are recommended in the treatment of moderate to severe AD associated with Parkinson disease or vascular dementia. This recommendation is not applicable for vascular dementia alone.
  - Ensure establishing clear goals for treatment and how to assess for cognition and possible side effects (eg, gastrointestinal, genitourinary).
  - Cholinesterase inhibitors do not provide long-term benefit as they do not prevent hospitalization/institutionalization.
- With sudden changes in cognition/function/behaviour search for causes of delirium
  - Dementia is a risk factor for delirium.
- Assess for behavioural challenges, for example anxiety, insomnia, depressive symptoms.
  - Management is best with nonpharmacologic techniques when possible.
- Driving: Assess both cognition and visual-spatial skills, when doubt exists send for driving examination.
  - Safety to drive is based on functional "assessment," **not** on the diagnosis of any particular medical condition.
  - Physicians do not take away license, but they should report to provincial motor vehicle licensing authority if they believe someone is unfit for driving and the authorities will assess.
    - Physicians must report patients who have a medical condition that makes it dangerous to drive or patients who continue driving despite being warned of the risk.
  - *CMA Driver's Guide* is a good resource.

Lifestyle

- Individualized exercise program is beneficial.
- Refer to community resources (eg, adult day care, Alzheimer's Society, social worker)
- Assess risk for falls and household safety.
- Inquire about advance directive.
- Caregivers are often called the hidden patient—assess needs and supports of caregiver!

3. Severe

- Goals of management: (1) improving quality of life (patient and caregiver), (2) maintaining optimal function, and (3) providing maximum comfort.
- Assess needs for help with activities of daily living (ADLs) and living situation.
- Assess every 3 to 4 months: Cognition, function, behaviour, medical and nutritional status, caregiver's safety and health.
- Assess for behavioural challenges: For example, anxiety, insomnia, and depressive symptoms.
  - Management is best with nonpharmacological techniques when possible.
  - When there is change in behaviour, search for causes; do not assume it is a progression of dementia.
- Pharmacotherapy
  - "Start slow and go slow"
  - Risperidone 1 mg/day and olanzapine 5 to 10 mg/day improve symptoms, associated with increased risk of death in this patient population.
  - Lorazepam may be used short-term for behavioural emergencies.
  - Depression can be treated with SSRI.

Bibliography

Canadian Task Force on Preventive Health Care. Recommendations on screening for cognitive impairment in older adults. *CMAJ*. 2015;188(1):37-46.

Carnahan R, Lund B, Perry P, et al. The anticholinergic drug scale as a measure of drug-related anticholinergic burden: associations with serum anticholinergic activity. *J Clin Pharmacol*. 2006;46(12):1481.

Chen A, Tran C. Geriatric medicine. In: Pabani F, Rosenthal E, Goldlist BJ, et al, eds. *Toronto Notes* 2015. 31st ed. Toronto, ON: Toronto Notes for Medical Students; 2015:GM1-GM18.

Chertow H, Massoud F, Nasreddine Z, et al. Diagnosis and treatment of dementia: Mild cognitive impairment and cognitive impairment without dementia. *CMAJ*. 2008;178(10):1273.

CMA driver's guide: Determining medical fitness to operate motor vehicles. 8th ed. 2012. Available from: https://www.cma.ca/En/Pages/drivers-guide.aspx.

Feldman H, Jacova C, Robillard A, et al. Diagnosis and treatment of dementia: 2. Diagnosis. *CMAJ*. 2008;178(7):825.

Fitzpatrick-Lewis D, Warren R, Ali M, et al. Treatment of mild cognitive impairment: A systematic review and meta-analysis. *CMAJ*. 2015;3(4):E419-E427.

Gauthier S, Patterson C, Chertow H, et al. Recommendations of the 4th Canadian Consensus Conference on the diagnosis and treatment of dementia (CCCDTD4). *Can Geriat J*. 2012;15(4):120-126.

Guidelines and Protocols aAdvisory Committee. Cognitive impairment: Recognition, diagnosis and management in primary care. 2016. Available from: http://www2.gov.bc.ca/assets/gov/health/practitione-pro/bc-guidelines/cogimp-full-guideline.pdf.

Herrmann N, Gauthier S. Diagnosis and treatment of dementia: 2. Diagnosis. *CMAJ*. 2008;179(12):1279.

Hogan D, Bailey P, Black S, et al. Diagnosis and treatment of dementia: 4. Approach to management of mild to moderate dementia. *CMAJ*. 2008;179(8):787.

Hogan D, Bailey P, Black S, et al. Diagnosis and treatment of dementia: 5. Nonpharmacologic and pharmacologic therapy for mild to moderate dementia. *CMAJ*. 2008;179(10):1019.

Incapability assessments: A review of assessment and screening tools final report. Centre for Research on Personhood in Dementia, University of British Columbia. British Columbia: 2009. Available from: http://www.trustee.bc.ca/documents/STA/Incapability_Assessments_Review_Assessment_Screening_Tools.pdf.

Moore A, Patterson C, Lee L, et al. Fourth Canadian Consensus Conference on the Diagnosis and Treatment of Dementia: Recommendations for family physicians. *Can Fam Physician*. 2014;60:433-438.

Patterson C, Feighter J, Garcia A, et al. Diagnosis and treatment of dementia: 1. risk assessment and primary prevention of aAlzheimer disease. *CMAJ*. 2008;178(5):548.

Priority topics and key features with corresponding skill dimensions and phases of the encounter. 2010. Available from: http://www.cfpc.ca/uploadedFiles/Education/Priority%20Topics%20and%20Key%20 Features.pdf.

Mental Capacity and Competency

Priority Topic 64

KEY POINTS

- It is important to differentiate capacity from competency. Mental capacity implies a clinical status established by a health care professional whereas mental competency refers to a legal status as judged by a legal professional.
- Clues of possible cognitive impairment decline include concerns from family/ friends, difficulty managing medications, showing up on the wrong date for appointments, changes in behaviour, for example, decline in personal hygiene.
- Consider capacity when diagnoses are made which are associated with a higher likelihood of cognitive decline, for example, CVA, dementia, mental illness. However, a particular medical diagnosis does *not* indicate incompetency.
- Capacity may change over time and should be seen in the context of specific domains including, medical, cognitive and functional. This will impact the competency of the patient when assessed in a legal context.
  - Competence is situation-specific, for example, competence to care for self, to sign out AMA, to stand trial, sign a POA, change a will, and to make financial decisions. Moreover, financial competence for CEO of company differs from financial competency to run a household.
- To be incompetent in one area does not necessarily imply incompetence in another. For example, a patient may be competent to make care decisions but not financial decisions.

ASSESSMENT

- Standardized screening tests for cognitive decline are available (see Dementia Priority Topic 23)
- Assessing capacity and competence
  - Clinical interviewing for assessment of capacity is the gold standard
  - Type of questions depends on type of competence being assessed
  - Collect relevant collateral information as required
  - Patients can be referred for further assessment (eg, safety in kitchen cooking assessment)
  - For financial competency, questions could include: If you go to the store to buy milk and eggs how much do you expect that would cost? And who helps you pay bills?

LEGAL

- If a patient is not competent to make a decision, there is a hierarchical list of the legal substitute decision maker.
  - This varies by province—be aware of the legislation in your jurisdiction
  - There may be provisions for emergency situations.

- Think about the need to assess competence when patient is making decisions, for example, filling out documents such as advance directive.
  - Encourage patients to fill out documents prior to onset of impairment or early in progressive conditions

Bibliography

Incapability assessments: a review of assessment and screening tools final report. Centre for Research on Personhood in Dementia, University of British Columbia. British Columbia: 2009. Available from: http://www.trustee.bc.ca/documents/STA/Incapability_Assessments_Review_Assessment_Screening_Tools.pdf.

MacKay M. Financial and personal competence in the elderly: The position of the Canadian Psychiatric Association. *Can J Psy.* 1989;34:829.

Priority topics and key features with corresponding skill dimensions and phases of the encounter. 2010. Available from: http://www.cfpc.ca/uploadedFiles/Education/Priority%20Topics%20and%20Key%20Features.pdf.

Disability

Priority Topic 28

- Monitor, diagnose, and treat patients with disability.
- Assess all spheres of function including emotional, physical, and social (finances, employment, family).
- Assess patients with chronic medical conditions for disability.
- Use multifaceted management to minimize impact of the disability and prevent functional deterioration, for example, orthotics, lifestyle modification, time off work, community support, social workers, OT/PT, pharmacist.
  - Consider short- and long-term disability leave in your plan.
- Offer primary prevention strategies for patient at risk for disability (eg, exercises, braces, counselling, work modification, hand rails, lighting).
- Risk factors for disability: Elderly, mental illness, manual labour, chronic conditions, and frailty assessment.

FALLS

- More than one-third of people over 65 have a fall per year; significant morbidity and mortality are associated with falls.
- Differential diagnosis for falls:
  - Visual impairment, peripheral neuropathy, CVA, TIA, joint instability, deconditioning, medications effects, environmental or home hazards, orthostatic hypotension.
- Risk factors: Previous falls, balance impairment, decreased muscle strength, visual impairment, more than four medications or psychoactive drugs, gait impairment and walking difficulty, depression, dizziness or orthostasis, functional limitations, age >80 years, female, incontinence, cognitive impairment, arthritis, diabetes, pain.
- Assessment
  - Integrate fall assessment into complete history and physical assessment.
  - Quick screen: Ask about falls in the past year and problems with gait or balance, if yes do further assessment.
    - Ask about surrounding circumstances, associated symptoms and assess list of medications, acute and chronic medical problems, mobility level and cognitive and functional level.
  - Physical examination: Gait, sensory (hearing and vision), orthostatic vital signs, neurological and musculoskeletal assessment, depression and cognitive impairment screen, review appropriateness of footwear and gait aids.

- Prevention
  - Screen and treat osteoporosis if indicated.
  - Vitamin D 800 to 1000 IU/day (NNT 14 to prevent one fall).
  - Individualized exercise program (strength, gait, and balance) and gait aids.
  - Home safety assessment and modifications for high-risk individuals, for example, anti-slip shoe devices and hip protectors.
  - Gradual withdrawal of psychotropic medications (where appropriate).
  - Treat pain effectively.

Bibliography

Al-Aama T. Falls in the elderly: spectrum and prevention. *Can Fam Physician.* 2011;57:771.

Assessment of falls in the elderly. 2011. Available from: http://bestpractice.bmj.com/best-practice/monograph/880/diagnosis/differential-diagnosis.html.

Evidence-based best practices for the prevention of falls. 2009. Available from: http://www.phac-aspc.gc.ca/seniors-aines/publications/pro/injury-blessure/falls-chutes/chap4-eng.php.

Priority topics and key features with corresponding skill dimensions and phases of the encounter. 2010. Available from: http://www.cfpc.ca/uploadedFiles/Education/Priority%20Topics%20and%20Key%20Features.pdf.

Rao S. Prevention of falls in older patients. *Am Fam Physician.* 2005;72:81-8:93-94.

Palliative Care

Priority Topic 70

DEFINITION

"Palliative care is an approach that improves the quality of life of patients and their families facing the problem associated with life-threatening illness, through the prevention and relief of suffering by means of early identification and impeccable assessment and treatment of pain and other problems, physical, psychosocial and spiritual"

—World Health Organization

PRINCIPLES OF PALLIATIVE CARE

- Indicated for all patients with terminal conditions (not just cancer).
- Goal—To enhance quality of life.
- Early discussions and planning with multidisciplinary support and involvement of family/friends.
- Address/clarify patient wishes for end-of-life issues: Intubation, resuscitation, use of antibiotics, home versus hospital versus hospice. Review patient wishes often.
- Identify and address possible causes of requests for hastened death: Poor symptom management, depression, isolation, fear of dying, anxiety, and spiritual distress.
- Consider the whole patient (grief, sadness, loss, fear) and provide support to the patient and family.
  - The FIFE tool (Feelings—Ideas—Functions—Expectations) may be useful for this purpose.

MEDICATIONS

- Review medications according to changes in goals of therapy.
  - Stop medications no longer compatible with goals.
- Monitor for side effects of medication, anticipate and manage side effects.

- **Pain**: Use oral route if possible
  - Prescribe long-acting medications with short-acting for breakthrough pain
  - Add adjuvant pain medications (NSAIDs, steroids, bisphosphonates, cannabinoids)
- **Nausea**: Anticholinergics (eg, scopolamine), 5HT3 antagonists (eg, ondansetron), prokinetic (eg, metoclopramide), antihistamines (eg, dimenhydramine-less effective)
- **Dyspnea**: Position and increase air circulation, opiates are drug of choice, oxygen based on symptom improvement, manage cough/secretions/anxiety
- **Constipation**: Hydration, osmotic agents (PEG-tasteless and well tolerated), motility agents (senna), lubricating agents (docusate, glycerin suppository)

Bibliography

The Foundation for Medical Practice Education. End of life: chronic disease and transition of care. *BPLP*. 2011;19(2):2-4.

Information for health care professionals: Compassionate care. 2011. Available from: http://www.hrsdc .gc.ca/eng/publications_resources/health_care/ei_ccb.shtml.

Position statement—issues related to end of life care. 2015. Available from: http://www.cfpc.ca/uploaded Files/Resources/Resource_Items/Health_Professionals/CFPC%20Position%20Statement_Palliative %20Care_ENGLISH.pdf.

WHO definition of palliative care. 2011. Available from: http://www.who.int/cancer/palliative/definition/en/.

CHAPTER 13

Travel Medicine

Travel Medicine

Priority Topic 93

GENERAL TRAVEL/SAFETY ADVICE

(Refer to www.travel.gc.ca for more country-specific travel information. Also refer to your local travel clinic.)

- Accidents (wearing seatbelts) and vehicular trauma risks
- Safe sex practices
- Safe travel for women, pregnant women, children, immunocompromised patients, and those with chronic disease
- Drink water from only clean sources (no ice cubes, brush teeth with bottled water)
- Food: Only eat peeled or cooked fruit/vegetables; avoid street food, unpasteurized dairy, raw meat/seafood
- Proper hand washing and use of antiseptic gels/washes
- Sunscreen/sun protection
- Avoid intoxication and illicit drugs
- Use insect repellent and sleep under nets where appropriate
- Travel insurance and medical insurance

RISK ASSESSMENT: "FIVE Ws"

- Who—Healthy? Allergies? Medications? Age? Pregnancy? Breastfeeding? Reproductive age?
- Where—The exact location(s) you are travelling to (urban/rural, low-medium-high risk) and where you will be staying?
- What—What exact activities will you be doing there?
- When—When are you leaving and when are you coming back?
- Why—Group travel? Visiting family/friends? Military? Religious?

MEDICATIONS

- Ensure the patient has enough medication for their trip.
- Medication should always travel with the patient. If required for narcotics or needles, a letter from the physician documenting the need and number of medications and supplies should always be with the patient.
- A list of medications, their indications, and allergies should be kept in the patient's wallet.
- Ensure that the patient has an adequate understanding of how to manage medications and their chronic illnesses (thus eg, when to use steroid cream for psoriasis flares, when to use a PRN antibiotic + prednisone prescription for a COPD exacerbation).

VACCINATIONS

- For travel-specific vaccination, check online at travel.gc.ca since it varies from time to time and country to country.
- Always check that routine vaccinations are up to date: Hepatitis B, tetanus, MMR, pertussis, etc.

IN A RECENTLY RETURNED TRAVELLER

- In patients returning from travel with illness or a fever of unknown origin, take into account the risk of an infection acquired abroad that may have lain dormant or have an atypical presentation.
- For up-to-date information on geographic and seasonal patterns of disease and travel advisories, check the Web site for the United States Centers for Disease Control and Prevention (www.cdc.gov/travel) or Foreign Affairs Canada (travel.gc.ca).

COMMON CONDITIONS ASSOCIATED WITH TRAVEL

Motion Sickness

- Treatment
  - Lifestyle measures: Deep, controlled breathing; look forward to the distant horizon
  - Medications: Scopolamine (anticholinergic, 0.6 mg po 0.5 to 1 hour before travel or 1.5 mg patch 6-8 hours before travel) or dimenhydrinate

Jet Lag

- Symptoms: Insomnia, fatigue, generalized weakness, poor memory, difficulty concentrating, dysphoria, GI disturbance
- Worsened by travelling multiple time zones and travelling west to east (easier to lengthen a day than to shorten it)
- Treatment
  - Lifestyle measures: Intrinsic clock resets by 1-1½ h/day; light exposure optimization; seek out bright light in the morning after eastward travel and in the evening after westward travel; can use sunglasses to simulate darkness; may even shift sleep 1 to 2 hours earlier/later a few days before the trip; keep daytime naps <30 minutes
  - Medications: Melatonin 0.5 to 3 mg at local bedtime nightly if falling asleep *earlier* than at home; melatonin 0.5 mg during second half of night if adapting to later time

Altitude Sickness

- Patients may exhibit symptoms above 10,000 feet including dizziness, headache, SOB, change in mentation, somnolence, insomnia, hallucinations, nausea, vomiting, and decreased urinary output (major concern is developing cerebral edema).

- Slow and gradual ascent (<500 m/day) is recommended.
- If symptomatic, stop and descend until symptoms resolve (300-1000 m generally sufficient, but variable).
- Treatment: Dexamethasone 4 mg po/IM/IV q6h (if moderate/severe) and/or acetazolamide 250 mg bid (if mild); supplemental oxygen; hyperbaric oxygen; acetaminophen/ibuprofen if only mild headache.
- Prophylactic treatment: Acetazolamide 125 mg po bid 24 to 48 hours prior to ascent until 48 hours after peak altitude or symptoms disappear.

Traveller's Diarrhea

- Most common problem for travellers to developing countries
  - Usually a self-limiting problem → No treatment necessary (see also Table 13-1).

TABLE 13-1	Traveller's Diarrhea: Severity and Management	
SEVERITY OF ILLNESS	SYMPTOMS	TREATMENT
Mild–moderate	<3 bowel movements (BM)/day and no blood	Peptobismol, loperamide, oral rehydration (OR)
Moderate–severe	3-5 BM/day and no blood	OR and antibiotics (ciprofloxacin or azithromycin)
Severe	6+ BM/day or blood in stool ± fever	OR and antibiotics (ciprofloxacin or azithromycin)

  - Common pathogens: Enterotoxigenic *Escherichia coli* (ETEC), *Campylobacter*, *Salmonella*
- ETEC/cholera oral vaccine (Dukoral) has been shown to provide moderate, short-term protection against diarrhea caused by ETEC and cholera caused by *Vibrio cholerae*. It is not recommended as a complete prevention strategy as not everyone will be fully protected by the vaccine.

Bibliography

Chen YA, Tran C (eds). *The Toronto Notes*. 27th ed. Toronto, ON: Toronto Notes for Medical Students; 2011.

Committee to Advise on Tropical Medicine and Travel, Health Canada. Statement on New Oral Cholera and Travellers' Diarrhea Vaccination. http://www.phac-aspc.gc.ca/publicat/ccdr-rmtc/05vol31/-asc-dcc-7/index-eng.php. Accessed March 19, 2012.

DynaMed [Internet]. Ipswich (MA): EBSCO Information Services. 1995. Record No. 116210, Acute altitude illnesses; [updated 2014 Dec 15, cited 2016 Aug 28]; [about 13 screens]. Available from http://search.ebscohost.com.cyber.usask.ca/login.aspx?direct=true&db=dnh&AN=116210&site=dynamed-live&scope=site.

Dynamed [Internet]. Ipswich (MA): EBSCO Information Services. 1995. Record No. 115827. Melatonin for jet lag; [updated 2010 Jun 02, cited 2016 Nov 27]; [about 3 screens]. Available from http://search.ebscohost.com.cyber.usask.ca/login.aspx?direct=true&db=dnh&AN=115827&site=dynamed-live&scope=site.

Sack RL. Jet lag. *N Engl J Med*. 2010;362:440-447. doi 10.1056/NEJMcp0909838 Public Health Agency of Canada. Travel Medicine. http://www.phac-aspc.gc.ca/tmp-pmv/index-eng.php. Accessed March 19, 2012.

Zhang LL, Wang JQ, Qi RR, et al. Motion sickness: Current knowledge and recent advance. *CNS Neurosci Ther*. 2016;22(1):15-24.

MOSQUITO-BORNE DISEASE

1. **Malaria**

- Mosquito-borne parasitic disease caused by *Plasmodium* species: *P. falciparum* (most common + lethal) or *P. vivax, P. ovale, P. malariae, and P. knowlesi*. Results in infection/lysis of hepatocytes and RBCs.

- Clinical features
  - Starts 8 days to months post *Anopheles* mosquito bite
  - Paroxysmal/cyclical fever and chills (timing of fevers can help in diagnosing species)
  - Abdominal pain, diarrhea, headache, hepatosplenomegaly, thrombocytopenia, cerebral involvement—seizures/coma
- Investigations: Thick/thin blood smear (Giemsa stain)
- Prevention: Use treated bed-nets, avoid mosquitos, avoid dusk-dawn activities, use insect repellent with DEET and chemoprophylaxis
- Treatment/chemoprophylaxis
  - Chloroquine: Possibly safe in pregnancy, but cannot be used in most areas of Central America, Subsaharan African, or Southeast Asia due to resistance
  - Mefloquine: Possibly safe in pregnancy, some resistance in Southeast Asia
  - Doxycycline: Contraindicated in pregnancy and in children <8 years old
  - Atovaquone/proguanil (Malarone): Contraindicated in pregnancy
  - Primaquine: Contraindicated in pregnancy, reserved for areas with high *P. vivax*; must have negative lab test for G6PD before initiating per CDC

2. **Zika**

- Arbovirus
- Countries affected: Caribbean, Central America and Mexico, South America, Southeast Asia, Ocean Pacific Islands, and limited areas in North America (including parts of Florida) and West Africa
- Incubation: 3 to 12 days
- Three-fourths of people with virus are asymptomatic
- Transmission: Mosquitoes (*Aedes* species), sex
- Symptoms last 2 to 7 days
- Signs and symptoms
  - Maculopapular rash: Starts on face, spreads to body
  - Conjunctivitis
  - Eye pain
  - Pruritis
  - Headache
  - Weakness, lethargy
  - Myalgias, arthralgias
  - Arthritis
    - Hands, feet
  - Low grade fever (<38.5°C)
- Labs
  - RNA PCR: Serum, urine, CSF, amniotic fluid, or placental tissue
    - Detectable in serum for 3 to 5 days after symptom onset
    - Detectable in urine for up to 10 days after symptom onset
    - Unknown how long RNA remains detectable in amniotic fluid, so may only indicate current and not past fetal infection
  - Serology (ELISA): IgM
    - Positive as early as 5 days after symptom onset
    - False-positive with other flaviviruses such as dengue, West Nile, Yellow Fever, and Yellow Fever vaccination
    - May repeat q2 to 3 weeks for diagnostic increase (expect fourfold)
    - Confirmatory test: Zika plaque reduction
  - Both PCR and serology recommended by PHAC within 10 days of symptom onset
  - >10 to 14 days after symptom onset, do only serology

- Treatment
  - Supportive: Rest, hydration, antipyretics, analgesics
- Complications
  - Thrombocytopenia
  - Guillain-Barre syndrome
  - Meningoencephalitis
  - Fetal
    - Microcephaly (1% risk in first trimester)
    - Arthrogryposis (joint contractures)
    - Hydrops fetalis
    - Demise
    - IUGR
    - Placental insufficiency
- Management in pregnancy
  - Serial U/S q3 to 4 weeks
  - Microcephaly can be detected as early as 15 weeks
- Prevention
  - Abstinence or barrier contraceptives for anyone whose partner recently travelled to a Zika-prone area.
    - Women should wait 2 mo after return from Zika-prone area to conceive
    - May wait 6 mo to conceive if male partner travelled to Zika-prone area
  - Personal protective measures to Zika.
  - Women who are pregnant or thinking of becoming pregnant should avoid travel to Zika-prone areas.

3. **Chikungunya**
- Arbovirus, transmitted by *Aedes* mosquito
- Areas affected: Subtropical and tropical Africa, South Asia, Southeast Asia, Central America, South America, Indian Ocean islands
- Symptoms (3 to 7 days after infection)
  - Acute febrile illness (often >39°C)
  - Polyarthralgia/polyarthritis: Bilateral, symmetric, usually hands and feet +/− other joints
  - Maculopapular or petechial rash
  - N/V
  - Back pain
  - Conjunctivitis
  - H/A
  - Often self-limited, <10 days
- Complications (rare)
  - Neurologic (most common): Menigoencephalitis, Guillain-Barre, seizure
  - Others: Cardiac (peri- or myocarditis), renal (acute renal failure), ocular (retinitis, uveitis, optic neuritis), lymphadenopathy
- Investigations
  - Reverse transcriptase PCR: Detectable days 1 to 8.
  - Serology: IgM for acute infection.
  - Rule out dengue, as co-infection is common and requires more aggressive management.
- Treatment: Supportive, no antiviral available

4. **Dengue**
- Arbovirus, transmitted by *Aedes* mosquito
  - Vertical and transplant/blood transfusion transmission rare but reported
- Endemic to: Southeast Asia, Western Pacific, South and Central America, Eastern Mediterreanean, Africa
- Signs and symptoms
  - Often asymptomatic
  - Fever after 4 to10 day incubation period
  - N/V
  - Headache (classically retro-orbital)
  - Rash: Begins as facial or generalized flushing/erythema, then morbilliform or maculopapular eruption
  - Myalgias
  - Warning signs for severe dengue
    - Abdo pain
    - Vomiting
    - Mucosal bleeding: Nosebleeds, gums, petechiae
    - Lethargy
  - Severe dengue
    - Respiratory distress
    - Hemorrhage: Can be vaginal or gastrointestinal
- Investigations
  - CBC: Low WBCs; low platelets; high hematocrit if plasma leaking
  - Consider based on symptoms: renal panel, LFTs, U/A, lactate, cardiac enzymes, ECG, CXR
  - Dengue virus PCR: Needs to be collected in first 1 to 5 days of symptoms
  - Dengue antigen (NS1): First 1 to 6 days of symptoms
  - Viral culture: Needs to be collected in first 1 to 5 days of symptoms
  - Serology: IgM (acute, detectable as early as day 3 postinfection), IgG (may be detectable by day 7 of symptoms, may see fourfold increase in acute infection)
- Treatment: Supportive: monitoring, antipyretics, analgesics, blood transfusion, rehydration
  - Many require hospital admission
  - No antiviral available

Bibliography

Centres for Disease Control and Prevention. Yellow Book 2016. http://wwwnc.cdc.gov/travel/yellowbook /2016/infectious-diseases-related-to-travel/malaria. Accessed August 28, 2016.

DynaMed [Internet]. Ipswich (MA): EBSCO Information Services. 1995. Record No. 161709, Chikungunya fever; [updated 2016 Sep 15, cited 2016 Nov 28]; [about 11 screens]. Available from http://search.ebscohost.com.cyber.usask.ca/login.aspx?direct=true&db=dnh&AN=161709&site=dyna med-live&scope=site.

DynaMed [Internet]. Ipswich (MA): EBSCO Information Services. 1995. Record No. 116824, Dengue; [updated 2016 May 08, cited 2016 Nov 28]; [about 28 screens]. Available from http://search.ebscohost .com.cyber.usask.ca/login.aspx?direct=true&db=dnh&AN=116824&site=dynamed-live&scope=site.

Government of Canada. Zika virus. Updated 17 Nov 2016. Available at http://healthycanadians.gc.ca /diseases-conditions-maladies-affections/disease-maladie/zika-virus/index-eng.php.

Government of Canada. Zika virus infection: Global updated. Updated 17 Nov 2016. Available at https://travel.gc.ca/travelling/health-safety/travel-health-notices?_ga=1.243158210.114673946.1468261315.

Public Health Agency of Canada. Canada Communicable Disease Report: Volume 42-5, 5 May 2016. Available at http://www.phac-aspc.gc.ca/publicat/ccdr-rmtc/16vol42/dr-rm42-5/ar-01-eng.php.

Hepatitis

Priority Topic 45

DEFINITION

Inflammation of the liver. The condition can be self-limiting or progress to acute failure, or fibrosis or cirrhosis. Chronic hepatitis is defined as hepatitis persisting for >6 months.

ETIOLOGY

Hepatitis viruses (most cases of hepatitis worldwide), toxins, alcohol, medications, some industrial organic solvents, and plants, and autoimmune diseases

Causes of noninfective hepatitis:

Alcohol	Excessive intake
Autoimmune	Idiopathic
Drug-induced	Acetaminophen, INH, tetracyclines, antiepileptics, phenytoin

Transmission of infective hepatitis:

Hepatitis A/E	Fecal-oral
Hepatitis B/C	Blood/sexual

ACUTE HEPATITIS

Symptoms

Flu-like illness, RUQ pain, jaundice, pruritus, change in bowel habit, arthralgia, fatigue, fever, nausea/vomiting

Risk Factors

IVDU, travel to hepatitis-endemic areas, contaminated foods (hepatitis A), blood/bodily fluid contacts, alcohol intake, pharmacological history, toxic ingestions, high-risk sexual activity, blood transfusion prior to 1990, newborn from infected mother, tattoos, HIV+

Prevention

Vaccinate individuals at high risk of hepatitis A/B and offer postexposure prophylaxis for hepatitis A/B along with harm reduction measures where indicated.

No vaccine is available for Hepatitis C. Diagnose and treat early for improved cure and complication rates.

Investigations

- Liver function tests (see Table 13-2)
  - Raised AST/ALT from liver damage; if >1000 increased likelihood of viral/drug-induced
  - ALP + GGT raised is likely cholestasis
- PT/INR (sensitive for impaired hepatic function)
- Bilirubin
- Ultrasound should be performed if obstructive cause is being considered
- "ToAST with alcohol" —Alcohol-related hepatitis: AST:ALT > 2:1
- "virAL"—Viral-related hepatitis: ALT >5x normal

TABLE 13-2	Hepatitis: Liver Function Testing		
TEST	**NORMAL**	**HEPATOCELLULAR**	**OBSTRUCTIVE**
Direct bilirubin (conjugated)	0-5 mmol/L	▲	▲
Total bilirubin	2-20 umol/L	▲	▲
ALT	10-40 u/L	▲	Transient ▲
AST	15-40 u/L	▲	–
Alk phos	30-155 u/L	▲	▲▲▲

CHRONIC HEPATITIS

Definition: Serum transaminases increased for 6 months from any cause: autoimmune, infective.

Rule out obstructive causes for elevated enzymes with ultrasound +/− ERCP.

At risk of ascites, cirrhosis, and hepatocellular carcinoma.

VIRAL HEPATITIS

Hepatitis A

- Etiology: Fecal-oral transmission with 4 to 6 week incubation period
- Prognosis
  - Self-limiting
  - Possible relapse but never chronic
  - Can acutely cause hepatic failure and death

Hepatitis B (see Table 13-3)

- Etiology: Maternal → fetal, sexual contact, blood-borne transmission, IVDU
- Prognosis
  - May be self-limiting or chronic
  - Age at infection is inversely related to risk of chronic infection
  - Cirrhosis develops in 15% to 20% of cases with chronic hepatitis B
  - Hepatocellular carcinoma (HCC) develops in 10% to 15% of cases with chronic hepatitis B

TABLE 13-3	Hepatitis B Seromarkers			
	HBsAg (surface antigen)	HBsAb (surface antibody)	HBeAg (core antigen)	HBeAb (core antibody)
Acute hepatitis B	+	−	+	−
Chronic (high infectivity)	+	−	+	−
Chronic (low infectivity)	+	−	−	+
Resolved	−	+/−	−	+/−
Immunization	−	+	−	−

- Infectivity/transmissibility is assessed using HBeAg or HBV DNA (PCR)
- Carrier state/active infection is assessed by continued presence of HBsAg
- Past infection or immunization is assessed by anti-HBs

Hepatitis C

- Aetiology: Blood-borne transmission (IVDU), blood transfusion prior to 1992, body fluids
- Clinical manifestations occur about 2 months after infection
- Diagnosis: Positive serum HCV-RNA (positive 2 weeks postinfection). Note: serum HCV-RNA (viral load) levels inversely correlate with response to treatment.
- Prognosis
  - Acute or chronic: Chronic hepatitis C develops in 80% of those exposed
  - Of those who develop chronic hepatitis C, 20% go on to develop cirrhosis
  - Of those who develop cirrhosis, 1% to 4% goes on to develop HCC (hepatocellular carcinoma)
- Chronic hepatitis C
  - Refer for specialist care.
  - Consider treatment with antivirals—especially if liver fibrosis/cirrhosis, consistently raised liver enzymes, age <50, hepatitis C genotype 2 or 3.
  - HCV-RNA should be measured at conclusion of 3 months of treatment then 3-6 months after treatment is completed.

- If patient is not a candidate for treatment, monitor for HCC: ultrasound and serum alfa-fetoprotein levels.

Hepatitis D

- Coinfection with hepatitis B only (cannot have hepatitis D without having hepatitis B)
- Treat with interferon
- Transplant for end-stage disease

Hepatitis E

- Rarely seen in North America, usually a self-limiting disease
- Etiology: Fecal-oral transmission
- Consider in patients returning from endemic areas with hepatitis symptoms
- High mortality rate in pregnant patents

JAUNDICE

(Supplementary Topic)

- Definition: A yellow pigmentation of the skin, conjunctivae, and other mucous membranes caused by hyperbilirubinemia
  - Signs and symptoms: Dark urine and pale stools, RUQ pain, pruritus
  - Investigations: CBC, bilirubin, liver enzymes and function tests, amylase

TABLE 13-4	Differential Diagnosis for Causes of Jaundice
UNCONJUGATED (INDIRECT) HYPERBILIRUBINEMIA	CONJUGATED (DIRECT) HYPERBILIRUBINEMIA
Hemolysis Drugs Neonatal Gilbert/Crigler–Najjar syndromes	Hepatocellular disease Primary sclerosing cholangitis Primary biliary cirrhosis Sepsis Gallstones Biliary stricture Malignancy Metastases

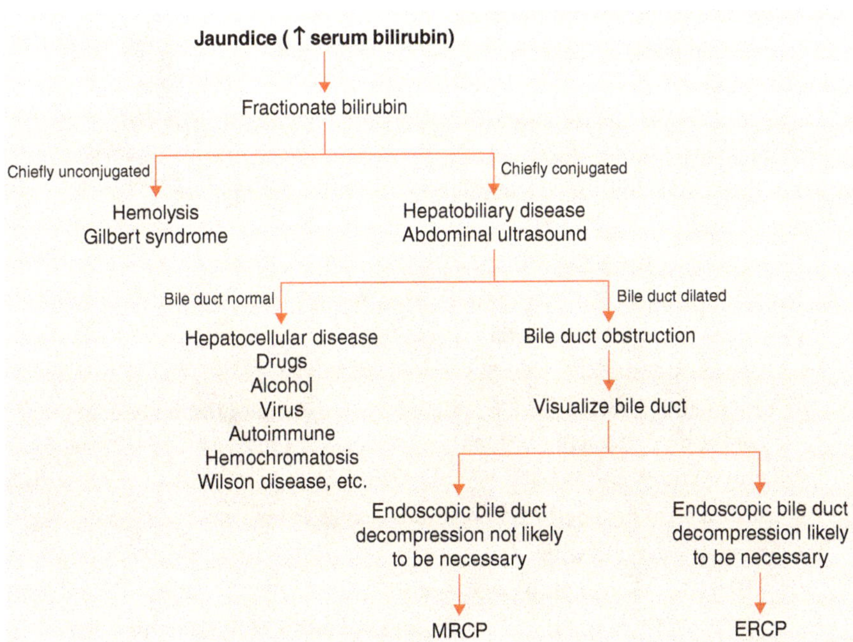

FIGURE 13-1:   Approach to jaundice. Source: Chen YA, Tran C (eds). *The Toronto Notes*. 27th ed., 2011.

Bibliography

Chen YA, Tran C (eds). *The Toronto Notes*. 27th ed. Toronto, ON: Toronto Notes for Medical Students; 2011.

Immigrant Health

Priority Topic 48

- Foreign born individuals account for almost 20% of the Canadian population.
- Immigrants are eligible for healthcare coverage under the Canada Health Act. However, there are sometimes specified wait times of up to 90 days and this is an active area of federal legislation and controversy.

Preimmigration Health Examination

- All immigrants undergo an Immigration Medical Examination (IME) preceding arrival in Canada. The purpose of the IME is to assess the potential burden of illness and limit number of public health risks. It is not designed to provide clinical preventive screening. The first visit examination should therefore include deficits from the IME examination.
- The IME includes:
  - Complete physical examination including vision and hearing screen
  - CXR (age 11 and older) to screen for TB
  - Syphilis serology
  - Urinalysis (age 5 and older), dipstick for protein, glucose, blood, and if positive, microscopy
  - HIV testing (age 15 and older, as well as for children who have received blood or have a known HIV+ mother)

The First Visit—Once in Canada

- The patient–doctor communication and relationship can be more challenging. Modify your approach when possible to accommodate cultural differences.
- Language—If necessary have an interpreter present during visits. Be aware of the limitations of nonmedical and family interpreters. Be aware of existing interpreter services in your area, including professional telephone interpreter services such as CanTalk.
- Document all findings. Take note of cultural/ritualistic scarring versus scars from possible torture.
- When patient presents with illness, inquire about the use of alternative therapies/herbal remedies.
- Other items to include in new immigrant first visit examination:
  - Tuberculosis
    - Test if from a country with high prevalence
    - Investigations: CXR; PPD/Mantoux test (not a marker of disease activity); sputum for acid fast bacteria
    - Symptoms/signs: Night sweats, weight loss, fatigue, chronic cough, hemoptysis
    - Treatment (empiric): RIPE (rifampin, INH, pyrazinamide, ethambutol) + vitamin B_6. Preferably, refer to a TB treatment clinic.
  - Other infectious diseases
    - Malaria—Do not routinely screen/test only if symptoms.
    - Screen for the following:
      - Hep B/C—Screen using serology
      - HIV—If from a country with high rates and immigrated to Canada before age 15
      - Intestinal parasites

- ◦ Chronic diseases—Consider screening for the following:
  - ▫ DM
  - ▫ Iron deficiency anemia
  - ▫ Sickle cell disease
  - ▫ Thalassemia
- Mental health
  - ◦ Depression: Immigrants are at a higher risk than the general public. Monitor for and link new immigrants with resources that can aid in transition to Canada
  - ◦ Torture/abuse—Inquire about past history as appropriate
- Women's health—Discuss contraceptive options, cervical cancer screening, and immunization for HPV
- Routine screening—Bring patient up to date with Canadian screening guidelines (mammography, FIT testing for colon cancer, etc.)
- Vaccination
  - ◦ Assess vaccination status and plan a schedule to bring patient up to date
  - ◦ The following vaccinations should be considered:
    - ▫ Hepatitis A/B
    - ▫ If patient tests positive for sickle cell or beta-thalassemia:
      - Pneumococcal (polysaccharide and conjugated)
      - *Haemophilus influenzae*
      - Meningococcal
- Influenza
- Varicella—High rate of adult VZV in temperate climates
- If vaccination status unknown:
  - ◦ Start on primary immunization schedule according to age
  - ◦ No concerns about adverse events for revaccination for MMR, polio, *H. influenzae* B, pneumococcal, meningococcal, hepatitis A/B, varicella, influenza

Bibliography

Citizenship and Immigration Canada. http://www.cic.gc.ca/english/department/what.asp. Accessed November 18, 2012.

The Foundation for Medical Practice Education. New Immigrants and refugees: screening and health care. *Educational Module.* 2011 Nov;19(12). www.fmpe.org. Accessed November 18, 2012.

Health Canada, Healthy Living, Just for You—Immigrants. http://www.hc-sc.gc.ca/hl-vs/jfy-spv/ immigrants-eng.php. Accessed November 18, 2012.

Pottie K, Greenaway C, Feightner J, et al. Evidence-based clinical guidelines for immigrants and refugees. *Can Med Assoc J.* 2011;183(12):E824-E925. http://www.cmaj.ca/cgi/collection/canadian_guidelines_for_immigrant_health. Accessed November 18, 2012.

CHAPTER 14

Social Medicine/Psychology

Domestic Violence

Priority Topic 30

DEFINITION

Violence is any action, inaction, or threat, regardless of intent or intensity that results in either physical or psychological injury to an individual, family, or community.

- No lower limit of harm, thus no minimum intensity to violence.
- Good intent (discipline) does not transform violence to nonviolence.
- Psychological injury often has greater and more long-lasting consequences for people living with violence or the ongoing threat of violence.

RISK FACTORS

- Low socioeconomic status
- Pregnancy
- Disability
- Age 18 to 24
- History of abuse
- Substance abuse

MECHANISM OF VIOLENCE

Fear: Fear is the power tool used to control others, thus violence is the manifestation of fear that is intended to control another.

Control: Controlling individuals prefer the position of having power over others. Their actions maintain a differential of power typically through degradation, isolation, and impoverishment. The tenuous position of power is maintained with the constant atmosphere of fear.

CYCLE OF VIOLENCE

1. Tension build up: Here an individual gradually ramps up the fear and threats to establish control.
2. Violent outburst: The episode of violence with anger, verbal, emotional, or physical abuse.

3. Honeymoon phase: Declaration of remorse and promises of love and better times to come.

4. The honeymoon ends and soon the ramping up begins the next turn of the cycle but this time the cycle is shorter and reaches a higher level more quickly ending with more severe violence.

MANAGEMENT

Recognize: Identify unhealthy relationships where violence and abuse can occur

Relate: Assess the stage of readiness for change

Refer: Offer choices:

- Determine immediate and long-term risk to patient and children → Ask about weapons in home.
- Make safe exit plan for all involved → Safe place to go, essentials together if needing a quick exit.
- Provide options for community resources, shelters, experts, and programs.
- Reassure that the patient is not to blame.
- Support the adult victim but do not make decisions for them or tell them what they must do.
- Make clear documentation of all events.
- In children and elderly if abuse is suspected, confirmed or witnessed it must be reported.

Bibliography

Doctors Opposing Violence Everywhere (DOVE). *Clinical Practice Guideline.* Accessed January 2015.

http://www.cfpc.ca/uploadedFiles/Education/Priority%20Topics%20and%20Key%20Features.pdf. Accessed June 5, 2016.

Towards Optimizing Practice (TOP)—Motivational Interview with Survivors of Violence. *Clinical Practice Guidelines.* January 2015.

Rape/Sexual Assault

Priority Topic 78

- Between 50% and 80% of sexual assaults from someone known to survivor
- Immediate care includes legal, medical, and psychosocial
- May present to emergency department or to family physician's office where a referral could be made depending on:
  1. Availability of another site for assessment
  2. Time available to complete the evaluation
  3. Experience with evaluation and treatment
  4. Ability to collect and preserve appropriate evidence

HISTORY

- Critical to ensure survivor knows she is safe and not to blame. History is taken in a gentle, nonjudgmental way and recorded in patient's exact words.
- Document the patient's identifying information. Include the date, time, location, and specific circumstances of the assault.
- Document any use of restraints (eg, weapons, drugs, alcohol).

- Document the patient's gynecological history (including most recent consensual sexual encounter).
- Limit documentation to observation and other necessary medical information (ie, avoid recording hearsay).

PHYSICAL EXAMINATION

- Consent from survivor should be obtained for each step of examination to allow survivor to gain a sense of control and may be a legal requirement.
- Examine entire body. In the absence of major trauma collection of evidence is done concurrently with the physical examination.
- Collector must be trained and familiar with sexual assault kit (used up to 72 hours).
- Drug facilitated sexual assault must be considered when patient reports amnesia or "that something sexual happened".
- Alcohol is the most common substance associated with sexual assault.
- Chloral hydrate, Gamma hydroxybuterate, ketamine, and benzodiazepines are detectable in urine up to 72 hours.

INVESTIGATIONS

- Urine and serum β-hCG (5% risk of pregnancy)
- A complete STI screen:
  - HIV
  - Serum VDRL or rapid plasma regain
  - Urine PCR for gonorrhea, chlamydia
  - HBsAg + HBcIgM, HCV—not routinely recommended
  - Wet mount preparation for detection of sperm (motile up to 6 hours)

MANAGEMENT

- Major trauma requires immediate attention and takes priority over further forensic evaluation.
- Emergency contraception should be given to all women of child bearing age, for example, plan B which is effective within 12 hours, up to 5 days
- Hep B vaccination (if not immune).
- HIV prophylaxis may be started based on risk assessment. (HIV serology is to be checked at baseline, 6 weeks, 3, and 6 months.)
- Prophylaxis against gonorrhoea, chlamydia, trichomoniasis (azithromycin 1 g po once + metronidazole 2 g po once + ceftriaxone 250 mg IM once).
- Victims often present with disbelief, anxiety, fear, and guilt; thus provide psychological support. Counselling should be offered to all involved parties.
- Avoid "second rape" feeling when possible—defined as secondary victimization from legal, medical, and mental health systems.
- Long-term issues experienced include depression, PTSD, variety of medical and psychosocial issues including chronic pelvic pain, headaches, IBS, alcohol and drug abuse, and sleep disorders, thus provide close and periodic long-term follow-up.

Bibliography

http://www.cfpc.ca/uploadedFiles/Education/Priority%20Topics%20and%20Key%20Features.pdf. Accessed June 5, 2016.

Luce H, Schrager S, Gilchrist V. Sexual assault of women. *Am Family Physician*. 2010:81(4):489-495.

Violent/Aggressive Patient

Priority Topic 98

- All healthcare workers, especially general practitioners and staff in emergency departments, are likely to encounter aggression and violence. This behaviour may be caused by a medical illness, a psychiatric illness, or drug intoxication or withdrawal.

- Some patients try to use aggression as means of achieving a particular goal, such as being seen earlier or obtaining drugs.

- Medical illness may result in behaviour disturbance. It can also coexist in patients with mental health, drug and alcohol problems, or other conditions.

- Medical conditions which can cause aggression:
  - Hypoxia, hypercarbia—Pneumonia, worsening chronic airway disease
  - Hypoglycaemia—Diabetes, malnourished alcoholic
  - Cerebral insult—Stroke, tumour, seizure, encephalitis, meningitis, trauma
  - Sepsis—Systemic sepsis, urine infection in the elderly
  - Metabolic disturbance—Hyponatremia, thiamine deficiency, hypercalcemia
  - Organ failure—Liver or renal failure
  - Withdrawal—Alcohol, benzodiazepines
  - Drug effects—Amphetamine, steroids, alcohol, prescribed medications, and interactions

PREVENTION

- Signs should make clear that aggression and violence are not tolerated.
- A functioning duress system and protocols for responding.
- The assessment area should have no dangerous objects.

ASSESSMENT

- Look for clues that the behaviour disturbance may be due to an organic cause.
- A general physical examination including:
  - Measure the pulse, blood pressure, and temperature
  - Basic blood tests such
  - Clues that a psychiatric cause is likely

DE-ESCALATION

- Use an empathic nonconfrontational approach, but set boundaries.
- Listen to the patient, avoid excessive stimulation.
- Recruit family, friends, and case managers to help.
- Address medical issues especially pain and discomfort.
- Try to ascertain what the patient actually wants and the level of urgency.

PHARMACOLOGICAL MANAGEMENT

- Diazepam 5 to 10 mg oral or intravenously. Max 30 mg per event.
- Lorazepam 2 mg. Max 10 mg in 24 hours. Parodoxical reactions.
- Midazolam 5 to 10 mg intramuscularly. Max 20 mg per event. Rapid onset.
- Olanzapine 5 to 10 mg oral. Max 30 mg per event.
- Haloperidol 5 to 10 mg intramuscularly. Max 20 mg per event.
- Acute dystonia—Benztropine 2 mg oral or intramuscularly or intravenously

Bibliography

Fulde G. Managing aggressive and violent patients. *Australian Prescriber.* 2011;34(3). Accessed
   July 15, 2016.

http://www.cfpc.ca/uploadedFiles/Education/Priority%20Topics%20and%20Key%20Features.pdf.
   Accessed June 5, 2016.

Stress

Priority Topic 87

1. Symptoms that could be attributed to stress could be physical or emotional:
   - Anxiety, back pain, constipation or diarrhoea, depression, feeling tired,
     headaches, high blood pressure, relationship problems, shortness of breath,
     stiff neck, trouble sleeping, upset stomach, weight gain or loss
2. Assess the impact of the stress on patient's function (ie, coping vs not coping,
   stress vs distress).
3. In patients not coping with stress, look for and diagnose, if present, mental illness
   (eg, depression, anxiety disorder).
   - Screen for major depression, eating disorder, general anxiety disorder, panic
     disorder, acute stress disorder, PTSD, and panic disorder.
4. In patients not coping with the stress in their lives,
   - Clarify and acknowledge the factors contributing to the stress.
   - Explore their resources and possible solutions for improving their situations.
5. In patients experiencing stress, look for inappropriate coping mechanisms
   (eg, drugs, alcohol, eating, violence).
   - Must screen for substance abuse, alcohol abuse, eating disorders, and
     over-working.

Bibliography

http://www.aafp.org/afp/2006/1015/p1385.html. Accessed January 3, 2017.

http://www.cfpc.ca/uploadedFiles/Education/Priority%20Topics%20and%20Key%20Features.pdf.
   Accessed June 5, 2016.

Crisis Management

Priority Topic 19

- Four per cent of primary care visits involve psychiatric or social crises.
- Crisis is defined as "when a person is confronted with a critical incident or
  stressful event that is perceived as overwhelming despite the use of traditional
  problem-solving and coping strategies."
- Physicians can assist patients by:
  - Evaluating the nature of the problem, determine patient's mental status
  - Ensuring the safety of the patient and others
  - Aid patient in developing an action plan to minimize distress and obtaining
    patient commitment
  - Follow-up with patient on progress and possibly provide additional support
- Steps for the physician in crisis management:
  1. Reassure the patient that it is safe to discuss crisis
     - Establish report by active listening and nonverbal skills

2. Evaluate crisis severity and patient status
   - Psychiatric and medical statuses.
   - May have to contact family member for additional information.
   - Assessing psychiatric status is important because depression, schizophrenia, bipolar disorder, borderline personality disorder, and substance abuse or dependency greatly increases suicide risk.
   - When dealing with an unanticipated medical crisis, assess the environment for needed resources, stay calm and ask for help.
3. Ensuring the safety of the patient and others
   - There is increased risk of suicide and homicide with a history of aggressive behaviour to self or others, criminal behaviour, abuse or witness to domestic violence as a child, low intelligence, neurologic impairment, hostility, substance abuse or dependency, and perceptions of threat or of someone else controlling one's thoughts.
   - If the patient is homicidal, the physician must ensure the safety of the patient and of potential victims.
4. Develop action plan
   - Assist in developing constructive response and plan to crisis.
   - First reassure patient, then teach relaxation techniques (deep breathing); may consider use of short-term pharmacological therapies (eg, anxiolytics and hypnotics)
   - The action plan goal is to restore emotional stability, and must incorporate realistic and positive steps.
   - Offer appropriate community resources (counsellor, etc).
5. Follow-up improves the patient's likelihood of adherence to the action plan and provides patients with a lifeline.

Bibliography

http://www.cfpc.ca/uploadedFiles/Education/Priority%20Topics%20and%20Key%20Features.pdf. Accessed June 5, 2016.

Kavan MG, Guck TP, Barone EJ. A practical guide to crisis management. *Am Fam Physician.* 2006;74(7):1159-1164.

Family Issues
Priority Topic 37

- Routinely ask about family issues to understand their impact on the patient's illness and the impact of the illness on the family.
- Explore family issues periodically and at important lifecycle points:
  - Bader's family lifecycle stages
- Leaving home:
  - Establishing personal independence
  - Beginning the emotional separation from parents
- Commitment to the couple relationship:
  - Establishing an intimate relationship with partner
  - Further development of emotional separation from parents
- Learning to live together
  - Dividing the various couple roles in an equitable way
  - Establishing a new, more independent relationship with family and friends

- Parenting the first child
  - Opening the family to include a new member
  - Dividing the parenting roles
- Living with the adolescent:
  - Increasing the flexibility of the boundaries to allow the adolescent(s) to move in and out of the family system
  - Refocusing on midlife marital and career issues
- Launching children: The empty nest phase:
  - Accepting the multitude of exits from and entries into the family system
  - Adjusting to the ending of parenting roles
- Retirement:
  - Adjusting to the end of the wage-earning roles
  - Developing new relationships with children, grandchildren, and each other
- Old age:
  - Dealing with lessening abilities and greater dependence on others.
  - Dealing with losses of friends, family members, and eventually each other.
  - In the normal aging process, there is often a decline in physiologic function, however, treatment of diabetes mellitus, hypertension, and glaucoma and other debilitating conditions can prevent significant future morbidity.
  - It is important that physicians weigh the potential harms of screening before screening older patients. It is essential to consider family preferences regarding treatment if a disease is detected, and the patient's functional status, comorbid conditions, and predicted life expectancy.

Bibliography

Elsawy B, Higgins KE. The geriatric assessment. *Am Fam Physician.* 2011;83(1):48-56.

http://www.cfpc.ca/uploadedFiles/Education/Priority%20Topics%20and%20Key%20Features.pdf. Accessed June 5, 2016.

Poon V, Bader E. *Individual and Family Life Cycles:* Predicting Important Transition Points. 2014. Family and Community Medicine University of Toronto.

Bad News

Priority Topic 9

Bad news defined as "any news that drastically and negatively alters the patient's view of her or his future."

- Physicians may be judged on attitude, clarity of the message, privacy, and ability to answer questions when giving bad news. It becomes not an isolated skill but a set of communication skills.

The ABCDE mnemonic of bad news:

- **A**dvance preparation: Familiarize yourself with the family, history, given enough time, prepare both mentally and physically by rehearsing how you will deliver the news.
- **B**uild a therapeutic environment/relationship: Foreshadow bad news with *"I am afraid I have some bad news,"* use touch where appropriate, avoid humour, and assure patient you will be available.
  - Possibly have family members present. Must obtain patient consent before involving family members.
- **C**ommunicate well: Find out what the patient already knows. Speak frankly but compassionately, ask if the patient understands and encourage questions by listening.
  - Add a summary at the end because patients may not remember all the information.

- **D**eal with patient and family reactions: Be empathetic while assessing the emotional reaction of patient; avoid being defensive for or criticizing colleagues.
- **E**ncourage and validate emotions: Explore what the news means to the patient, offer realistic hope, and provide interdisciplinary care as needed for further care. Take care of own emotions and emotions of staff.

After giving bad news, arrange scheduled follow-up opportunities to evaluate patient's impact and understanding.

Bibliography

http://www.cfpc.ca/uploadedFiles/Education/Priority%20Topics%20and%20Key%20Features.pdf. Accessed June 5, 2016.

Vandekieft GK. Breaking bad news. *Am Fam Physician*. 2001;64(12):1975-1978.

Difficult Patient

Priority Topic 27

- Prevalence of difficult patient is 15% of most practices.
- A high level of trust and communication are required to maintain a successful patient–doctor relationship.
- The physician–patient relationship is of primary importance in the overall healthcare delivery model.
- In difficult patient interactions consider that difficulties may be traced to patient, physician, or healthcare system.
  - Patient factors include psychiatric disorders, personality disorders, or subclinical behavioural traits.
  - Physician factors include overwork, poor communication skills, low level of experience, and discomfort with uncertainty.
  - Healthcare system factors include productivity pressures, change in healthcare financing, fragmentation of visits, and availability of outside information that challenge the physician's authority.
- A considerable number of patients who are labelled difficult meet Axis II criteria for diagnosis of personality disorder.
- When confronted with difficult patient interactions, seek out and update, when necessary, information about the patient's life circumstances, current context, and functional status.
- Management of such patients routinely should begin with tactful assessment of patient's distress. With screening for depression, anxiety, substance abuse, and somatoform disorder.
- Take steps to end physician–patient relationship when it is in the patient's best interest or when the patient is threatening or demanding.

Bibliography

Haas LJ, Leiser JP, Magill MK, et al. Management of the difficult patient. *Am Fam Physician*. 2005;72(10): 2063-2068.

http://www.cfpc.ca/uploadedFiles/Education/Priority%20Topics%20and%20Key%20Features.pdf. Accessed June 5, 2016.

http://www.cpso.on.ca/CPSO/media/uploadedfiles/policies/policies/policyitems/ending_rel.pdf?ext=.pdf. Accessed September 5, 2016.

CHAPTER 15

Preparation for the SOO

The SOO—Overview, Nine Helpful Questions and How to Attack It

The SOO is a 15-minute simulated office oral examination. There are four SOOs that each examinee must complete as part of the CFPC examination, and there are two problems incorporated into each SOO. The SOO is **not** only a medical aspect but also an oral examination. It is your job to identify and manage each problem both socially and medically. The marking grid for the SOO can be divided in 11 sections (see Table 15-1)—only 4 of them are medical!!

TABLE 15-1	Simplified SOO Marking Grid
PROBLEM 1	**PROBLEM 2**
1. Identification—*medical*	5. Identification—*medical*
2. Illness experience	6. Illness experience
3. Management—*medical*	7. Management—*medical*
4. Finding common ground	8. Finding common ground
Overall SOO social and developmental context	
9. Identification of the issues	10. Integration of issues into interview/problems
11. Overall interview process and organization	

The "9 SOO things" listed below should help with the nonmedical sections.

"9 SOO THINGS" to include:

You do not have to ask these questions in any particular order but always try to ask all nine questions in each SOO.

1. Timeline of the symptoms (ie, how long have you been battling this problem?— Gives a sense of the impact on their life.)

2. What are you (the patient) worried this is? (Cancer, heart attack, brain tumour ….)

3. Family:
    - Married—Doing well and good relationship?
    - Kids—Doing well and good relationship?

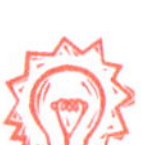

9 SOO Questions

1. Timeline
2. What are you worried about (cancer?, etc)
3. Family
4. Social support (friends, religion, etc)
5. Job and finances
6. Disease self-limited or lifelong
7. Physical examination
8. Elderly: Will, advance directives, etc.
9. Family meeting

Tip: Feel free to write a few things down during the SOO (they provide you with a blank paper and pen/pencil in the examination room)—it might help you summarize and make your management plan. It also can help you be a bit more personable if you aren't a person that can remember names—write it on your paper and use their name once or twice during your interview.

- Mom/dad—Alive and good relationship?
- Siblings—Doing well and good relationship?
- In-laws—Doing well and good relationship?

4. Social supports (family/friends/activities/religion)—Ask about each of the four areas.
5. Job and finances.
6. Tell patient if the disease/problem is a lifelong illness or self-limited.
7. Always state you're going to bring them back for a physical examination—mention what you want to do and be fairly specific, for example, "I want to bring you back for a physical and I'm going to do" … Have a differential of two to three diagnoses for each medical problem and list the testing you'd like to do/order to exclude/include each diagnosis.
8. If the patient is an elderly make sure to ask about a will, power of attorney, and advanced directive.
9. Always offer to have a family meeting or to talk to their family about whatever problem the patient is having or social situation, etc.

HOW TO ATTACK THE SOO—A SUGGESTED APPROACH

The SOO is not a re-enactment of a typical first encounter between a patient and their family physician. It is meant to demonstrate the various aspects that contribute to the patient's overall problem(s) and well-being, and some of the factors that contribute to the development of a therapeutic bond between a patient and family physician. It may seem out of place to ask many of the questions when you are meeting a patient for the first time. If you want to do well on the SOO, you must incorporate some of these questions into your approach (see Table 15-2).

TABLE 15-2	SOO—Steps to Organizing Your Attack	
STEPS TO ORGANIZE YOUR ATTACK		**9 SOO THINGS**
1. Introduce yourself, and state the patients' name.		
2. **HINT/CLUE 1:** The patient gives away problem 1 in their opening statement of why they came to the doctor.		
3. Attack the SOO by starting with the first problem and asking all the pertinent medical questions including Q1 and Q2 from the 9 SOO things. If you have a tentative diagnosis be sure and mention it.		1 and 2
4. Move onto social questions: How's the family (married, parents, in-laws, etc.)? finances? Etc. ….		3, 4, and 5
5. **HINT/CLUE 2:** At approximately 5 minutes (10 minutes remaining) the patient will give a hint/clue to the second problem.		
6. Start on problem 2—Often this is a social or psychiatric problem. If you haven't already, start questioning the patient about supports, and finances/job (questions 4 and 5). Make sure to still include any medical questions related to this problem. Also, if you have a tentative diagnosis, be sure and mention it.		1, 2, 3, 4, and 5
7. At 3-4 minutes left (the patient will give you a signal) summarize! An example: "It looks like we have two issues going on here, let's make a plan for each of these together."		
8. Make a management plan for each problem including a physical examination, lab testing, arranging a family meeting, prognosis for the disease/reassurance ….		6, 7, 8, and 9

Be aware, you may stumble on the second problem before the second clue is given (when you start asking the social questions after problem 1). This can result in being unsure of the exact second problem, as they won't give you the hint/clue if you've already found the problem—but remember, if it's social and there is a lot going on in the patient's life, you do not need a specific name for the problem. Example "you have two issues: one is your poor diabetes control and the second is your social situation." Additionally, the plan for most social problems is often the similar—family meeting, social work/counselling, offer follow-up, make them aware of community resources or support groups, etc.

CHAPTER 16

Short Answer Management Problems (SAMPs)[1]

1. Karen is a 32-year-old woman who presented in emergency with a 12-hour history of increasing abdominal pain centred around the epigastrium. She states she has nausea, no vomiting, and no change in bowel habits. She states the pain is 7/10 and "seems to go straight through to the back." On examination of the abdomen, you note guarding in the epigastrium.
   a. What is essential to be ruled out in this particular presentation? Pregnancy
   b. Name five initial lab investigations you would like to perform:
      i. AST, ALT, ALP, GGT, amylase/lipase, bilirubin: direct and indirect; WBC, Hb, glucose, and β HCG, urinalysis: leukocytes, nitrites, RBCs; urea, and creatinine.
   c. With a presentation of acute epigastric pain list five possible differential diagnoses:
      i. Biliary/liver: Cholecystitis, cholangitis, cholelithiasis, and hepatitis
      ii. Pancreas: Pancreatitis, pancreatic mass/malignancy
      iii. Gastric/GI: Gastritis, gastric ulcer, esophagitis, and obstruction
      iv. Vascular: Aortic dissection, mesenteric ischemia
      v. MI, pneumonia
   d. If lipase is noted to be elevated, name the five causes for this elevation:
      i. Alcohol, gallstones, idiopathic, traumatic, drug-induced, hypertriglyceridemia, polyarthritis nodosa, vascular disease, pancreas divisum, hypercalcemia, and infections/toxins
   e. Name one criteria or index that can be used as a predictive tool for the severity of acute pancreatitis:
      i. Ranson's criteria, Glasgow Prognostic Criteria (Imrie's criteria), Balthazar CT severity Index, the extrapancreatic inflammation on CT score.

---

[1]These SAMPs were created especially for this book. They reflect the style of the exam and include current accepted practice, but are not taken directly from any other source.

Bibliography

British Medical Journal Best Practice (Dec, 2015). Acute Pancreatitis: Diagnostic Criteria. http://bestpractice
.bmj.com/best-practice/monograph/66/diagnosis/criteria.html/. Accessed Feb 11, 2017.

Penner RM. Evaluation of the adult with abdominal pain. In: UpToDate, Post TW (eds), UpToDate,
Waltham, MA. *UpToDate*. http://www.uptodate.com/contents/evaluation-of-the-adult-with-
abdominal-pain. Accessed Feb 12, 2017.

Vege S. Clinical manifestations and diagnosis of acute pancreatitis. In: UpToDate, Post TW (eds),
UpToDate, Waltham, MA. *UpToDate*. http://www.uptodate.com/contents/clinical-manifestations-
and-diagnosis-of-acute-pancreatitis. Accessed Feb 11, 2017.

2. A 51-year-old man presents to your office with a 1-year history of vague abdominal pain not localized, with persistent diarrhea, and just generally feeling fatigued. He states that he is unsure of any weight loss. Denies any nausea or vomiting. Has not noted any blood in his stool. Abdominal examination is benign.

   a. List five potential differential diagnoses for his abdominal pain:

      i. Colorectal Ca, ulcerative collitis, Crohn disease, diverticulosis, lactose intolerance, coeliac disease, and irritable bowel syndrome.

   b. Patient has a colonoscopy performed and biopsy of inflammation is positive for Crohn disease. Please identify three clinical features that distinguish Crohn disease from ulcerative collitis:

      i. Involvement of the small bowel, sparring of the rectum, absence of gross bleeding, presence of perianal disease, presence of granulomas, presence of fistulas.

   c. List three classes of medications that are used to treat Crohn disease:

      i. Oral 5-aminosalicylates (eg sulfasalazine), glucocorticoids (eg prednisone), immunomodulators (methotrexate), biologics (eg infliximab)

   d. What are the colorectal cancer screening guideline recommendations currently for frequency of FOBT/FIT testing for normal risk patients ages 50 to 74?

      Screening testing should be performed ever 2 years.

Bibliography

Canadian Task Force on Preventive Health Care. Recommendations on screening for colorectal cancer in
primary care. *CMAJ*. 2016;188(5):340-348.

Farrel R, Peppercorn M. Overview of medical management in mild to moderate Crohn disease in adults.
In: UpToDate, Post TW (eds), UpToDate, Waltham, MA. *UpToDate*. https://www.uptodate.com/
contents/overview-of-the-medical-management-of-mild-to-moderate-crohn-disease-in-adults.
Accessed February 12, 2017.

Peppercorn M, Kane S. Clinical manifestations, diagnosis and prognosis of Crohn disease in adults. In:
UpToDate, Post TW (eds), UpToDate, Waltham, MA. *UpToDate*. https://www.uptodate.com/contents/
clinical-manifestations-diagnosis-and-prognosis-of-crohn-disease-in-adults. Accessed February 12, 2017.

3. A 29-year-old woman presents to your outpatient clinic with persistent nausea and vomiting for the past week. You subsequently perform a urine pregnancy test and identify that she is pregnant. She is severely dehydrated and has lost approximately 8 pounds, or 6% of her bodyweight, over this past week.

   a. What is this patient most likely diagnosis?

      Hyperemesis gravidarium

   b. List three possible other differential diagnoses for this condition?

      i. GI: Appendicitis, hepatitis, pancreatitis, biliary disease, and obstruction

      ii. Urinary tract: Pyelonephritis

      iii. Metabolic conditions: Diabetic ketoacidosis, Addison disease

   c. If this was mild nausea and vomiting in early pregnancy what lifestyle changes or diet changes would you recommend? List 3

      i. Diet: Eat small frequent meals, avoid spicy foods, avoid fatty foods, and avoid strong odour food.

      ii. Lifestyle: Frequent naps, shorten work day.

d. If lifestyle/diet changes were not sufficient list three classes of medication that could be used for nausea/vomiting in pregnancy?

Serotonin antagonists, dopamine antagonists, and H1 antagonist with vitamin B$_6$

Bibliography

Smith J, Refuerzo J, Ramin S, et al. Treatment and outcome of nausea and vomiting in pregnancy. In: UpToDate, Post TW (ed), UpToDate, Waltham, MA. *UpToDate*. https://www.uptodate.com/contents/treatment-and-outcome-of-nausea-and-vomiting-of-pregnancy. Accessed Feb 13, 2017.

4. A 27-year-old man presents to your primary health clinic due to a pulsating headache over his left temple. He states that he has been nauseas and forced to lie in a dark quite room for the past day to try and mitigate the symptoms. He denies any prodromal symptoms. He states that this happens about 6 times per year.

a. What is the most likely diagnosis?

Migraine without aura

b. Name four characteristics that are part of the diagnostic criteria for this condition?

Unilateral location, pulsating quality, moderate to severe intensity, aggravated by routine physical activity, nausea/vomiting, photophobia, and phonophobia

c. List five potential triggers for this condition?

Emotional stress, hormones in women, not eating, weather, sleep disturbances, odours, neck pain, lights, alcohol, smoke, sleeping late, heat, food, exercise, and sex

d. Name four classes of medications that can be used to treat this condition?

Triptans, NSAIDs, acetaminophen, ergots, antiemetics/dopamine receptor blockers, *dexamethasone—reduces rate of early recurrence

Bibliography

Bajwa Z, Smith J. Acute treatment of migraines in adults. In: UpToDate, Post TW (ed), UpToDate, Waltham, MA. *UpToDate*. https://www.uptodate.com/contents/acute-treatment-of-migraine-in-adults. Accessed February 13, 2017.

Cutrer F, Bajwa Z. Pathophysiology, clinical manifestations, and diagnosis of migraines in adults. In: UpToDate, Post TW (ed), UpToDate, Waltham, MA. *UPToDate*. https://www.uptodate.com/contents/pathophysiology-clinical-manifestations-and-diagnosis-of-migraine-in-adults. Accessed February 13, 2017.

5. A 28-year-old woman has been suffering from knee and shin pain for the past 2 weeks. She notes that she has increased the number of kilometers, she has been running recently as she has a goal of running a marathon at the end of the year. Your clinical impression is that she has a stress fracture.

a. List four risk factors for stress fractures?

History of previous stress fracture, low level of physical fitness, increasing volume or intensity of a physical activity, female gender and menstrual irregularity, low BMI, low calcium diet, old age, prolonged glucocorticoid use, and poor biomechanics (eg, limb length discrepancy)

b. Name three possible differential diagnoses?

Tendinopathy, muscle strain, ligament sprain, medial tibial stress syndrome (shin splints), neoplasm, and infection (osteomyelitis)

c. Conservative management is chosen in this case. List five recommendations for her conservative management?

Acute pain control (NSAIDs), protection of the fracture site (ie, splinting or reduced weight bearing), reduction or change in activities so pain not present, gradual resumption of activities AFTER pain free, ensure proper nutrition—with particular attention to vitamin D and calcium, and flexibility and strengthening exercises (physiotherapy).

d. In which patients diagnosed with a stress fracture would you consider a bone scan? List three:

Unexplained stress fractures (ie, no change in physical activity), recurrent stress fractures, family history of osteoporosis, regular use of glucocorticoids, and eating disorders

e. According to the clinical practice guideline for the diagnosis and management of osteoporosis, what lifestyle modifications should we encourage with everyone above 50? List three:

Regular active weight-bearing exercise, calcium 1200 mg daily, vitamin D 800 to 2000 IU daily, and fall prevention strategies.

Bibliography

deWeber K. Overview of Stress Fractures. In: UpToDate, Post TW (ed), UpToDate, Waltham, MA. *UpToDate*. https://www.uptodate.com/contents/overview-of-stress-fractures. Accessed February 13, 2017.

Papaioannou A, Morin S, Cheung AM, et al. Clinical practice guidelines for the diagnosis and management of osteoporosis in Canada: summary. *CMAJ*. 2010;182:1864-1873.

6. A 65-year-old man presents to the emergency department with an acute shortness of breath over the previous 12 hours. His history is of note for coronary artery disease with a CABG, diabetes, hyperlipidemia, obesity, and has a 35-pack year history of smoking.

a. Give five differential diagnoses for this man's presentation?

Heart failure, MI, chronic kidney disease, COPD, pneumonia, asthma, pulmonary embolism, diabetic ketoacidosis, anemia, exercise intolerance

b. List five lab investigations you would include in your initial workup?

WBC, haemoglobin, glucose, urea, creatinine, potassium, d dimer, arterial blood gas, troponin, and creatinine kinase

c. X-ray findings are suspicious for COPD—Spirometry is performed. What are the diagnostic criteria for COPD from spirometry?

Postbronchodilator FEV 1/FVC < 0.7

d. Name five classes of medication utilized in the treatment?

Short-acting bronchodilator, short-acting anticholinergic, long-acting anticholinergic, short-acting beta-2 agonist, long-acting beta-2 agonist, inhaled corticosteroid.

Bibliography

Ferguson G, Make B. Management of stable chronic obstructive pulmonary disease. In: UpToDate, Post TW (ed), UpToDate, Waltham, MA. *UpToDate*. https://www.uptodate.com/contents/overview-of-stress-fractures. Accessed February 13, 2017.

O'Donnell DE, Aaron S, Bourbeau J, et al. Canadian Thoracic Society recommendations for management of chronic obstructive pulmonary disease – 2010 update. *Can Respir J*. 2010; http://www.respiratoryguidelines.ca/guideline/chronic-obstructive-pulmonary-disease. Accessed February 11, 2017.

7. A 12-month-old girl presents to you in emergency following a seizure at home, where the parents stated she just started spontaneously shaking. The parents stated the episode lasted approximately 2 minutes. She had a cough and runny nose for the previous 2 days. Her mother noted a temperature of 39.2°C the hour preceding. She is otherwise a healthy girl with immunizations up to date. She was a full-term SVD, no complications. On examination in the ER her temperature is 38.6°C, her throat is erythematous, ears clear bilaterally, and her neurological examination is grossly normal. Your provisional dx is febrile seizure.

a. List three of the generally accepted criteria for a febrile seizure?

A convulsion associated with a temperature greater than 38°C, child is older than 3 months but less than 6 years, absence of CNS inflammation or infection, absence of metabolic abnormality that could cause the seizure, no history of previous afebrile seizures.

b. True or false? Bacterial infections are more likely to cause febrile seizures than viral infections.

False

c. If the child had presented in status epilepticus what medication would you use to treat?

Per the CPS guidelines: Lorazepam buccal/pr 0.1 mg/kg, midazolam buccal 0.5 mg/kg or intranasal 0.2 mg/kg, diazepam 0.5 mg/kg.

d. List five differential diagnoses of the acute causes of status epileptics other than febrile seizure:

  i. Acute CNS infection—Bacterial/viral meningitis, encephalitis

  ii. Metabolic—Hyponatremia, hyperglycemia, hypoglycemia, hypocalcemia, anoxic injury

  iii. Epilepsy—Drug withdrawal/noncompliance, antiepileptic drug overdose

  iv. Drug overdose

Bibliography

Friedman JN. Emergency management of the pediatric patient with generalized convulsive status epilepticus. Canadian Pediatric Society, Acute Care Committee, *Pediatr Child Health*. 2011;16(2):91-97.

Millichap J, Millichap JG. Clinical features and evaluation of febrile seizures. In: UpToDate, Post TW (ed), UpToDate, Waltham, MA. *UpToDate*. https://www.uptodate.com/contents/clinical-features-and-evaluation-of-febrile-seizures. Accessed February 13, 2017.

8. A 52-year-old man has just completed his screening labs following an appointment at your office. His HbA1c is 6.3 and his fasting glucose was 6.9. You recall him into the office to discuss the results.

a. What is his diagnosis?

Prediabetes or impaired fasting glucose

b. List two lifestyle modifications that you would recommend?

Weight loss—5%, exercise 150 minutes/week

c. List five risk factors for diabetes:

  i. First-degree relative with type 2 DM, high risk populations (aboriginal, African, Asian, Hispanic), history of pre diabetes/gestational diabetes, metabolic syndrome, obesity, PCOS, OSA, drugs (steroids), and HIV/HAART

d. In 3 years' time, the patients HbA1c is 8.6%, blood pressure is 137/88, and Framingham risk score is 21%. What classes of medications should he be on at this time based solely on these figures?

Biguanides (Metformin) and ACE/ARB and statin

Bibliography

Canadian Diabetes Association Clinical Practice Guidelines Expert Committee. Canadian Diabetes Association 2013 clinical practice guidelines for the prevention and management of diabetes in Canada. *Can J Diabetes*. 2013;37 (suppl 1); http://guidelines.diabetes.ca/app_themes/cdacpg/resources/cpg_2013_full_en.pdf.

McCullough D, Robertson R. Risk Factors for type 2 diabetes mellitus. In: UpToDate, Post TW (ed), UpToDate, Waltham, MA. *UpToDate*. https://www.uptodate.com/contents/risk-factors-for-type-2-diabetes-mellitus. Accessed February 13, 2017.

9. A 30-year-old man presents to your clinic with unilateral testicular pain that has been increasing over the past 2 weeks. States his scrotum is excruciatingly tender and does note some urethral discharge. The only way he is able to get relief is with elevating his testicles. He does note he has had multiple sexual partners over the past 3 months.

a. What is the most likely diagnosis?

Epididymitis

b. In patients, *older* than 35 list the two most common infectious causes:

Pseudomonas, E. coli

c. What investigations would you perform in your workup?

Urethral swab of discharge for gram stain, urine (initial stream) for gonorrhoea and chlamydia, urine midstream for C&S, and urinalysis (leukocytes, nitrites, blood)

Bibliography

Eyre R. Evaluation of acute scrotum in adults. In: UpToDate, Post TW (ed), UpToDate, Waltham, MA. *Up ToDate*. https://www.uptodate.com/contents/evaluation-of-the-acute-scrotum-in-adults. Accessed February 13, 2017.

10. A 72-year-old man presents to your office because his wife is concerned about his ability to carry out his activities of daily living. She states over the past year, he has become progressively slower at performing tasks and all movements seem to take an exaggerated amount of time. On examination, you note he has difficulty rising from the chair and has a shuffling gate with no arm swing. He has no facial expression and a resting tremor. Clinical diagnosis is Parkinson disease.

a. List three of the diagnostic criteria for Parkinson disease:

Bradykinesia with at least one of the following: Muscular rigidity, resting tremor, postural instability unrelated to visual, cerebellar, and vestibular or proprioceptive dysfunction.

b. In patients with early Parkinson's name 2 classes of medications that can be used as first-line treatment?

Levodopa, dopamine agonists, and MAO-B inhibitors

c. List three risk factors for a more rapid progression of Parkinson disease:

Older age at onset, rigidity/hypokinesia as initial symptom, postural instability/freezing gait, male sex, poor levodopa response, dementia, and comorbidities (stroke, auditory deficit, vision impairment)

Bibliography

Grimes D, Gordon J, et al. Canadian Neurological Sciences Federation Canadian Guidelines on Parkinson's Disease. *Can J Neurol Sci*. 2012;39 (4 suppl 4). http://parkinsonclinicalguidelines.ca/sites/default/files/PD_Guidelines_2012.pdf

11. A 64-year-old woman presents to your office with pain in her hands and wrists bilaterally. She states this pain has been going on for about the last year. They are stiffest in the morning but the pain and stiffness tends to ease as she uses them more, probably 2 to 3 hours into the day. They are swollen and tender to the touch. On examination, erythema and swelling identified bilaterally in the MCP, PIP, and wrist joints. These areas are tender to palpation. You clinically suspect rheumatoid arthritis.

a. What investigations or labs would you like to perform to confirm you diagnosis? List four:

CRP, ESR, rheumatoid factor, anti-CCP, x-ray—Looking for diagnostic erosion of hands and feet, platelets, and Hb

b. Name four medications used to treat RA:

Hydroxychloroquine, methotrexate, sulfasalazine, cyclosporine, azathioprine, leflunomide, infliximab, etanercept, and anakinra; corticosteroids/NSAIDs provide symptom relief but do not affect disease course

c. Name three complications of untreated RA:

i. Anaemia, scleritis, deformities—Ulnar deviation etc. from continued joint erosion, pericarditis, and increased infection risk.

Bibliography

Bykerk VP, Akhavan P, Hazlewood GS, et al. Canadian Rheumatology Association recommendations for pharmacological management of rheumatoid arthritis with traditional and biologic disease-modifying antirheumatic drugs. *J Rheumatol.* 2012;39(8):1559-1582.

Moreland L, Cannella A. General principles of management of rheumatoid arthritis. In: UpToDate, Post TW (ed), UpToDate, Waltham, MA. *UpToDate.* https://www.uptodate.com/contents/general-principles-of-management-of-rheumatoid-arthritis-in-adults. Accessed February 13, 2017.

12. A couple, 28-year-old man and 29-year-old woman, present to your office with concerns about not being able to conceive a child despite having had unprotected intercourse approximately three times per week for the past 3 months. The female has not been on birth control for more than 1 year. Her cycles are a regular 28 days. She has no previous pregnancies, G0P0. The male has no problems achieving or maintaining an erection until ejaculation. They are hoping that you, as their GP, will refer them for fertility treatments.

    a. What percentage of couples would be expected to achieve pregnancy within 1 year?

    80% to 90%

    b. What lifestyle and education counselling would you provide for optimizing chances of conceiving and carrying a pregnancy? List three:

        i. Lifestyle: Folic acid 0.4 mg daily, smoking cessation, weight management, avoid alcohol/drugs.

        ii. Education: Optimal intercourse timing 6 days prior to ovulation, intercourse 2 to 3 times weekly.

    c. What would you advise them about a referral?

    Referral would not be warranted until after 1 year as both under the age of 30.

    d. What percentage of cases of infertility are male-factor related?

    1/3 of all cases.

Bibliography

Kuohung W, Hornstein M. Overview of infertility. In: UpToDate, Post TW (ed), UpToDate, Waltham, MA. *UpToDate.* https://www.uptodate.com/contents/overview-of-infertility. Accessed February 13, 2017.

13. A 62-year-old Caucasian man presents to the emergency department with excruciating pain to his left flank. It came on suddenly in the past 3 hours. He remembers a similar pain approximately 5 years previously and was diagnosed with a kidney stone at that time. He does not note any trauma to his flank. The rest of his history is notable for gout and obesity.

    a. What is the initial lab workup if you are considering a renal stone?

    Serum sodium, potassium, chlorine, creatinine, calcium, uric acid, phosphorous, urinalysis with pH—query hematuria, and stone analysis

    b. Calcium stones were identified. List four lifestyle management changes you would recommend:

        i. Increase fluid intake with goal of urine output >2 L, reduce salt intake (<2300 mg Na/d), decrease animal protein <2 meals/d and <6 to 8 ounces/d, moderate calcium intake (1000–1200 mg/d), moderate high oxalate foods <1000 mg/d, and increase citrated rich foods such as lemonade, orange juice.

    c. What is the primary urine abnormality in uric acid stone formers?

    Acidic urine with a pH <5.5

Bibliography

Paterson R, Fernandez A, Razvi H, Sutton R. Evaluation and medical management of the kidney stone patient. *Can Urol Assoc J.* 2010;4(6):375-379.

14. A 32-year-old woman develops a fever of 38.7°C on the mother/baby unit. She is 3 days postpartum for a full-term SVD complicated by a postpartum bleed with an approximate blood loss of 1 L secondary to retained products. She had a second-degree perineal tear which was repaired. She and her baby have done well postdelivery. You are called to the ward to assess due to the elevated temperature.

    a. What is the definition of postpartum fever?

    Fever greater than 38°C on any two of the first 10 days postpartum excluding the first 24 hours.

    b. List five differential diagnoses you have for the development of postpartum fever in any case:

    Urinary tract infection, wound infection, pelvic thrombophlebitis, DVT, mastitis, breast abscess, endometritis, drug reaction, and atelectasis, pneumonia

    c. What labs should be performed if your working diagnosis is endometritis? List three.

    Blood and genital cultures, WBC, Hb, platelets, urea, and creatinine,

    d. What is the prevalence of postpartum blues?

    85% of new mothers

    e. What are the risk factors for postpartum blues?

    History of depression, family history of depression, inadequate social support, psychosocial stress, and pregnancy loss.

Bibliography

Berens P. Overview of postpartum care. In: UpToDate, Post TW (ed), UpToDate, Waltham, MA. *UpToDate.* (https://www.uptodate.com/contents/overview-of-postpartum-care. Accessed February 13, 2017.

15. A 56-year-old woman presents to you in the emergency department with left leg swelling and pain. She is notable for having just returned to Vancouver from 9-hour flight from Australia. She does note having received hormone replacement therapy as she was going through menopause.

    a. What is your differential diagnosis of unilateral leg oedema, warmth, and pain? List four:

    Muscle strain, deep vein thrombosis, arterial occlusion, ruptured popliteal cyst, venous insufficiency, cellulitis, and lymphangitis.

    b. What are the three elements of Virchow triad:

    Endothelial damage, hypercoagulability, and venous stasis

    c. Your patient has a Well's score of 4.5 what investigation should be performed based off this score?

    Doppler U/S of leg

    d. What preventative measures could have been discussed and enacted prior to this patients flight? List two:

    Compression stockings, exercise leg muscles while in flight, stay well hydrated, avoid constricting clothing around the legs/waist

Bibliography

Kearon C, Akl EA, Ornelas J, et al. Antithrombotic therapy for vte disease: Chest guideline and expert panel report. *Chest.* 2016;149(2):315-352.

Teeple L. Acute venous thomboemblosim: Diagnosis, Treatment and Prevention. The Foundation for Medical Practice Education. 2010;18.8:1-10.

16. A 22-month-old boy presents to you in emergency. One day history of fever peaking at 39.5°C, poor feeding, lethargic, nausea, and vomiting with neck stiffness. You clinically suspect meningitis.

    a. What are the most likely pathogens in this 22-month-old? List two

    S. Pneumonia, *H. Influenza*, and *N. Meningitidis*

  b. Name one of the physical examination signs for meningeal irritation:

     i. Kernig sign, Brudzinski sign

  c. What imaging may be required prior to the complete workup for meningitis being completed?

    CT Head should be performed if concerns regarding increased intracranial pressure present before a lumbar puncture as that could cause brain herniation.

  d. Empiric treatment recommended by CPS—List two antibiotics:

    Ceftriaxone or cefuroxime and vancomycin

Bibliography

Le Saux N. Guidelines for the management of suspected and confirmed bacterial meningitis in Canadian children older than one month of age. *Paediatr Child Health.* 2014;19.3:141-146. http://www.cps.ca/documents/position/management-of-bacterial-meningitis.

17. A 9-year-old boy presents to your clinic accompanied by his mother. This is your third meeting with them both. She is quite concerned with regard to his academic performance at school and the number of notes/meetings; she gets called in to with regard to his disruptive behaviour. School assessment provided by his teacher notes he has significant impairment; not able to follow instructions, cannot sustain attention, is easily distracted and often forgetful of daily activities. The mother has similar concerns with regard to his behaviour at home. His mother states these symptoms have been ongoing for more than a year. You note he fidgets often as he sits in the examination room, often blurts out answers and often tends to talk excessively. His neurological examination is normal. You diagnose him with attention deficit hyperactivity disorder.

  a. Often people diagnosed with ADHD have common comorbid psychiatric conditions. List three:

    i. Oppositional defiant disorder, conduct disorder, depression, anxiety, developmental disorders/learning disability, substance abuse, Tourette, and personality disorder.

  b. Why are extended-release pharmacological formulations preferred over instant-release medications? List two reasons:

    i. Improve adherence, reduce stigma (child doesn't have to take medications at school), reducing problems schools having to have controlled substances on site, improved pharmacokinetics. Less likely to be diverted.

  c. Medical therapy and psychosocial interventions are the most effective way to treat ADHD. List three interventions:

    i. Psychoeducation, behavioural interventions, social interventions, psychotherapy, and educational/vocational accommodations.

Bibliography

Canadian Attention Deficit Hyperactivity Disorder Resource Alliance (CADDRA): Canadian ADHD Practice Guidelines, Third Edition, Toronto ON; CADDRA, 2011. https://www.caddra.ca/pdfs/caddraGuidelines2011.pdf.

Feldman M, Blanger S. Extended-release mediations for children and adolescents with attention-deficit hyperactivity disorder. *Paediatr Child Health.* 2009;14:9. http://www.cps.ca/documents/position/extended-release-medications-ADHD.

18. A 63-year-old patient who has been suffering from long-term depression has confided in you that he is having thoughts of self-harm.

  a. What are the risk factors for suicide? List five

    Think SAD PERSONS: Sex, Age >60 or <18, Depression, Previous Attempts, Ethanol Abuse, Rational thinking loss, Suicide in family, Organized plan, No spouse/lack of supports, Serious Illness/pain

b. What are the nonpharmacologic first-line treatments for depression? List two:

Cognitive therapy/cognitive behavioural therapy, interpersonal therapy, regular exercise

c. List five side effects of SSRI pharmacotherapy:

Anxiety, nausea, insomnia, agitation, tremor, headache, and sexual dysfunction.

Bibliography and References: See Chapter 6 Psychiatry.

19. A 35-year-old woman presents to your office with burning on urination, urgency, and increased frequency. She states that she has had UTIs in the past and had the same deep burning sensation. She is an otherwise healthy lady. No current medications or significant medical history. You suspect another urinary tract infection.

a. What physical examinations should you perform?

Temperature, heart rate, assess for CVA tenderness, and suprapubic tenderness.

b. In this case what would be in your differential for dysuria? List four

Cystitis, urethritis, vulvovaginitis, mechanical/chemical irritation secondary to sexual activity, neurogenic or psychogenic conditions, and inflammatory disease

c. What are the elements of the validated UTI Score for uncomplicated cystitis?

Dysuria, leukocytes on urine dipstick, nitrites on urine dipstick

d. What are the first-line treatments for uncomplicated cystitis?

tmp/smx and macrobid

Bibliography: See Chapter 3 Infectious Diseases.

20. A 16-year-old boy presents to your clinic because he is quite distressed with regard to his acne and is becoming quite self-conscious about his appearance. It has been getting progressively worse over the past year despite no acute changes to his hygiene. You note that he does have 15 to 20 closed comedones on the face with mild erythema. No signs of scarring.

a. Advise two lifestyle changes that he could put into practice today?

Wash face once daily with a mild soap and a water-based or soapless cleanser, avoid scented products; shaving: go over areas lightly once if possible and follow the grain of the hair.

b. Name two topical treatments that could be used on this young man's acne.

Benzoyl peroxide, retinoids, and clindamycin

c. If topical treatments were not effective the next modality would be oral antibiotics? Name one

Tetracycline or doxycycline.

d. Isotretinoin therapy requires what two extra safeguards when prescribing to women of reproductive age?

Pregnancy test before and during treatment and two forms of birth control while on treatment.

Bibliography and References: See Chapter 2: Internal Medicine

Index

CPSIA information can be obtained
at www.ICGtesting.com
Printed in the USA
BVHW010011100821
613622BV00008B/86